The Sigma Nu Fraternity
Medical Book Collection
At The University of Rhode Island Library
Zeta Rho Chapter
Adversis Major-Par Secundis

Caring
for the
Older Woman

CURRENT TOPICS IN OBSTETRICS AND GYNECOLOGY

Series Editor
Morton A. Stenchever, MD
Professor and Chairman
Department of Obstetrics and Gynecology
University of Washington
School of Medicine
Seattle, Washington

Controversies in Reproductive Endocrinology and Infertility
Michael R. Soules, MD

Caring for the Older Woman
Morton A. Stenchever, MD
George Aagaard, MD

Caring for the Exercising Woman
Ralph W. Hale, MD

Caring for the Older Woman

Edited by
Morton A. Stenchever, MD
Professor and Chairman
Department of Obstetrics and Gynecology
University of Washington
School of Medicine
Seattle, Washington

George A. Aagaard, MD
Dean Emeritus and Professor
Departments of Medicine and Pharmacology
University of Washington
School of Medicine
Seattle, Washington

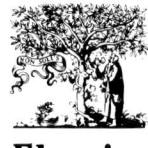

Elsevier
New York • Amsterdam • London

*To our wives,
Diane and Lorna*

No responsibility is assumed by the Publisher for any injury and/or damage to persons or property as a matter of products liability, negligence, or otherwise, or from any use or operation of any methods, products, instructions, or ideas contained in the material herein. No suggested test or procedure should be carried out unless, in the reader's judgment, its risk is justified. Because of rapid advances in the medical sciences, we recommend that the independent verification of diagnoses and drug dosages should be made. Discussions, views, and recommendations as to medical procedures, choice of drugs, and drug dosages are the responsibility of the authors.

Elsevier Science Publishing Co., Inc.
655 Avenue of the Americas, New York, New York 10010

Sole distributors outside the United States and Canada:
Elsevier Science Publishers B.V.
P.O. Box 211, 1000 AE Amsterdam, the Netherlands

© 1991 by Elsevier Science Publishing Co., Inc.

This book has been registered with the Copyright Clearance Center, Inc.
For further information, please contact the Copyright Clearance Center, Inc., Salem, Massachusetts.

This book is printed on acid-free paper.

Library of Congress Cataloging-in-Publication Data:

Caring for the older woman / edited by Morton A. Stenchever,
George Aagaard.
    p. cm.—(Current topics in obstetrics and gynecology)
    Includes index.
    ISBN 0-444-01549-3 (alk. paper)
    1. Geriatric gynecology. 2. Aged women—Diseases.
I. Stenchever, Morton A. II. Aagaard, George. III. Series.
    [DNLM: 1. Aging. 2. Genital Diseases, Female—in old age.
3. Women. WP 140 C277]
RG103.C27 1991
618.97'81—dc20
DNLM/DLC
for Library of Congress   91-15711
                                                                                    CIP

Current printing (last digit):
10 9 8 7 6 5 4 3 2 1

Manufactured in the United States of America

Contents

Preface / vii
Contributors / ix

Chapter 1
The Role of the Gynecologist in the Care of the Older Woman / 1
Morton A. Stenchever, MD

Chapter 2
Ethical Issues in the Care of the Geriatric Patient / 7
Nancy Jecker, PhD and Albert Jonsen, PhD

Chapter 3
Biology of Aging and the Human Female / 21
George M. Martin, MD

Chapter 4
Alterations of Host-Defense Mechanisms and the Susceptibility to Infections / 37
Gurkamal Chatta, MD and David C. Dale, MD

Chapter 5
Aging and Pharmacotherapeutics / 57
George Aagaard, MD

Chapter 6
Preventive Health Care of the Older Woman / 65
Wylie Burke, MD, PhD and Wendy H. Raskind, MD, PhD

Chapter 7
Hypertension / 121
George Aagaard, MD

Chapter 8
Genitourinary Changes and Incontinence / 139
Morton A. Stenchever, MD

Chapter 9
Problems of Loss of Pelvic Support / 157
Morton A. Stenchever, MD

Chapter 10
Vulva and Vaginal Conditions / 171
Morton A. Stenchever, MD

Chapter 11
Gynecologic Malignancies in the Elderly / 183
Morton A. Stenchever, MD

Chapter 12
Hormone Replacement / 205
Morton A. Stenchever, MD

Index / 219

Preface

This series, *Current Topics in Obstetrics and Gynecology*, is designed to raise issues of current interest to obstetricians and gynecologists and other physicians and professionals involved in the care of women. Since the population is aging and many women are living more than one third of their lives in the postmenopausal period, an important issue to them and their health-care providers is appropriate care. Just as young girls cannot be considered "little women" in their health needs, neither can older women be treated in exactly the same manner as younger ones.

Physicians, in general, and obstetricians and gynecologists, in particular, are in an excellent position to continue caring for women as they age. However, to do this properly they must learn to prioritize the health issues important to this class of women, and must be able to provide this care in as competent and as empathetic a manner as they did the care of women in their reproductive years.

This volume, *Caring for the Older Woman*, attempts to provide the health-care provider with information about the aging process in general, changes in the immune state, general health-care information (including preventive medicine measures), specific up-to-date information on the treatment of hypertension (one of the most common chronic conditions to afflict the elderly), data on the response of the elderly to therapeutic measures, and the gynecological issues and conditions specific to older women. In addition, ethical issues important to the care of this age group are considered.

The authors are experienced practitioners in the care of older women—one a gynecologist (Morton A. Stenchever, M.D.) and the other an internist (George Aagaard, M.D.) with a career interest in hypertension and therapeutics. The contributors are all recognized experts in their specific disciplines.

It is our hope that this volume will not only help the practitioner care for the older woman, but will also make it possible for her or him to continue enjoying the doctor–patient relationship with persons in their later years. As the number of these patients increases, so will the opportunities available to the physician. Older women deserve excellent and specialized care so that they may continue to enjoy life to the fullest measure of their physical and emotional capabilities.

Morton A. Stenchever, M.D.

George Aagaard, M.D.

Contributors

George A. Aagaard, MD
Dean Emeritus and Professor, Departments of Medicine and Pharmacology, RG-23, University of Washington School of Medicine, Seattle, Washington

Wylie Burke, MD
Department of Medicine—PMC, ZB-30, University of Washington, Seattle, Washington

Gurkamal S. Chatta, MD
Professor, Department of Medicine, University of Washington, Seattle, Washington

David C. Dale, MD
Professor, Department of Medicine, University of Washington, Seattle, Washington

Nancy S. Jecker, PhD
Assistant Professor, Department of Medical History and Ethics, University of Washington, Seattle, Washington

Albert R. Jonsen, PhD
Professor and Chairman, Department of Medical History and Ethics, University of Washington, Seattle, Washington

George M. Martin, PhD
Professor and Adjunct Professor, Department of Pathology, University of Washington School of Medicine, Seattle, Washington

Wendy H. Raskind, MD, PhD
Assistant Professor, Department of Internal Medicine, University of Washington, Seattle, Washington

Morton A. Stenchever, MD
Chairman, Department of Obstetrics and Gynecology, University of Washington School of Medicine, Seattle, Washington

Chapter 1

The Role of the Gynecologist in the Care of the Older Woman

Morton A. Stenchever, MD

The practice of gynecology has been changing for the last several years. These changes have not only occurred because of the changing, or *perceived* changing, needs of gynecologic patients but also for a variety of other reasons, including medical and technological advances, changes in the style of practice, and changes in who is actually doing the practice of the specialty.

People are living longer, and women in particular are enjoying greater longevity. Because of this, there is a rapidly increasing number of individuals in the older age groups. Table 1.1 reflects the fact that both men and women are demonstrating greater longevity in many of the developing and developed countries of the world. This change was noted to be quite substantial between 1965 and 1983.[1] We can only assume that this trend will continue. While the increase has been noted in both sexes, it is particularly significant for women. Furthermore, if one looks at the percentage of the total population in different age groups, it can be seen that, in 1980, 11% of the population of developed countries were in the age group of 64 years and older (Table 1.2).

If one projects population totals into the next century, by the year 2025, 23% of the population of developed nations and 12% of developing nations will be in the over-60 age group (Table 1.3). World Health Association figures would indicate that by the year 2000 there will be 251 million women over the age of 45 in the developed countries, and 468 million in this age group in the developing nations.[2]

As the number of elderly increase both in numbers and in percentage of population, medical needs of this group will also increase. The type of services necessary will be varied and the need for physicians to deliver these services will increase. Gynecologists have always been recognized as physicians concerned with women's health-care needs, and should be in an excellent position to continue to offer medical services to women beyond the reproductive years. Currently, it is estimated by the American College of Obstetricians and Gynecologists that only about 1% of women beyond the age of 60 consider their gynecologist their primary physician. This may be due to a number of reasons, including the following patient perceptions: that gynecologists are only interested in issues of women's health that relate to reproduction; that gynecologists, because of their training, are only comfortable in offering services related to the reproductive organs and their usual period of function; or that the style of

Table 1.1 Life Expectancy at Birth (Years) in Selected Countries in 1965 and in 1983*

	\multicolumn{4}{c}{Life expectancy at birth}
	Men		Women	
Country	1965	1983	1965	1983
Angola	34	42	37	44
Argentina	63	66	69	73
Bangladesh	45	49	44	50
Brazil	55	61	59	66
China	55	65	59	69
Cuba	65	73	69	77
India	46	56	44	54
Indonesia	43	52	45	55
Japan	68	74	73	79
Jordan	49	63	51	65
Korea, Rep. of	55	64	58	71
Mexico	58	64	61	68
Nigeria	40	47	43	50
Pakistan	46	51	44	49
Sudan	39	47	41	49
Sweden	72	75	76	80
USA	67	72	74	79
USSR	65	65	74	74

* Adapted from the World Bank: *World Development Report 1985*. London, Oxford University Press, 1985. Used by permission.

gynecologic practice is not conducive to addressing the health-care needs of the older woman. On the other hand, the gynecologist is the physician to whom the younger woman turns for most of her health-care needs during her reproductive years. Since she is generally comfortable receiving services from an individual who is trained in the health-care needs of women, it seems reasonable that she would continue to feel comfortable obtaining services from such an individual even when her reproductive years are completed. Therefore, this chapter will address the opportunities that the gynecologist has in offering continuing health care to the older woman. Several of the areas noted will be expanded upon in later chapters of this book.

Table 1.2 Estimated Age Composition of Population (in Percentages) in 1980*

Age group (years)	Developed countries	Developing countries	World total
0–14	23	39	35
15–44	45	44	44
45–64	21	13	15
>64	11	4	6

* Adapted from the World Health Organization: *World Health Statistics Annual*. Geneva, 1983. ISBN 92-4-067831X. Used by permission.

Table 1.3 Projected Age Structure as Percentage of Population*

	Developed countries age group		Developing countries age group	
Year	<15	>60	<15	>60
1975	25	15	41	6
2000	21	18	33	7
2025	20	23	26	12

* From the United Nations World Assembly on Aging, Vienna, 1982; The Vienna International Plan of Action on Aging, 1982. Used by permission.

Primary Care Goals for Older Women

Hormone Replacement

Most health authorities now believe that hormone-replacement therapy should be offered to all postmenopausal women who lack a contraindication for such therapy. Estrogen replacement has been proven to prevent osteoporosis, more than likely helps to prevent cardiovascular disease, aids in preventing or has an ameliorating effect on pelvic relaxation problems, and generally promotes well-being. Since vasomotor symptoms of hot flashes and night sweats are common in women who are postmenopausal, estrogen replacement clearly improves this condition in most women, allowing them to enjoy a restful night of sleep and thereby preventing insomnia in many instances. In addition, vaginal dryness caused by withdrawal of estrogen from vaginal epithelium can be prevented by estrogen replacement. Many women report dyspareunia with this vaginal dryness, and find that estrogen replacement relieves this. With these changes, libido frequently improves. Estrogen replacement will often improve subcutaneous connective tissue and its vascular supply, thereby improving skin texture and avoiding the cutaneous signs of aging for a considerable period of time. Gynecologists are not only adept at prescribing hormone-replacement therapy, and at understanding the consequence of utilizing such therapy, but they are also trained to manage the potential complications that can arise when such therapy is utilized (Chapter 12). Therefore, they are ideally suited to be the physicians to offer such therapy.

Screening for Breast Disease

Gynecologists are generally well-trained in the evaluation of the human breast for function and abnormalities, and are most able to offer preventive and diagnostic counseling for breast disease. The gynecologist can offer patients several services in this respect. These include the utilization of the American Cancer Society guidelines for mammographic screening for women in the over-50 age group, teaching of self breast examination to patients, and annual physician examinations. With the combination of annual mammography and the performance of self breast examination, the discovery of breast cancer should be earlier in its natural history; therefore, treatment should begin earlier when the prognosis may be better. The gynecologist should perform diagnostic studies, such as aspiration of breast cysts and excisional biopsies, and should offer proper referrals in the event that more serious problems are noted (Chapter 11).

Screening for General Medical Problems

The gynecologist can, as the primary physician for women, perform a complete history annually and carry out a physical examination to include blood pressure, general physical examination, and pelvic examination. In addition, a variety of screening programs aimed at conditions more common to the older patient can be offered. These may include stool guaiac for occult GI bleeding, rectal examination, which (if carried out properly) should detect a large number of lesions of the lower colon, sigmoidoscopy in women over 50 (particularly those who are symptomatic or at high risk for colon cancer), and a variety of other laboratory tests. The use of routine laboratory screening during annual physical examinations is discussed in Chapter 6.

Screening for Abuse

It has been estimated that at least 500,000 elderly women per year are victims of abuse.[3] This may be at the hands of a spouse, another family member, or others either known to the individual or strangers. Elderly women are often victimized because of their dependent role in a household or society in general. The gynecologist seeing these patients for an annual evaluation and other healthcare needs is in an excellent position to question them about whether or not anyone is hurting them and to counsel them as to their legal rights and the protection afforded them under the law. Certainly, if evidence of injury is noted during the physical examination, the patient should be questioned with respect to how this came about. Open-ended questions offered in a nonjudgmental manner are useful. For instance, "Has anyone hurt you recently or in the past? Has anyone used abusive language toward you? Have you been the victim of a robbery or other crimes?"

Evaluation and Treatment of Urinary Incontinence

Many elderly females are incontinent. This may take the form of dribbling of urine or of frank loss of urine. The gynecologist is well-trained to evaluate such problems. A careful history and physical exam will often offer evidence of incontinence, and the type of problem that the patient has. Office cystometrics, urinalysis, culture, and the ordering of special workups, such as cystometric and urodynamic studies and cystoscopy, may be helpful. Many elderly women take medications for a variety of reasons, and often these may have an effect on the urinary tract. The gynecologist is in an excellent position to sort these circumstances out and to offer advice (whether it be medical or surgical) as to correction of a problem that the patient may find both socially disturbing and limiting (Chapter 8).

Management of Grief and Loss

Every individual will suffer loss. This is greatly accentuated in the elderly. The individual may lose a spouse or other close loved one, such as an adult child or a close friend. Frequently, an acute grief reaction can be initiated by the loss of a pet. Many elderly individuals live alone and have only a dog or a cat or some other pet to keep them company. When such a creature dies, the grief reaction can be quite acute. A grief reaction may also be initiated if the individual loses a job or other activity which they enjoy and which gets them out of the household situation.

The grief reaction may also be initiated if the individual must face the loss of an organ, particularly one of emotional importance, such as a breast or the uterus. Roberts has defined four phases that an individual will generally go through when faced with the loss of an important organ, such as an eye, limb, breast, or the uterus.[4] The first is *impact*. During this phase the individual may not hear that the physician has said the organ must be removed and on a subsequent visit or by telephone call may indicate to the physician that she has no recollection whatsoever of having been told that she needs such surgery. This is a denial process but will soon be overcome, allowing the patient to go on to the next stage, which is *retreat*. During this stage, the patient may seek alternatives to the removal of the organ. Consultations with other physicians may take place, and actually should be encouraged. Following this is the stage of *acknowledgment*, during which the patient has accepted that the operation must take place but is swept up in technical considerations of how the operation will be performed, the type of anesthesia to be used, and how she will feel when it is over. The final stage, *reconstruction*, is one in which the patient has accepted that the surgery will be performed and now wishes to know what she will be like and how others will view her when the operation is completed. If a spouse or other close individual is available, often the opinion which that individual holds is important during this reorganization phase. Physicians would do well to understand these phases and help the patient through each of them, rather than imposing a procedure on a patient before she is prepared. It may be possible to avoid depression and other emotional instability if these steps are allowed to occur.

The Management of Impending Death

All patients will eventually face death, and for the elderly this is a very likely happening. Kubler-Ross defined five stages that the patient usually goes through in accepting the inevitability of death.[5] The first is *denial*, during which stage the patient may not hear that she is facing a likely demise and may speak to the physician as though this has not been said. However, after the patient passes through this phase, the next stage, that of *anger*, is often very frustrating for the patient, her family, and her physicians. During the anger stage, the patient is likely to rebuff in an angry or argumentative fashion any information or comments made by family or professionals. Since this is irritating to these individuals, the tendency is to isolate the patient and not interact with her. This is the exact opposite of what the patient wishes, and the physician must continue to relate to the patient understanding that the anger is part of the process and will pass.

The third stage is *bargaining*, during which time the patient, in the hopes that good actions and deeds may buy time (perhaps from God), will set her house in order. Often she will reestablish attachments to her religious beliefs and make peace with friends and relatives with whom she has been quarreling. Often, steps may be taken that involve fiscal matters, such as adjusting her estate and preparing a will. A *depression* state may take place at any time during this process, at which time the patient will demonstrate all of the classic findings of depression, including a negative outlook, a feeling of total remorse, frequently accompanied by loss of appetite and of interest in others and in her usual activities.

The final state is that of *acceptance*. This is often described as the period when the patient is too sick to fight any longer. However, many patients who are not suffering, but know the inevitability of their demise, reach this state. It is probably the time when all of the preparation that the patient is capable of has taken place and many of the conflicts have been worked out. While many patients die before they attain this state, in those who last long enough it is often observed.

The physician must understand the stages through which the patient must pass and be prepared to deal with her at each step along the way, offering advice, comfort, and understanding.

While the discussion in this chapter has been aimed at the gynecologist in the hopes of outlining a number of areas in which the gynecologist can continue to be of service to aging women, it is recognized that physicians who have assumed the role of the gynecologist in caring for women would also be of optimum service to these individuals by following these guidelines. Certainly, family physicians and internists can fulfill these needs; in many cases, nurse clinicians will be able to address many of them as well.

References

1. World Bank: *World Development Report.* London, Oxford University Press, 1985.
2. *World Health Statistics Annual.* Geneva, 1983.
3. Select Committee on Aging: Domestic violence against the elderly. Hearings before the Sub-Committee of Human Services House of Representatives, April 21, 1980. Washington, D.C., U.S. Government Printing Office, 1980.
4. Roberts SL: *Behavioral Concepts in the Critically Ill Patient.* Englewood Cliffs, New Jersey, Prentice-Hall, 1976.
5. Kubler-Ross E: *On Death and Dying.* New York, Macmillan, 1969.

Chapter 2

Ethical Issues in the Care of the Geriatric Patient

Nancy S. Jecker, PhD, and Albert R. Jonsen, PhD

In the years ahead, physicians will serve an increasing number of elderly patients.[1] This will be true not only for physicians with special expertise, interest, or commitment to geriatric care, but for physicians of diverse specialties, skills, and interests. The fact that life expectancy for women is on average 7.5 years higher than for men[2] means that women will be disproportionately represented in the oldest and fastest growing age groups. To meet new demands, physicians will clearly need to hone medical skills and knowledge concerning care of the aged, and care of the aged female, in particular. Beyond this, physicians will be challenged to fine-tune medical ethical principles to suit a new patient population, reconceptualize dominant attitudes toward the elderly, and strengthen their commitment to care for older patients.

This chapter focuses on ethical aspects of clinical geriatric care. Our strategy for charting these issues will be threefold. First, we sketch a series of cases that bring to the fore important medical ethical questions involving care of elderly patients. Second, we note alternative conceptions about the aged and clarify how these can affect the interpretation and application of medical ethical principles. Finally, we propose ways in which age is objectively and subjectively significant and suggest how physicians might differentiate between the real significance of age and ageist assumptions.

Cases Illustrative of Geriatric Ethical Issues

A currently favored approach for assessing ethical issues of the following kind is to frame them in terms of competing ethical principles. In the first pair of cases, an initial framing of ethical issues can be made in terms of traditional principles of autonomy and beneficence.[3] Autonomy refers to the capacity to act on the basis of principles that are one's own. This implies an absence of internal constraints, such as fear, duress, or impaired cognitive functioning, as well as an absence of external constraints, such as coercion or threats by others. By contrast, the principle of beneficence enjoins us to promote a person's best interests. This may require either actions that produce benefits, the omission of actions that produce harm, or the avoidance of harm that is not outweighed by benefits. The related concept of paternalism specifies that beneficence is appropriate even in situations where it conflicts with respecting a person's autonomous choice. Although professionals and nonprofessionals alike are under a duty to refrain from actions that harm others, physicians possess a special duty to do good for patients. For example, failure to benefit a stranger when one is in a position to do so is less morally serious than failure on the part of a physician to benefit his or her own patient.

Case One

Mrs. A, a 76-year-old woman with diabetes, has already had a below-the-knee amputation and refuses to consent to similar surgery on her other leg. Recently, she has had repeated hospital stays for sepsis of this leg and other complications. She now is brought to the emergency room in an obtunded state due to hyperosmolar coma. Following discussions with Mrs. A's son, surgery is performed on the leg. Mrs. A recovers and, with rehabilitation, adjusts well to a second prosthesis. Medicare billings total more than $62,000.[4]

Case Two

Mrs. B, age 85, was treated 5 years earlier for basal cell carcinoma of the vulva by local excision. She was depressed about her condition, seemed to respond negatively to the information given her, and wondered aloud repeatedly, "Why should this happen to an old woman who just wants to live out her last years in peace?" Now, metastatic lesions have been discovered. The physician considers chemotherapy, but decides against it and decides not to tell Mrs. A of the findings, believing that it would be more than she could bear. "At her age, she doesn't have much time left even if we arrested the disease," reasons the physician; "Why make her last months miserable with futile treatment or with the knowledge that she is dying?"[5]

The cases of Mrs. A and Mrs. B dramatize the potential conflict between autonomy and beneficence. In the first case, it appears that Mrs. A's best interests are promoted by amputating her leg in order to prevent spreading of sepsis. But this is done against her wishes in a situation where, due to coma, she is unable to protest. Here, the principle of beneficence prevails against the principle of autonomy. Hence, the conflict is resolved in accordance with the principle of paternalism.

In the second case, Mrs. B's preferences are also not determinative of treatment. Mrs. B's physician presumably judges that the deleterious effects of disclosing medical information would be overwhelming and may result in inappropriate and cruel prolonging of Mrs. B's suffering. Unlike in Mrs. A's case, in this case there may or may not be an actual conflict between the patient's wishes and serving the patient's best interests. By assigning priority to beneficence, the physician dissipates the tension between competing principles and precludes the possibility of practical conflict.

The second set of cases display conflicting, but different, ethical imperatives. Here, a central issue is quality of life and care of chronic diseases, rather than prolongation of life and treatment of potentially life-threatening conditions. Three competing conceptions of quality of life may be operative[6]: (1) quality of life understood as subjective satisfaction and as a patient's own subjective perception of life quality; (2) quality of life judged by an onlooker, such as a physician or family member, who assesses the patient's condition; and (3) quality of life interpreted as achievement of certain attributes a culture deems necessary for life quality, such as a certain level of physical or mental functioning.

Case Three

At age 90, Mrs. C is bedridden, blind, and has never fully recovered her mental faculties after striking her head in a fall. She is cared for in a comparatively inadequate nursing home. Except for an occasional respiratory infection and arthritic pain, she seems in no distress. She sometimes recognizes her husband, but his attempts to speak to her are usually unintelligible. Six years ago Mrs. C had given a talk at her church on the misery of prolonging the life of the dying elderly, particularly in nursing homes, and made an eloquent plea for "a dignified and simple way to choose death." Now her husband and physician face the problem of determining whether her present situation is a violation of the concept of "death with dignity" that she seemed to advocate.[7]

Case Four

Mrs. D is a 67-year-old retired store clerk who suffers from mild urinary stress incontinence. On this particular visit to her physician, she complains, in a whisper, of loss of sexual libido and discomfort during coitus, but says she prefers not to discuss it. She consistently finds discussing her sexual life or disclosing gynecological symptoms excruciatingly difficult. Two years earlier, she was treated surgically for vaginal phimosis, although she had never complained of the obvious discomfort caused from inspissated smegma collecting beneath the prepuce. Her doctor is now uncertain whether to insist upon discussing her sexual concerns or to accept her clearly expressed wish to terminate the discussion.

In Mrs. C's case, historical evidence suggests that life quality does not meet Mrs. C's own subjective standards, and both her physician and spouse are concerned to respect this subjective measure as far as possible. Mrs. D more clearly conveys a present dissatisfaction with her quality of life. Since Mrs. D is extremely reluctant to discuss sexual issues, the mere broaching of them raises the suspicion that her sexual discomfort and loss of libido matter deeply to her. In both Mrs. C's and Mrs. D's cases, patients or physicians or family members may forfeit their own assessment of life quality by succumbing to cultural stereotypes and values. For example, Mrs. D or her physician may not expect a 67-year-old woman to enjoy a regular and active sexual life. The concern Mrs. C's husband and physician voice about the quality of Mrs. C's life in a nursing home may be based, in part, on the fact that Mrs. C's life falls below accepted cultural standards of what qualifies as a worthwhile life.

These ethical aspects obviously warrant further discussion. For example, what we have said so far clearly has implications for clinical ethical decisions concerning Do Not Resuscitate (DNR) orders and withdrawal of care. However, we now turn our attention to some unique issues in geriatric medical ethics. Our aim will be to underscore the myriad ways in which ethical principles may be vitiated when negative attitudes toward aging impinge upon treatment decisions.

Negative Conceptions of the Elderly

Properly balancing medical ethical principles and standards is part of sound ethical decision-making, but not the whole of it. In geriatric care, in particular, the attitudes of both physicians and patients toward aging may have a pernicious influence on clinical decisions. Even if important ethical considerations are clarified, the interpretation and application of these considerations can be sullied at the start by negative stereotyping by the elderly themselves or by others. Such stereotyping can infect the entire assessment and place in jeopardy the very values ethical principles aim to protect.

Although controversy exists about the extent and manner in which negative attitudes toward the elderly operate in clinical decision-making,[4,8-12] there is mounting evidence that: (1) age is a risk factor for inadequate treatment[13]; (2) variations in patterns of care are related to age[14-16]; and (3) scarce medical resources are less likely to be distributed to older or female patients who are equally medically needy.[17-20] Moreover, despite the difficulty of documenting the precise nature and scope of these problems, to the extent that negative stereotyping is legion in the larger society, both physicians and patients may take for granted certain assumptions about the elderly and incorporate these into their treatment choices. We would do well, then, to explore negative conceptions of the elderly and see how they might influence ethical assessment.

"Ageism," a term first coined by Robert Butler in the late 1960s,[21] refers to a subjective experience of "deep seated uneasiness on the part of the young and middle-aged—a personal revulsion to and distaste for growing old . . . and fear of powerlessness, uselessness, and death." Whereas racism and sexism involve systematic stereotyping of and discrimination against people because of skin color and gender, ageism accomplishes this with chronological age. For example, elderly people are characterized as senile, physically weak and fragile, rigid in thought and manner, and old-fashioned in morality and skills. Attributing negative characteristics to older individuals enables younger individuals to distance themselves and subtly cease identifying with elders as human beings.

So defined, ageist attitudes impart a negative tinge to perceptions of the elderly made by the nonelderly. However, it is important to extend Butler's analysis to incorporate negative stereotypes the elderly *themselves* may harbor. Only then can we fully comprehend the magnitude of ageism and its potential to wreak havoc on otherwise careful ethical argument. Age bias directed at oneself involves internalizing negative attitudes toward aging and, therefore, rejecting personal traits and life events that make age salient (eg, qualities such as wrinkles or graying hair, and hallmark events such as birthdays or becoming a grandparent). A negative stance toward personal aging produces alienation by literally distancing a person from certain aspects of the self which are experienced as revolting and distasteful.

The following illustrations of ageist attitudes are culled from recent literature.

1. *The Equation of an Individual's Value with Life Years Remaining.* Because older individuals have, on average, fewer years remaining, the lives of elderly persons are deemed less valuable.

2. *The View That Life Has Already Been Lived.* Old age is regarded as "borrowed time" or "icing on the cake" because the old have already lived a full life.[22-25]

3. *The Hasty Generalization.* Declining physiological functions that are statistically concomitant with aging are assumed to be present in each aging individual. For example, since many nursing home residents are cognitively impaired, every resident is assumed to be.[8,26]

4. *The Sexual Standard.* Senescence is viewed as synonymous with loss of sexual libido and it is considered normal and desirable for regular sexual activity to cease in later years.[27]
5. *The Devaluation of Later Years.* Older years are thought to be of lower quality than younger years.[28]
6. *The View That Aging Is a Disease.* Age and disease are regarded as one process. Clinical changes associated with aging are negatively evaluated as "deterioration, disorganization, disintegration," even when there is nothing degenerative about these changes unless one assumes that young adulthood represents the paradigm of health.[29-33]

These ageist attitudes present difficulties when interposed between ethical principles and the concrete cases to which these principles apply. For example, an ageist stance can work against the application of an ethical principle or skew its proper interpretation. Ageist starting points can also parade as makeshift principles themselves, gaining legitimacy because of the widespread cultural norms they reflect. Finally, in an opposite fashion, the effort to avoid even the appearance of ageism can discourage frank probing of ways in which age is genuinely relevant.

Interpreting and Utilizing Ethical Principles

Autonomy and Beneficence

Having summarily stated examples of ageist attitudes, we are now in a position to assess how these attitudes can infiltrate otherwise acceptable ethical assessment. To this end, it will be useful to return to the four cases outlined earlier. With respect to each case, we should attempt to say exactly how attributions of ageist assumptions may impugn otherwise sound reasoning.

Let us consider, first, the case of Mrs. A, the 76-year-old with sepsis of the leg. One question that arises in connection with this case is the basis for the physician's decision to treat against the patient's prior wishes. Respecting Mrs. A's wishes would presumably call for not amputating the leg and allowing her to die (eg, from infection that may be present when she arrives at the emergency room in a coma). It may be fear of death, or the view that the death of one's patient constitutes a personal failure, that underlies the physician's decision to treat. One philosopher eloquently describes this as "the fear of one's own death as it peers out at one from the face of debilitated patients. . . . A physical, stomach-wrenching fear [that] can cause some to withdraw and 'do nothing' and others to continue aggressive therapy beyond the point of making sense."[34] If fear of death is operative, the antidote is mustering courage: the courage to confront ethical decisions. Courage can be aided by consulting with colleagues or an ethics committee or by education. But, in the end, it must emanate from within, from self-awareness and from letting go of fear.

An alternative explanation of the outcome in Mrs. A's case would occur if we attribute to her physician an ageist viewpoint, such as that because a greater proportion of elderly people are cognitively impaired, Mrs. A must be. If this assumption is entertained, the physician may reason in the following way. "The principle of autonomy requires that I respect my patient's capacity to make her own rational choice about treatment. But the scope of this principle is obviously limited to persons who actually possess the capacity for autonomous choice. Mrs. A is old and probably not in full possession of this capacity. Her persistent refusal to accept my recommendation for appropriate treatment is further evidence of an impaired state. Hence, my responsibility as her physician is to promote her interests to the best of my ability." The upshot of this reasoning may be a consultation with family members that excludes Mrs. A, followed by an agreement between the physician and family concerning the treatment course that best promotes Mrs. A's interests.

In this case, ageism stands in the way of sound ethical reasoning. The application of the principle of autonomy is obstructed, because the physician is inclined to judge that older people are not in possession of the capacity for autonomous choice. What makes this judgment unwarranted is that it may or may not apply to Mrs. A. Unless and until Mrs. A is evaluated for competency and diagnosed as incompetent, she should not be assumed to be so. Being old is associated with a greater frequency of cognitive impairment, but that does not imply that this particular individual is cognitively compromised. Second, even if informal assessment provides some evidence of incompetence, competence is task-specific. For example, incompetence in performing mathematical calculations or remembering the day of the week may not be germane to assessing competence to decide between treatment options. What is critical in the latter case is just that Mrs. A fully comprehend the nature of the options before her and the risks and benefits associated with each. Finally, although consulting with family members may be advisable, so long as Mrs. A is competent, the decision rests with her, not with her son or other family members.

In connection with the first case, it is also important to focus on the statement that the costs of care for Mrs. A totaled $62,000 in Medicare funds. To what extent should her physician take this into account? Suppose that, rather than treating against Mrs. A's wishes, the physician is considering not treating on the following grounds. "An investment of public monies in Mrs. A will probably yield a lower return than alternative investments of Medicare dollars. That money can be better spent elsewhere."

Even if the decision not to treat is ethically sound, this reasoning does not support it. Such reasoning can be faulted on several grounds. First, it displays the ageist view that an individual's worth is simply a function of life years remaining. But surely this assumption does not reflect our considered judgments. For example, the murder of an older person is not considered less of a crime than the murder of a younger person, nor does it receive a lighter penalty.[35] This suggests that we regard all persons as possessing an underlying worth and dignity, regardless of the number of future years a person will live. Second, the physician's role is to advocate the patient's interests, not to decide how public resources should be distributed. Dispersing Medicare funds is a decision rightly made at the level of public policy by the larger society and not left to the discretion of individual practitioners. Although physicians do not owe more care than a patient is legally or ethically entitled to receive, care supported by public funding should not be withheld on the grounds that dispersing it is unjust. Physicians who oppose present policies should enter into public debates, but they should not usurp a decision that rightly rests with the public at large.[36-40]

Finally, let us consider how ageist assumptions may enter into Mrs. A's *own* decision to forgo care. Suppose we attribute to *her* a poor self-image and lack of self-esteem and the consequent belief that, at her age, she does not deserve publicly funded medical care aimed at prolonging life. How might this belief skew the outcome of Mrs. A's deliberations? Suppose Mrs. A does wish to continue living; however, she declines treatment because she judges that a woman of her age does not *deserve* to have her life extended.

Here, it is helpful to begin by focusing on the ageist assumption itself and exposing it as unfounded. To do this, we need to explain why it is wrong to suppose that after reaching the marker of a "full life span," individuals have no claim to life-extending care. To begin with, it is far from clear to what a "full life span" refers or whether it refers to the same thing for every individual. Second, even assuming that this considerable difficulty can be surmounted, a further difficulty remains—namely, that although having lived a full life span may make a person's death easier to accept *in hindsight,* it hardly makes any *manner* of death acceptable.[41,42] In the case of an individual like Mrs. A who desires to live and whose future holds out the hope of many good years, it would be wrong to deny routine antibiotic care simply because she is old. Although Mrs. A's claim to medical care is not unlimited, Mrs. A should reject the idea that old age per se makes her ethically ineligible for routine treatment.

Let us turn now to the case of Mrs. B, the 85-year-old with recurrent carcinoma. In this case, it is important to distinguish between the process of weighing competing ethical principles, on the one hand, and the process of guarding against ageist assumptions inimical to these principles, on the other hand. To illustrate this, let us suppose that Mrs. B entertains the ageist assumption that since she does not have much time left, it follows that her life is not worth much. If we suppose that Mrs. B is apprised of her situation, this assumption will be inimical both to autonomy and to beneficence. It is contrary to both because it undervalues the importance of all of Mrs. B's interests, including her capacity to make self-directed choices. For example, on these grounds, Mrs. B will be considerably less motivated to protect her own welfare and to struggle with making an autonomous choice between options. She will be less likely to protect any of her interests should they be threatened by others.

Next, suppose that we assign to Mrs. B's physician the view that 85-year-olds are cognitively impaired and so stand in need of special protection. On these grounds, the choice is made to withhold information about Mrs. B's condition from her. The outcome of this reasoning favors beneficence, but ageism itself does not *support* beneficence. Mrs. B's best interests are not protected by ageist assumptions, because her interests include being treated with respect, but ageism prompts others to regard her as childlike and incompetent. Mrs. B's interest in developing and sustaining self-esteem and self-confidence are also ill-served. Hence, even where ageism leads to favoring one ethical principle rather than another it fails to *uphold* ethical principles.

Finally, suppose that ageist assumptions are not held by either Mrs. B or her physician. How should the principles of beneficence and autonomy be weighed against one another? To begin with, the physician should make a careful assessment as to whether his suspicion that knowledge of recurrent cancer would "be more than Mrs. B could bear" is genuinely warranted. If she is diagnosed as depressed, this factor should be taken into consideration. It may be decisive, but it is not necessarily decisive. This will depend on how depressed the patient is diagnosed as being. It may be possible, for example, to bring a mild depression under control to the point where, with counseling and assistance, Mrs. B is able to face her situation and make autonomous choices. Alternatively, if Mrs. B is not clinically depressed but is nonetheless anxious and fearful about facing death, she should be told of the situation and assisted.

What about the other argument, suggested by the physician's remark that it is best "not to make her last months miserable with futile treatment or the knowledge that she is dying"? First, it will be important to probe the medical judgment that chemotherapy for this patient would be "futile." Although the efficacy of chemotherapy in older patients is controversial, there is evidence to suggest that its value has been understated.[13,43] It may well be that the choice is between gaining a small benefit (eg, a few months' more time purchased at the price of an unpleasant chemotherapy regime versus not undergoing therapy and perhaps dying sooner). If the choice can be framed appropriately in this way, then confronting the patient with options may be crucial to clarifying the patient's values and goals. For example, Mrs. B may wish to be alive a few more months to witness the birth of her first great-grandchild or to attend the wedding of her only granddaughter. Protecting her true interests may not be possible without exploring with her where her interests lie.

Even if we accept the suggestion that beneficence as well as autonomy support disclosing information to a competent patient, it is still important for the physician to make efforts to prevent the knowledge of terminal illness from making Mrs. B's last months miserable. For instance, it would be appropriate for the physician to tell Mrs. B about her situation while concomitantly attending to her emotional needs. One physician, who works with terminally ill geriatric cancer patients,[44] recommends that palliative care at this point include the following:

1. *Empathy:* acknowledging the patient's emotional reaction.
2. *Legitimation:* affirming that the patient's emotions are legitimate by underscoring the fact that these emotions are common and reasonable emotions to experience under the circumstances.
3. *Support:* explicit affirmation by the physician that he or she will be with the patient and provide care throughout the entire course of the illness.
4. *Partnership:* offering assistance in decision-making.
5. *Respect:* expressing regard for the patient—for example, by an honest compliment praising the patient's openness, courage, or honesty.

Quality of Life

As caring for large numbers of elderly patients becomes a central mission of health-care professionals, the present emphasis on acute care and crisis intervention is likely to shift to chronic care and to improving the patient's quality of life. The three remaining ageist assumptions are: (4) the sexual standard, (5) the devaluation of later years, and (6) the view that age is a disease. These pose special problems for clinical decisions involving chronic conditions that threaten the quality of a patient's life without presenting a threat to life itself.

For example, Mrs. D, who finds coitus painful and experiences a loss of libido, may be prevented from seeking assistance because she falsely believes that old age is synonymous with loss of libido or that her discomfort during intercourse is nature's way of telling her that sex at her age is no longer possible. Simple medical treatment, such as estrogen therapy or vaginal cream, may ameliorate her discomfort and make sexual activity more enjoyable.[45] Yet even if

Mrs. D combats her embarrassment and discusses her difficulties with her physician, ageist assumptions may keep her from following through and complying with her doctor's recommendations.[46]

It is important to begin by spelling out the reasons for rejecting the ageist stereotype Mrs. D holds. First, although deprivation of sexual stimulation can result in loss of erotic desire, senescence need not be accompanied with deprivation of sexual stimulation. Although physiological changes in genitalia in postmenopausal women can make coitus uncomfortable (eg, by shrinkage in the diameter of the introitus and diminished secretion of vaginal fluid), these conditions can be treated and sexual activity made possible. Finally, sexual activity in later years is desirable for the same reason it is desirable at any age: it improves the quality of a person's life, eg, by imparting a sense of well-being and vitality and by strengthening feelings of love for another human being. On these grounds, it is important to do what is possible to make sexual relations possible for elderly patients who wish them. One way of doing this is to unmask ageist assumptions. Otherwise, even if aging does not actually interfere with sexual functioning, a view of aging that rejects sexuality as inappropriate prevents sexual relations from occurring.[47] Another way of making sexual relations possible is to perform medical procedures, such as surgery, in a way that preserves capacity for intercourse wherever possible. Finally, practical issues should be addressed: if nursing home resident romances develop, opportunities for privacy and intimacy should be afforded; for elderly patients with special disabilities, such as stroke, a footboard or trapeze can assist mobility.[48-51]

Physicians should also be aware that ageist standards can be an especially heavy burden for the older woman. In our society, women are encouraged to believe that loss of youth represents loss of beauty and that physical beauty is an important gauge of personal worth. Moreover, women are often considered sexually ineligible much earlier than men. Whereas men remain eligible sexual partners as long as they can perform coitus, women are at a disadvantage because their sexual candidacy often depends upon meeting much stricter standards related to looks and age.[52] To the extent that Mrs. D or her spouse internalize these cultural standards, the likelihood of rich and meaningful intimacy is reduced.

Whereas Mrs. D appears in relatively good health, the case of Mrs. C—the bedridden, blind, and cognitively impaired 90-year-old—challenges us to identify the extent to which an acceptable quality of life is possible with multiple serious impairments. Mrs. C is especially vulnerable to becoming the victim of ageist assumptions, because she is not in a position to defend herself against them. The devaluation of life, because it is the life of a 90-year-old, or the related pejorative assumption that aging itself is a pathology, may impede ethically responsible care.

One way for Mrs. C's physician to improve the quality of Mrs. C's daily life is by assisting with locating a more adequate nursing home or extended-care facility. Alternatively, home care may be a feasible option if a spouse or offspring is able to assist with care, perhaps in conjunction with community-based assistance. In considering how to improve Mrs. C's situation, it is important to recall the distinction made earlier, between subjective satisfaction with life, the evaluation of life quality by third parties, and the evaluation of life quality implied by society's values. The pleasure of life in old age, even life with multiple impairments, is liable to be misjudged by those who are neither old nor impaired.[53]

Finally, it is important to distinguish between the views espoused by Mrs. C 6 years earlier, and her present subjective satisfaction.

Despite the fact that no specific treatment decision faces Mrs. C's physician, it is important to consider what role quality of life judgments should have in future decisions. While quality of life is sometimes an acceptable basis for limiting treatment, the judgment of life quality would ideally come from patients themselves. However, even though this is not possible in Mrs. C's case, poor life quality may nonetheless be an acceptable ground for limiting future care.[54] This will be so if the quality of Mrs. C's life falls below a minimal threshold and the intervention would only preserve this condition.[55] The minimal threshold would include, for example, loss of qualities necessary for human interaction. In the process of making such an assessment, it is important to denude ageist stereotypes hidden beneath the surface of seemingly benign judgments. As far as possible, third-party assessments should reflect the subjective standard patients themselves would apply if they were able.

The Salience of Age

> That direct stare which passes between the young and the old is high up among the classic confrontations. It prefaces one of the great dialogues of opposites, and contains a frank admission of helplessness on either side, for nothing can be done to blot out the detail of what has been, or block in the detail of what is to come. On the one side is the clean sheet and on the other the crammed page....[56]

Defusing ageist assumptions is not the only reason to attend specifically to medical ethical issues in geriatrics. It is also important to take stock of the multitude of ways in which having lived a long life distinguishes a person. It would be a mistake to suppose that age is never appropriately salient or that the old are no different from the young.

Caring for the elderly places special responsibilities on physicians, because diagnosis and communication with the elderly is more likely to pose a challenge. The elderly are more likely than other age groups to present with atypical or altered symptoms that make diagnosis difficult. They are more likely to present with qualities that make effective communication difficult, such as dementia (10%), impaired hearing (22%), and visual handicaps (15%).[29] In addition, as a group, elderly people have a high incidence of noncompliance. For example, one study revealed that 43% of elderly patients were noncompliant with their medication regimens and 90% of these patients underused their medication.[57] In another study, 59% of participating outpatients over 60 years of age had taken medications incorrectly, with 26% of the errors considered dangerous.[58] These and other medical factors set the elderly apart from other age groups and place upon physicians a duty to attend to special needs. For example, once a prescription is written for an elderly patient, the physician's responsibilities are not discharged. Physicians are additionally responsible to confirm compliance; enlist others to assist with medication where appropriate; maintain simple and short therapeutic regimens where possible; monitor compliance in nonobtrusive ways if indicated; facilitate compliance by compensating for problems, such as diminution of senses, confusion, and memory loss; and communicate effectively the importance of medication, especially in asymptomatic patients.[59]

In addition to these and other physiological differences that are sometimes present in old age, the subjective experience of aging distinguishes the elderly. Although the subjective experience of aging is not the subject of medicine, appreciating it is part of treating the patient as a full person. Medicine mistakenly objectifies patients when it regards them as bodies with symptoms, rather than attending to the inner experience of being in a particular body. Likewise, medicine mistakenly objectifies older patients when it stereotypes the elderly or imposes a predetermined meaning upon old age, rather than comprehending aging in the individual.

A patient's subjective experience of aging is evoked by augmenting objective medical methods with methods that aim to interpret patients' subjective life. Employing such an approach in medical history taking, for example, involves interpreting the chronological fact of age not only by asking, "How old are you?" but also by asking, "What is life now like for you?"[60] Acknowledging subjective components of aging recognizes that a person's biography and personal history are part of what makes individuals what they are. By contrast, ignoring these dimensions falsifies a reality that is part of a person in his or her fullness.[22]

If medicine aims to enlarge its perspective and find a place for a subjective focus, the possibility of morally grounding the physician–patient relationship is made possible. Moral grounding hinges not only on articulating and interpreting moral principles, it is also a matter of human beings and human interactions realizing the values these principles protect. In medicine, the visible body and the objective data it produces easily loom large, occluding human subjective aspects that animate the body. A more humane approach to geriatric medicine requires laying bare personal and idiosyncratic human qualities that enlighten us about each other and enable us to discover one another as persons.

These possiblities are especially potent in the long-term care of elderly patients. The rewards of caring for geriatric patients are more likely to be found in the ongoing therapeutic relationship, than in dramatic cures or heroic outcomes.[61] Geriatric medicine thus holds out the hope of an alternative model for the physician–patient relationship and a new and richer medical ethic.

References

1. Pifer A, Bronte DL: Squaring the pyramid. *Daedalus* 1986;115:1–9.
2. Leslie LA: Changing facts and changing needs in women's health care. *Nurs Clin North Am* 1986;21:111–123.
3. Beauchamp TL, Childress JF: *Principles of Biomedical Ethics*, ed. 2. New York, Oxford University Press, 1983.
4. Wetle TT: Ethical aspects of decision making for and with the elderly, in Kapp MB, Pies HE, Doudera AE (eds.): *Legal and Ethical Aspects of Health Care for the Elderly.* Ann Arbor, Health Administration Press, 1985, pp 258–267.
5. Gadow S: Medicine, ethics, and the elderly. *Gerontologist* 1980;20:680–685.
6. Pearlman R, Jonsen A: The use of quality of life considerations in medical decision making. *J Am Geriatr Soc* 1985;33:344–352.
7. Veatch RM: *Case Studies in Medical Ethics.* Cambridge, Harvard University Press, 1977, pp 340–342.
8. Crockett W, Hummert ML: Perceptions of aging and the elderly. *Annu Rev Gerontol Geriatr* 1987;7:217–239.
9. Greene MG, Adelman R, Charon R, et al: Ageism in the medical encounter: An exploratory study of the doctor–elderly patient relationship. *Language and Communication* 1986;6:113–124.

10. Kosberg JI: The importance of attitudes on the interaction between health care providers and geriatric populations. *Interdiscipl Topics Gerontol* 1983;17:132–143.
11. Ward RA: The marginality and salience of being old: When is age relevant? *Gerontologist* 1984;24:227–232.
12. Damrasch SP, Fischman SH: Medical students' attitudes toward sexually active older people. *J Am Geriatr Soc* 1985;33:852–855.
13. Wetle T: Age as a risk factor for inadequate treatment. *JAMA* 1987;258:516.
14. Greenfield S, Blanco DM, Elashoff RM, et al: Patterns of care related to age of breast cancer patients. *JAMA* 1987;257:2766–2770.
15. Samet J, Hunt WC, Key C, et al: Choice of cancer therapy varies with age of patient. *JAMA* 1986;255:3385–3390.
16. Wagner A: Cardiopulmonary resuscitation in the aged. *N Engl J Med* 1984;310:1129–1130.
17. Eggers PW: Effect of transplantation on the medicare end-stage renal disease program. *N Engl J Med* 1988;318:223–229.
18. Held PJ, Pauly MV, Bovbjerg RB, et al: Access to kidney transplantation: Has the United States eliminated income and racial differences? *Arch Intern Med* 1988;148:2594–2600.
19. Kjellstrand CM: Age, sex, and race inequality in renal transplantation. *Arch Intern Med* 1988;148:1305–1309.
20. Kilner JF: Selecting patients when resources are limited: A study of U.S. medical directors of kidney dialysis and transplantation facilities. *Am J Public Health* 1988;78:144–147.
21. Butler RN: Age-ism: Another form of bigotry. *Gerontologist* 1969;9:243–246.
22. Callahan D: *Setting Limits: Medical Goals in an Aging Society.* New York, Simon & Schuster, 1987.
23. Callahan D: On defining a natural death. *Hastings Cent Rep* 1977;7:32–37.
24. Somerville MA: Should the grandparents die?: Allocation of medical resources with an aging population. *Law Med Health Care* 1986;14:158–163.
25. MacIntyre A: The right to die garrulously, in Purtill RL (ed.): *Moral Dilemmas.* Belmont, Wadsworth, 1985.
26. Leslie LA: Changing factors and changing needs in women's health care. *Nurs Clin North Am* 1986;21:111–123.
27. Starr BD: Sexuality and aging. *Annu Rev Gerontol* 1985;5:97–126.
28. Schelling TC: The life you save may be your own, in Chase S (ed.): *Problems in Public Expenditure Analysis.* Washington, D.C., Brookings Institution, 1968, pp 127–176.
29. Rowe JW: Health care for the elderly. *N Eng J Med* 1985;312:828.
30. Jecker NS: Towards a theory of age group justice. *J Med Philosophy* 1989;14:655–676.
31. Caplan A: The 'unnaturalness' of aging—A sickness unto death?, in Caplan A, Engelhardt HT, McCartney JJ (eds.): *Concepts of Health and Disease: Interdisciplinary Perspectives.* Reading, Massachusetts, Addison-Wesley, 1981.
32. Rosenfeld A: *Prolongevity.* New York, Knopf, 1976.
33. Gelein JL: Aged women and health. *Nurs Clin North Am* 1982;17:179–185.
34. Thomasma DC: Ethical judgments of quality of life in the care of the aged. *J Am Geriatr Soc* 1984;32:525–527.
35. Bell N: Ethical considerations in the allocation of scarce medical resources. Ph.D. dissertation, University of North Carolina, Chapel Hill, 1978.
36. Dyer AR, Brazil P: Cost-cutting at the bedside: A debate. *Hastings Cent Rep* 1986;16:5–8.
37. Angell M: Cost containment and the physician. *JAMA* 1985;254:1203–1207.
38. Morreim HE: Cost containment: Challenging fidelity and justice. *Hastings Cent Rep* 1988;18:20–25.
39. Jecker NS: Integrating medical ethics with normative theory. *Theor Med* 1990;11:125–139.

40. Daniels N: The ideal advocate and limited resources. *Theor Med* 1987;8:69–80.
41. Jecker NS: Disenfranchising the elderly from life-extending care. *Public Aff Q* 1988;2:51–68.
42. Jecker NS: Excluding the elderly: A reply to Callahan. *Rep Cent Philos Public Policy* 1987;8:12–15.
43. Begg CB, Cohen FL, Ellerton J: Are the elderly predisposed to toxicity from cancer chemotherapy? *Cancer Clin Trials* 1980;3:369–374.
44. Kinzel T: Relief of emotional symptoms in elderly patients with terminal cancer. *Geriatrics* 1988;43:61–66.
45. Breen JL, Lebow M, Boffard D: Practice of gynecology in the elderly. *Clin Ther* 1985;7:400–405.
46. Pucino F, Beck CL, Seifert RL, et al: Pharmacogeriatrics. *Pharmacotherapy* 1985;5:314–326.
47. Nadelson CC: Geriatric sex problems: Discussion. *J Geriatr Psychiatry* 1984;17:139–147.
48. Renshaw DC: Geriatric sex problems. *J Geriatr Psychiatry* 1984;17:123–138.
49. Meyers WA: Sexuality in the older individual. *J Am Acad Psychoanal* 1985;13:511–520.
50. Renshaw DC: Sex, age, and values. *J Am Geriatr Soc* 1985;33:635–643.
51. Thienhaus OJ: Practical overview of sexual function and advancing age. *Geriatrics* 1988;43:63–67.
52. Sontag S: The double standard of aging. *Occas Pap Gerontol* 1975.
53. Avron J: Benefit and cost analysis in geriatric care: Turning age discrimination into health policy. *N Engl J Med* 1984;310:1294–1301.
54. Lo B, Jonsen A: Clinical decision to limit treatment. *Ann Intern Med* 1980;93:764–768.
55. Jonsen AR, Seigler M, Winslade WJ: *Clinical Ethics,* ed. 2. New York, Macmillan, 1988.
56. Blythe R: *The View in Winter: Reflections on Old Age.* New York, Harcourt Brace Jovanovich, 1979.
57. Cooper JK, Love DW, Raffoul PR: Intentional prescription nonadherance (noncompliance) by the elderly. *J Am Geriatr Soc* 1982;30:329–333.
58. Shaw PG: Common pitfalls in geriatric drug prescribing. *Drugs* 1982;23:324–328.
59. Robertson W: The problem of patient compliance. *Am J Obstet Gynecol* 1985;152:948–952.
60. Gadow S: Introduction to Part II, in Gadow S, Cole T (eds.): *What Does It Mean To Grow Old?* Durham, Duke University Press, 1986.
61. Cassel CK: The meaning of health care in old age, in Gadow S, Cole T (eds.): *What Does It Mean To Grow Old?* Durham, Duke University Press, 1986.

Chapter 3

Biology of Aging and the Human Female

George M. Martin, MD

The demographic data, outlined by Dr. Aagaard in Chapter 5, reveal major gains in life expectancies for human populations, particularly for the female. We are now witnessing exponential increases in the proportions of those segments of our population who are over the age of 65, particularly those over the age of 80. Thus, to an increasing degree, gynecologists and other health professionals should be aware of the state of our knowledge concerning the biology of aging. I have attempted to provide, in this chapter, a concise review of this field as of 1989, including some discussion of topics particularly germane to the human female, such as the biology of reproductive aging and current views as to the reasons females generally outlive their spouses.

By way of introduction, I must caution the reader that a rigorous program of research on basic mechanisms of aging is of relatively recent vintage. The National Institute on Aging is one of the newest branches of the NIH, having been established in 1974. While we know a great deal about the phenomenology of aging, including age-related disease, we still have comparatively little understanding of fundamental mechanisms.

Some Definitions

Some gerontologists (particularly plant biologists) use the term *aging* to refer to all of the structural and functional alterations observable during the lifecourse, from birth to death.[1] Mammalian gerontologists, however, differentiate between such changes associated with development and those that follow sexual maturation and the emergence of a young adult phenotype. They often use the term *aging* synonymously with *senescence* (or, more properly, senescing). In this chapter, we shall define aging as a constellation of changes in structure and function of an organism (usually deteriorative but sometimes adaptive), generally beginning after sexual maturation, such that there is a slow, insidious, and progressive decline in the efficiency of homeostasis and a decreasing probability of a successful reaction to injury. In the language of thermodynamics, there appears to be an inexorable increase in entropy, or, put another way, an increase in the degree of molecular disorder. In any case, the net result, for large populations of organisms, is an exponential increase in the probability of

Figure 3.1. Schematic diagrams of death rates, over time, for a hypothetical population of nonaging organisms (A) and two populations exhibiting intrinsic biological aging, although with contrasting life spans.

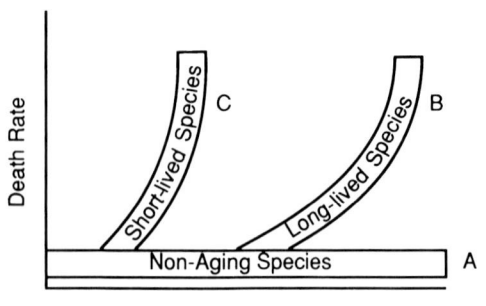

death per unit time. This is shown schematically in Figure 3.1. A hypothetical population of organisms that do not exhibit aging is represented by A in the figure, in which there is no change in the death rate over time. Populations exhibiting biological aging would follow trajectories indicated by B and C, the former representing a comparatively long-lived species in which the exponential rise in death rate is delayed and the initial slope is less steep in comparison with species C. These oversimplified diagrams refer to organisms with iteroparous types of reproduction—that is, repeated episodes of reproduction. Virtually all mammals are of that type. Organisms with semelparous types of reproduction ("big bang" reproduction)[2] typically exhibit, immediately following their single, massive reproductive effort, a very rapid and roughly synchronized structural and physiological deterioration, resulting in a pattern of approximately synchronized death of the population, often interpreted as "programmed" aging. Such patterns of aging are characteristic of certain species of migrating salmon, flowering plants, octopuses, and marsupial mice.

Evolutionary Biology and Aging

Why did aging evolve in biological systems? After all, given such incredible biological achievements as embryogenesis and the development of central nervous systems capable of higher cognition, the design of molecular machinery suitable for the indefinite maintenance of an adult structure would seem facile by comparison. Most evolutionary biologists believe that aging evolved on the basis of one or both of the following nonadaptive mechanisms (see Refs. 3 and 4 for reviews). Probably, the favored idea is that of antagonistic pleiotropy. According to that notion, various alleles at a number of genetic loci, selected because they confer enhanced reproductive fitness during the early phase of the life span, have negative effects late in the life span, when the force of natural selection is comparatively weak, since reproduction declines or ceases. One specific example cited in a classical paper by Williams[5] concerned genes with effects upon the efficiency of incorporation of calcium into bones of young organisms; he argued that alleles selected for enhanced efficiency might contribute to the development of calcific depositions in the arterial walls later in life, thus contributing to senescence. The second idea simply suggests that mutations with late-life effects accumulate during biological evolution because natural selection against such accumulations is not sufficiently strong.[6] There is some experimental evidence in fruit flies to support these ideas (see Ref. 7 for review). Whatever the mechanisms, in the last few years, two independent laboratories have shown that it is possible to indirectly select lines of long-lived flies by serially selecting for females exhibiting comparatively high fecundity *late* in the life span.[8,9] Both labs started with different isolates of genetically heterogeneous wild-type lines of *Drosophila melanogaster*. Many genes seem to be contributing to the increased life span.[10] A few of these genes are now being characterized. Could they prove to be of relevance to the life span of other species, including man? While it is indeed possible that there may be some common denominators, a priori, there are no compelling reasons why the specific kinds of antagonistically pleiotropic genes and accumulated mutations should be identical.[11,12] Furthermore, we must remember that all phenotypes are the result of the interactions of the genetic constitution and the environment. It is possible that the nature of a particular gene action, vis-à-vis its effect upon aging, could vary substantially in contrasting environmental settings.

How Many Genes?

The most obvious arguments that rates of aging are subject to genetic controls derive from observations on the variations of maximum life-span potentials of various species, including those within specific taxonomic groups. For example, there is more than a 30-fold difference in maximum life spans among mammalian species.[13] Note that I have emphasized *maximum* life span. It is well-established that, for many populations, *mean* life span is subject to wide fluctuations as functions of even modest alterations in environment, while, with the single exception so far of caloric restriction regimes (discussed below), effects of nonlethal alterations in environment on the maximum life span of a cohort appear to be relatively small. The maximum life-span potential indeed appears to be a constitutional feature of speciation.

How many genes might be involved in the determination of varying rates of aging and varying longevities among species and within a species? There are no satisfactory answers to this question. In the fruit-fly selection experiments noted above, while there were genetic elements contributing to long life span on all of the chromosomes of *Drosophila*, the total number of genes involved is unknown. Studies on the fossil remains of the hominid precursors of man (coupled with known correlations between brain size and longevity and estimates of rates of point mutation) have suggested that, during the comparatively rapid period of evolution to *Homo sapiens*, perhaps 200 to 300 genes were involved, supporting a polygenic basis for the modulation of life span.[14,15] There are reasons to believe, however, that the important changes in speciation involved chromosomal rearrangements rather than point mutations.[16] My own approach to this question involved a systematic analysis of the known mutations in man that had phenotypic effects that overlapped, to some extent, with the senescent phenotype of man, as we see it in the clinics and on the autopsy table.[17] The conclusion was that, as an upper limit, perhaps 7000 loci could be involved, assuming a total of 100,000 genes in man. Since, however, there was evidence of certain single-gene syndromes with rather profound, multiple effects upon the phenotype ("segmental progeroid syndromes"), such as the Werner syndrome,[18] it was speculated that only a small proportion of such loci (perhaps as few as 70 genes) might be of major importance in determining differential rates of aging in our species. That study is also subject to many uncertainties, however. Nonetheless, it is reasonable to conclude that the control of how we age is subject to rather complex genetic controls. Another conclusion, of special significance to the clinician, is that human beings, who are exceptionally heterogeneous in terms of both genetic and environmental influences, are likely to vary substantially in their patterns of aging. It is fair to say that no two individuals ever have aged, or ever will age, in precisely the same fashion. Thus, every time a clinician contemplates an intervention in a geriatric patient, he should consider that he (or she) is embarking upon a new experiment.

Molecular and Cell Biology of Aging

Rather than simply cataloging the numerous molecular and cellular alterations that occur in aging organisms, I shall review a selective subset of these within the framework of a few of the many theories of aging. For a more complete treatment, see Warner et al.[19] For the reader who wants to quickly learn the current status of "the bottom line," suffice it to say that there is no compelling evidence supporting a given theory of aging. Moreover, we are unlikely to discover a single mechanism or process of aging. Instead, one should think in terms of multiple processes of aging. At issue is exactly how many independent mechanisms are primarily involved. One interpretation of the caloric restriction experiments (see below) is that there may be comparatively few such processes. Such a conclusion is at odds with the evolutionary and genetic considerations discussed above. We will require a great deal more research to learn which interpretation is closer to the truth.

The Free Radical Theory of Aging

Chemical-free radicals are atoms or groups of atoms (eg, the hydroxyl ion) characterized by the presence of at least one unpaired electron. They are highly reactive moieties, capable of interacting with a variety of biologically important macromolecules. According to the free radical theory of aging, perhaps the currently most popular of the molecular theories of aging, such radicals are responsible for a host of oxidative alterations that are the root causes of cell alteration and cell death in aging aerobic organisms.[20,21] In all aerobic organisms, the cytochrome oxidase system of respiration evolved in order to quadrivalently reduce molecular oxygen. There is, however, a slight but significant "leakage" in the system, in which univalently reduced oxygen leads to the generation of active oxygen radicals.[22] While specific enzymatic protective mechanisms have presumably evolved to protect against such products (eg, the two major forms of superoxide dismutase, catalase, and glutathione peroxidase),[22] some degree of damage to cell organelles may nevertheless ensue, according to the theory. Moreover, there are numerous other biochemical reactions that produce active radicals as products of intermediary metabolism.

Under some circumstances, an attack by chemical-free radicals can lead to a chain reaction (eg, lipid peroxidation), resulting in extensive damage to the membranes of cells and cell organelles. Such reactions have been postulated

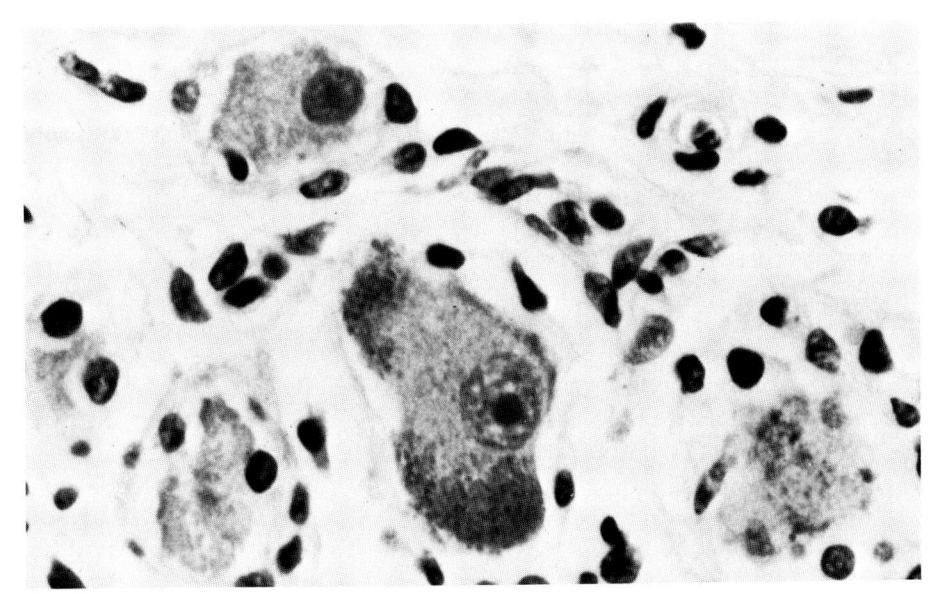

Figure 3.2. A light micrograph of a neuron of a spinal ganglion from an 88-year-old patient who died of Alzheimer's disease. There are masses of lipofuscin pigment within the cytoplasm that, with the H&E stain, appeared yellow-brown. These pigments also exhibit a characteristic fluorescence.

as the basis for the appearance, during aging, of lipofuscin pigments ("wear and tear pigments," "aging pigments").[23] These pigments (Figure 3.2) can be found in a number of cell types and in an amazing variety of aging organisms, ranging from fungi to man.[24] Its rate of accumulation appears to be related to intrinsic biological aging and not merely to chronological time.[25] Thus, it is a candidate for a biological marker of aging and may be interpreted as evidence in support of the free radical theory of aging. A relatively direct test of the theory, however, involving the treatment of experimental animals with antioxidants, has not resulted in convincing life-span extensions.[26] Life spans have been clearly increased, however, via caloric restriction.[27] This was initially interpreted by some as evidence in support of the free radical theory, as the assumption was that the metabolic rate of the calorically restricted animals was reduced. Direct measurements, however, have failed to show reductions in oxygen uptake per lean body mass.[28,29] Thus, the only experimental method that has been shown to enhance life span does not appear to alter the metabolic rate and, hence, the flux of oxygen-free radicals, although it is possible that caloric restriction could decrease the "leakiness" of the cytochrome oxidase system; direct measurements of the degree of univalent reduction of oxygen in control versus calorically restricted animals have not yet been carried out.

Somatic Mutational Theories of Aging

Somatic mutations are structural alterations in genes (either alterations in the primary nucleotide sequences of DNA or alterations in gene dosage) that occur in the cells of the body (soma). Their frequencies may or may not be correlated with mutations in the germ line. There are many different types of somatic mutation and these may result from a number of different molecular mechanisms.[30] One potential mechanism is in fact damage to DNA by active oxygen species. We know relatively little about the molecular details of such injury and its genetic consequences.

In model test-tube experiments, however, it has recently been shown that oxygen-free radicals, formed via the autoxidation of iron, are mutagenic, resulting in a preponderance of transversion types of point mutations (eg, substitution of adenine for thymine).[31] Do somatic mutations of any kind accumulate during aging in mammals? For the case of the peripheral blood T lymphocytes of man, there is evidence that mutations at the X-linked locus, hypoxanthine guanine phosphoribosyltransferase (HPRT), do indeed accumulate during aging.[32] No evidence for the accumulation of such HPRT mutations could be found in the somatic cells (renal tubular epithelium and interstitial fibroblasts of skeletal muscle) of very old mice, however.[33] Thus, the positive findings in man may simply be related to chronological time rather than to intrinsic biological aging, since the maximum life span of man is about 20 or 30 times that of the house mouse. Of course, it is difficult to make any generalizations at this time because so few genetic loci have been examined and in only a few cell types.

In the mutation research noted above, the lesions were presumably point mutations and intragenic deletions or rearrangements. Chromosomal mutations, involving larger scale mutations, do indeed accumulate in the tissues of aging mice at very high frequencies.[34] In addition, alterations in the numbers of chromosomes are seen. There are several possible etiologies for such aberrations, including free radical damage, viral-induced cell fusion, transposon-mediated rearrangements, premature centromere division (perhaps related to abnormalities in centromeric proteins), and gene amplification. With respect to the latter mechanism, it has been proposed that a variety of agents that interrupt DNA synthesis can result, via a sort of "stuttering" of reinitiation, in extra strands of DNA with resulting recombinational pathways leading to many different types of chromosomal lesions.[35] There have also been many studies showing increased frequencies of chromosomal aberrations in somatic cells from aging human subjects, mostly peripheral blood lymphocytes, including demonstrations of increased sensitivities of cells from older donors to agents that break chromosomes.[36]

A line of research that supports an important role of chromosomal pathology in aging comes from studies of a rare, but striking progeroid syndrome, the Werner syndrome (sometimes referred to as progeria of the adult). The disorder is inherited as an autosomal recessive and is characterized by a failure to undergo the usual adolescent growth spurt and the premature onset and rapid progression of greying of the hair, loss of hair, atrophic changes and ulceration of skin, ocular cataracts, osteoporosis, diabetes mellitus, several forms of arteriosclerosis, hypogonadism, and a susceptibility to neoplasia (particularly mesenchymal neoplasms).[18] Somatic cells from such subjects are prone to develop chromosomal deletions, inversions, and reciprocal translocations.[37] Intragenic mutations also appear to be predominately deletions.[38]

Arguments against a universal role for somatic mutations in aging come from experiments in insects.[39] For the case of recessive mutations, their effects upon life span could be tested in a species of wasps (*Habrobracon*), males of which may be either haploid or diploid. The life spans of haploids and diploids are the same but, in control experiments, ionizing radiation was much more effective in reducing life span in the haploids.[40] Thus, it seems unlikely that the accumulation of recessive mutations is of importance in the natural senescence of the wasp. A caveat, however, is that a number of critically important loci may in fact be diploid in the predominately haploid organism.

Protein Synthesis Error Catastrophe Theory

Although essentially "pronounced dead" by at least one distinguished gerontologist,[41] this particularly elegant idea still has not been rigorously tested, in my opinion, in certain critical settings—for example, in a variety of obligate postreplicative mammalian cells in vivo.

In his original formulation, Orgel[42] argued that errors in the synthesis of proteins that were themselves involved in the synthesis of other proteins would lead to an exponential increase in the subsequent error rates, leading to massive accumulations of abnormal proteins in the cells of very aged organisms. In a later publication, Orgel pointed out that such error catastrophes were by no means inevitable, a crucial variable being the efficiency with which proteolytic enzymes were able to recognize and degrade the abnormal protein synthetic machinery.[43] These ideas stimulated a great number of experiments, the bulk of which argue against the accumulation of biosynthetic errors during aging.[41] Abnormal proteins definitely accumulate; however, they result from posttranslational alterations.[44] One such type of alteration, the glycation of proteins, has recently been postulated to play an important role in aging and will be further discussed below.

Glycation of Proteins and DNA

Glycation is the currently preferred biochemical nomenclature for "nonenzymatic glycosylation" reactions. Glycations of proteins involve reactions between reducing sugars and the primary amino groups of proteins. The first product of the reaction is a comparatively labile Schiff base derivative of the protein. This slowly undergoes an isomerization reaction to form the relatively stable ketoamine adduct via an Amadori rearrangement.[45] The most familiar example to physicians would be the glycation of hemoglobins at the N-termini of their beta chains by glucose and its phosphorylated derivatives, assays for which are used for the monitoring of the level of control of diabetic patients.[46]

Cerami et al[47] have proposed that glucose-mediated glycations of proteins are major mediators of aging. His group has also emphasized the potential role of glycations of DNA in mutagenesis.[48]

Support for a role for glycation reactions in aging comes from the observations of reduced levels of glycated hemoglobins in long-lived, calorically restricted rodents.[49]

Clonal Senescence

Clonal senescence may be defined as the gradual attenuation of the growth of proliferating colonies of somatic cells (derived from single parental cells), culminating in populations of cells which are still viable, but "reproductively dead."[50] This is the basic phenomenology of the famous "Hayflick limit."[51] It is apparent that this phenomenon cannot be of relevance to the aging of most species of insects, since their somatic cells, with the exception of the lineages leading to the production of gametes, are obligately postreplicative. In mammals, however, the maintenance of the integrity of many tissues is dependent upon an orderly replacement of effete cells. Therefore, it is possible that the clonal senescence of certain critical cells types may contribute to the development of components of senescence. Furthermore, the senescent phenotype of mammals is characterized by a marked decline in proliferative homeostasis, with the appearance of tissue atrophy side by side with multiple foci of inappropriate proliferation.[52] It is, therefore, possible that aberrations in cell–cell interaction, consequent to clonal senescence, contribute to the precursors of age-related neoplasia.

That the phenomenon of clonal senescence, as studied in cell culture, may in fact be of relevance to cell aging in vivo is supported by three lines of evidence. Most important, perhaps, is the observation that the life spans of cultured somatic cells from a series of mammalian species of contrasting maximum lifespan potentials exhibit clear positive correlations with in vivo life spans.[53] Second, although there is considerable variance, cultured cells from older donors exhibit less growth potential than those from younger donors.[54,55] Finally, cultured somatic cells from patients with the striking progeroid disorder noted above (the Werner syndrome) exhibit marked deficiencies of growth potential.[54]

The mechanisms of the clonal senescence of normal diploid somatic cells are unknown. Two contrasting views are that it results from various forms of cell injury or that it represents a more physiological process, such as terminal differentiation resulting from regulated alterations in gene expression. Formally, the process appears to obey stochastic laws. The progeny of single cells show great variations in their growth potentials.[56,57] While the growth histories of mass cultures are quite predictable for given strains, the growth potential of an individual cell within a group of morphologically "young" cells (those that have not yet developed certain morphological alterations associated with senescent cells, notably greatly enlarged cytoplasmic masses) is not predictable.

The limited replicative life span of normal diploid somatic cells is dominant in crosses with cell lines of indefinite growth potentials.[58] Such experiments have defined four distinct complementation groups among such "immortal" cell lines, most of which are derived from cancer cells.[58] These exciting results are likely to prove of great importance in unraveling an important aspect of oncogenesis—the escape from a limited life span of at least a proportion of cells within a population of neoplastic cells.

There is some evidence that the dominance of the aging phenotype in culture may be related to specific alterations in gene expression and the appearance of specific proteins associated with the plasma cell membrane.[59-61] The block in the mitotic cell cycle of the senescent cells appears to be in late G_1,[62] but is potentially reversible, however.[63]

Neuroendocrine Mechanisms of Aging

The examples of rapid synchronized postreproductive death noted above for the case of some animal species with semelparous modes of reproduction suggest the possibility that some degree of neuroendocrine-regulated aging may be retained in iteroparous species. A number of gerontologists, in fact, believe that neuroendocrine alterations are of paramount and primary significance in the determination of the life spans of mammals. The conceptions have varied from positively acting "death hormones" (such substances have yet to be isolated)[64] to the notion of a gradual loss of sensitivity to feedback inhibition within the hypothalamus.[65] Finch[66] has pointed to the possibility of a neuroendocrine cascade of alterations leading to senescence.

Organ System Changes During Aging

Age-related alterations have been observed in all of the organ systems, as might be expected, given the above discussion of potentially pervasive cellular and molecular mechanisms of aging. The immune system has been covered in a separate chapter. Here we briefly review a few other key systems, concentrating upon what is known about major phenotypic changes in our own species. For more comprehensive coverage, textbooks such as Andres et al[67] should be consulted.

The Female Reproductive System

In comparison with other primates, the human female is unusual in undergoing menopause at a comparatively early phase of the overall life span (see Ref. 68 for review). Presumably, such early menopause evolved because it conferred an overall enhancement of reproductive fitness.

Although the complete cessation of menses is considered as a landmark qualitative marker of aging, there are signs of aging of the reproductive system beginning after the age of 30, including anovulatory cycles, spontaneous abortions, infertility, and the appearance of aneuploid progeny.[69] At the cellular level, the most dramatic feature of ovarian aging is the depletion of primary ovarian follicles (Figure 3.3). The ovary is essentially devoid of oocytes by the beginning of menopause.

Quite recently, epidemiologists have uncovered a statistically significant increased risk of relatively premature death, from all causes, among women

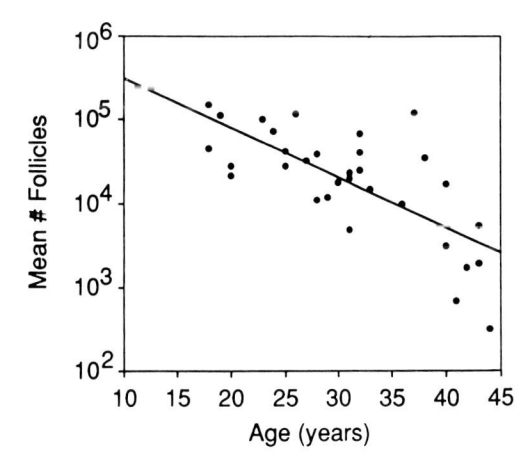

Figure 3.3. A replot of the data of Block,[87] showing an exponential decline in the numbers of human ovarian primordial follicles as a function of age.

with early natural menopause compared to a control group with natural menopause between the ages of 50 and 54.[70] Logistic regression analysis ruled out contributions of smoking, overweight, underweight, reproductive history and use of replacement estrogens. While these results will have to be confirmed with other population groups and longitudinal study designs, they are consistent with the proposition that rates of reproductive aging (in particular, the rates of loss of primordial follicles) may be coupled, to some degree, with aging rates in other systems.

Neuroendocrine System

In experimental rodents, there are many lines of evidence that document major alterations in the neuroendocrine milieu accompanying the transition to female infertility.[71] Measurements of circadian patterns of norepinephrine and serotonin turnover rates, alpha 1-adrenergic receptors, and the pulsatile release of leuteinizing hormone suggest a critical role for the suprachiasmatic-preoptic region of the hypothalamus, thought to be a master "pacemaker" of biological rhythms.

The dynamic coupling of aging of the neuroendocrine and reproductive systems can be modulated by environmental manipulations. Of potentially great clinical significance are observations for a "feedback" role of estrogens. Thus, physiological doses of estrogens can accelerate age-related alterations and, conversely, estrogen deprivation can delay the loss of reproductive function of aging rodents.[72,73]

Are there alterations of the suprachiasmatic nucleus of aging human subjects? The answer appears to be yes.[74] Such alterations could partially explain, for example, the sleep disturbances that are so commonly observed in older patients. The suprachiasmatic alterations, including cell loss, may be particularly striking in dementia of the Alzheimer's type. Although most clinicians have been taught to regard Alzheimer's disease as being distinct from normative aging, all of the classical histopathological stigmata of that disorder (neuritic plaques, neurofibrillary tangles, amyloid angiopathy) can be found, although to a lesser degree, in the hippocampus of older individuals who, by crude clinical criteria, appear to be cognitively intact.[75]

Special Senses

Physicians are well aware of age-related alterations in the visual and auditory systems, but are less well informed about alterations in the vestibular, gustatory, olfactory, and somatosensory systems.[76] About 80% of older subjects exhibit abnormalities in sense of smell and taste, presenting a major problem in the nutritional management of patients.

Cardiovascular System

This system, particularly the arterial components, can be considered the "Achilles' heel" of aging in our species. For those of us who manage to survive into the 90s, the vast majority will die as a result of major cardiovascular diseases.[24] We do not understand the cellular and molecular basis of this vulnerability, although progress has been made in elucidating such abnormalities as a diminished response to beta-adrenergic modulation.[77] As people age, there is a gradual increase in vascular stiffness, increases in systolic, diastolic, and mean arterial pressures, left ventricular hypertrophy, and decreases in early diastolic filling rates.[78] When subjected to maximal exercise, there is a diminution of the heart-rate response. In the absence of clinically detectable coronary artery disease, a normal cardiac output may be maintained via an enhanced end-diastolic volume (Starling mechanism); this is an excellent example of what may prove to be a large array of "second line" or "third line" compensatory mechanisms which aging organisms invoke in their constant attempts to maintain homeostasis.

Respiratory System

Significant age-related structural changes in the pulmonary system include: (1) loss of the alveolar elastic recoil; (2) alterations in chest wall structure with decreased respiratory muscle strength; (3) loss of alveolar surface area; (4) increase in the thickness of the media and intima of pulmonary arteries; and (5) decrease in the number of cilia lining the airways.[79] The functional consequences of these alterations include a decrease in the dynamic lung volumes, less uniform alveolar ventilation, a decreased response to hypoxia and hypercapnia, decreased vital capacity, and decreased arterial PO_2.[79] Chronic obstructive pulmonary disease is common by age 65 and the prevalence of pulmonary infections is increased in the elderly and the consequences of such infection are more serious.[80] Annual influenza vaccines are now recommended for subjects over the age of 65.

Urinary Tract

Pathologists are quite familiar with a number of anatomic alterations in the aged kidney. These include loss of tissue mass, progressive hyalinization (sclerosis) of glomerular units, diminished numbers of nephrons, thickened basement membranes of tubules and vasculature, interstitial fibrosis, arteriolosclerosis, and atherosclerosis. The functional consequences of these lesions include decreased renal blood flow, decreased glomerular filtration rate, impaired ability to concentrate or to dilute the urine, impaired reabsorption of glucose, and altered endocrine functions (renin-angiotensin; vitamin D metabolism; response to vasopressin).[81-83] A core problem in the interpretation of these alterations, vis-à-vis their relationships to underlying intrinsic aging processes, is the extent to which they may be secondary consequences of specific disease processes. (This difficulty is, of course, not unique to the kidney.) The fact that longitudinal studies of renal function have identified subsets of individuals who do not exhibit decrements of function with clinical testing, and who in fact appear to exhibit improvements of renal function, suggests to some workers that the alterations may, at least in part, be related to common age-related diseases.[81,84]

With respect to the common geriatric problem of urinary incontinence, it is certainly the case that intercurrent pathology of various types, when managed properly, can reverse the incontinence.[85] We need more research, however, on such questions as the possible underlying contribution of intrinsic aging of the urinary bladder smooth muscle and in its neural innervation.

Why Do Human Females Generally Outlive Their Spouses?

In the United States, the longevity differential between males and females, based upon life expectancy at birth, is currently about 7 years.[86] This female advantage is true in all of the developed countries. Is it related to an intrinsic biological advantage of the female or to differential life styles? There is no definite answer to this question.[86] We know that the human female is a somatic mosaic with respect to genes on the X chromosome; in some cells, she is operating on genetic information from the mother's X chromosome, while in others the X chromosome inherited from the father may be active. This could theoretically provide an advantage, in terms of the buffering of deleterious effects from certain classes of X-linked recessive genes, and in terms of a potentially more flexible metabolic repertoire. There is no hard evidence, however, that the female longevity advantage is a general property of mammalian species.

In contrast to the present uncertainty as regards genetic contributions to the longevity differential, we have plenty of evidence of a role for life-style differences, such as smoking behavior (although, for that particular example, there have been recent dramatic shifts in behavior in many cultures for both males and females).

References

1. Leopold AC: The biological significance of death in plants, in Behnke JA, Finch CE, Moment GB (eds.): *The Biology of Aging.* New York, Plenum Press, 1978, pp 101–114.
2. Diamond JM: Big-bang reproduction and ageing in male marsupial mice. *Nature* 1982; 298:115–116.
3. Rose MR: The evolution of animal senescence. *Can J Zool* 1984;62:1661–1667.
4. Kirkwood TBL: Comparative and evolutionary aspects of longevity, in Finch CE, Schneider EL (eds.): *Handbook of the Biology of Aging,* ed. 2. New York, Van Nostrand Reinhold, 1985, pp 27–44.
5. Williams GC: Pleiotropy, natural selection, and the evolution of senescence. *Evolution* 1957;11:398–411.
6. Medawar DB: *The Uniqueness of the Individual.* London, Methuen, 1957, pp 17–70.
7. Rose MR, Graves JL: Evolution of aging, in Rothstein M (ed.): *Review of Biological Research in Aging,* Vol 4. New York, Alan R. Liss, 1989, in press.
8. Rose MR: Laboratory evolution of postponed senescence in *Drosophila melanogaster. Evolution* 1984;38:1004–1010.
9. Luckinbill LS, Arking R, Clare MJ, Cirocco WC, Buck SA: Selection for delayed senescence in *Drosophila melanogaster. Evolution* 1984;38:996–1003.
10. Luckinbill LS, Graves JL, Reed AH, Koetsawang S: Localizing genes that deter senescence in *Drosophila melanogaster. Heredity* 1988;60:367–374.
11. Martin GM, Turker MS: Minireview: Model systems for the genetic analysis of mechanisms of aging. *J Gerontol* 1988;43:B33–39.
12. Martin GM: Genetic modulation of the senescent phenotype in *Homo sapiens. Genome* 1989;31:390–397.
13. Altman PL, Dittmer DS: Life spans: Mammals, in *Growth: Biological Handbook.* Washington, D.C., Fed Am Soc Exp Biol, 1962, pp 445–450.
14. Cutler RG: Evolution of human longevity and the genetic complexity governing aging rate. *Proc Natl Acad Sci USA* 1975;72:4664–4668.

15. Sacher GA: Maturation and longevity in relation to cranial capacity in hominid evolution, in Tuttle R (ed.): *Antecedents of Man and After,* Vol 1.—*Primates: Functional Morphology and Evolution.* The Hague, Mouton, 1975, pp 417–441.
16. Wilson AC, White TJ, Carlson SS, Cherry LM: Molecular evolution and cytogenetic evolution, in Sparkes RS, Comings DE, Fox CF: *Molecular Human Cytogenetics,* Vol 7. New York, Academic Press, 1977, pp 375–393.
17. Martin GM: Genetic syndromes in man with potential relevance to the pathobiology of aging, in Bergsma D, Harrison DE (eds.): *Genetic Effects on Aging, Birth Defects,* Vol 14, No. 1. New York, Alan R. Liss, 1978, pp 5–39.
18. Salk D, Fujiwara Y, Martin GM (eds.): Werner's syndrome and human aging. *Adv Exp Med Biol,* Vol 190. New York, Plenum Press, 1985.
19. Warner HR, Butler RN, Sprott RL, Schneider EL (eds.): Modern biological theories of aging, in *Aging,* Vol 31. New York, Raven Press, 1987.
20. Harman D: Aging: A theory based on free radical and radiation chemistry. *J Gerontol* 1956;11:298–300.
21. Harman D: Free radical theory of aging: Role of free radicals in the origination and evolution of life, aging, and disease processes, in Johnson JE Jr, Walford R, Harman D, Miquel J (eds.): *Free Radicals, Aging, and Degenerative Diseases.* New York, Alan R Liss, 1986, pp 3–49.
22. Fridovich I: The biology of oxygen radicals. *Science* 1978;201:875–880.
23. Tappel AL: Vitamin E and free radical peroxidation of lipids. *Ann NY Acad Sci* 1972;203:12–28.
24. Martin GM: Interactions of aging and environmental agents: The gerontological perspective, in Baker SR, Rogul M (eds.): *Environmental Toxicity and the Aging Processes,* Vol 228, *Prog Clin Biol Res.* New York, Alan R. Liss, 1987, pp 25–80.
25. Martin GM: Cellular aging—Postreplicative cells: A review (Part II). *Am J Pathol* 1977;89:513–530.
26. Balin AK: Testing the free radical theory of aging, in Adelman RC, Roth GS (eds.): *Testing the Theories of Aging.* Boca Raton, Florida, CRC Press, 1982, pp 137–182.
27. Weindruch R, Walford RL: *The retardation of aging and disease by dietary restriction.* Springfield, Illinois, Charles C. Thomas, 1988.
28. Masoro EJ, Yu BP, Bertrand HA: Action of food restriction in delaying the aging process. *Proc Natl Acad Sci USA* 1982;79:4239–4241.
29. McCarter R, Masoro EJ, Yu BP: Does food restriction retard aging by reducing the metabolic rate? *Am J Physiol* 1985;248:E488–490.
30. Martin GM, Fry M, Loeb LA: Somatic mutation and aging in mammalian cells, in Sohal RS, Birnbaum LS, Cutler RG (eds.): *Molecular Biology of Aging: Gene Stability and Gene Expression.* New York, Raven Press, 1985, pp 7–21.
31. Loeb LA, James EA, Waltersdorph AM, Klebanoff SJ: Mutagenesis by the autoxidation of iron with isolated DNA. *Proc Natl Acad Sci USA* 1988;85:3918–3922.
32. Trainor KJ, Wigmore DJ, Chrysostomou A, Dempsey JL, Seshadri R, Morley AA: Mutation frequency in human lymphocytes increases with age. *Mech Ageing Dev* 1984, 27:83–86.
33. Horn PL, Turker MS, Ogburn CE, Disteche CM, Martin GM: A cloning assay for 6-thioguanine resistance provides evidence against certain somatic mutational theories of aging. *J Cell Physiol* 1984;121:309–315.
34. Martin GM, Smith AC, Ketterer DJ, Ogburn CE, Disteche CM: Increased chromosomal aberrations in first metaphases of cells isolated from the kidneys of aged mice. *Isr J Med Sci* 1985;21:296–301.
35. Schimke RT, Sherwood SW, Hill AB, Johnston RN: Overreplication and recombination of DNA in higher eukaryotes: Potential consequences and biological implications. *Proc Natl Acad Sci USA* 1986;83:2157–2161.
36. Esposito D, Fassina G, Szabo P, De Angelis P, Rodgers L, Weksler M, Siniscalco M: Chromosomes of older humans are more prone to aminopterine-induced breakage. *Proc Natl Acad Sci USA* 1989;86:1302–1306.

37. Salk D, Au K, Hoehn H, Martin GM: Cytogenetics of Werner's syndrome cultured skin fibroblasts: Variegated translocation mosaicism. *Cytogenet Cell Genet* 1981;30:92–107.
38. Fukuchi K, Martin GM, Monnat, RJ Jr: The mutator phenotype of Werner syndrome is characterized by extensive deletions. *Proc Natl Acad Sci USA* 1989;86:5893–5897.
39. Maynard Smith J: Theories of aging, in Krohn PL (ed.): *Topics in the Biology of Aging.* New York, John Wiley, 1965, pp 1–35.
40. Clark AM, Rubin MA: The modification by x-irradiation of the life span of haploids and diploids of the wasp, *Habrobracon* SP. *Radiat Res* 1961;15:244–253.
41. Rothstein M: Evidence for and against the error catastrophe hypothesis, in Warner HR, Butler RN, Sprott RL, Schneider EL (eds.): *Modern Biological Theories of Aging, Aging,* Vol 31. New York, Raven Press, 1987:139–154.
42. Orgel LE: The maintenance of the accuracy of protein synthesis and its relevance to ageing. *Proc Natl Acad Sci USA* 1963;49:517–521.
43. Orgel LE: The maintenance of the accuracy of protein synthesis and its relevance to ageing: A correction. *Proc Natl Acad Sci USA* 1970;67:1476.
44. Adelman RC, Dekker EE (eds.): Modification of proteins during aging, in *Modern Aging Research,* Vol 7. New York, Alan R. Liss, 1985.
45. Watkins NG, Thorpe SR, Baynes JW: Glycation of amino groups in protein: Studies on the specificity of modification of RNase by glucose. *J Biol Chem* 1985;260:10,629–636.
46. Gallop PM: Biological mechanisms in aging: Post-translational changes in cells and tissues, in *Biological Mechanisms in Aging.* NIH publication no. 81-2194, Washington, D.C., United States Government Printing Office, 1981, pp 397–453.
47. Cerami A, Vlassara H, Brownlee M: Glucose and aging. *Sci Am* 1987;256:90–96.
48. Lee AT, Cerami A: Elevated glucose 6-phosphate levels are associated with plasmid mutations in vivo. *Proc Natl Acad Sci USA* 1987;84:8311–8314.
49. Masoro EJ, Katz MS, McMahan CA: Evidence for the glycation hypothesis of aging from the food-restricted rodent model. *J Gerontol* 1989;44:B20–22.
50. Martin GM, Sprague CA, Norwood TH, Pendergrass WR, Bornstein P, Hoehn H, Arend WP: Do hyperplastoid cell lines "differentiate themselves to death"?, in Cristofalo VJ, Holečková E (eds.): *Cell Impairment in Aging and Development, Adv Exp Med Biol,* Vol 53. New York, Plenum Press, 1975, pp 67–90.
51. Hayflick L, Moorhead PS: The serial cultivation of human diploid cell strains. *Exp Cell Res* 1961;25:585–621.
52. Martin GM: Proliferative homeostasis and its age-related aberrations. *Mech Ageing Dev* 1979;9:385–391.
53. Rohme D: Evidence for a relationship between longevity of mammalian species and life-spans of normal fibroblasts *in vitro* and erythrocytes *in vivo. Proc Natl Acad Sci USA* 1981;78:5009–5013.
54. Martin GM, Sprague CA, Epstein CJ: Replicative life-span of cultivated human cells: Effects of donor's age, tissue and genotype. *Lab Invest* 1970;23:86–92.
55. Schneider EL, Mitsui Y: The relationship between *in vitro* cellular aging and *in vivo* human age. *Proc Natl Acad Sci USA* 1976;73:3584–3588.
56. Martin GM, Sprague CA, Norwood TH, Pendergrass WR: Clonal selection, attenuation and differentiation in an in vitro model of hyperplasia. *Am J Pathol* 1974;74:137–153.
57. Smith JR, Whitney RG: Intraclonal variation in proliferative potential of human diploid fibroblasts: Stochastic mechanisms for cellular aging. *Science* 1980;207:82–84.
58. Pereira-Smith OM, Smith JR: Genetic analysis of indefinite division in human cells: Identification of four complementation groups. *Proc Natl Acad Sci USA* 1988;85:6042–6046.
59. Lumpkin CK Jr, McClung JK, Pereira-Smith OM, Smith JR: Existence of high abundance antiproliferative mRNA's in senescent human diploid fibroblasts. *Science* 1986;232:393–395.

60. Pereira-Smith OM, Fisher SF, Smith JR: Senescent and quiescent cell inhibitors of DNA synthesis: Membrane-associated proteins. *Exp Cell Res* 1985;160:297–306.
61. Stein GH, Atkins L: Membrane-associated inhibitor of DNA synthesis in senescent human diploid fibroblasts: Characterization and comparison to quiescent cell inhibitor. *Proc Natl Acad Sci USA* 1986;83:9030–9034.
62. Rittling SR, Brooks KM, Cristofalo VJ, Baserga R: Expression of cell cycle-dependent genes in young and senescent WI-38 fibroblasts. *Proc Natl Acad Sci USA* 1986;83:3316–3320.
63. Gorman SD, Cristofalo VJ: Reinitiation of cellular DNA synthesis in BrdU-selected nondividing senescent WI-38 cells by simian virus 40 infection. *J Cell Physiol* 1985;125:122–126.
64. Denckla WD: Role of the pituitary and thyroid glands in the decline of minimal O_2 consumption with age. *J Clin Invest* 1974;53:572–587.
65. Dilman JM: Age associated elevation of hypothalamic threshold to feedback control, and its role in development, aging, and disease. *Lancet* 1971;1:1211–1219.
66. Finch CE: The regulation of physiological changes during mammalian aging. *Q Rev Biol* 1976;51:49–83.
67. Andres R, Bierman EL, Hazzard WR: *Principles of Geriatric Medicine.* New York, McGraw-Hill, 1985.
68. Harman SM, Talbert GB: Reproductive aging, in Finch CE, Schneider EL (eds.): *Handbook of the Biology of Aging,* ed. 2. New York, Van Nostrand Reinhold, 1985, pp 457–510.
69. Gosden RG: *Biology of Menopause: The Causes and Consequences of Ovarian Ageing.* London, Academic Press, 1985.
70. Snowdon DA, Kane RL, Beeson WL, et al: Is early natural menopause a biologic marker of health and aging? *Am J Public Health* 1989;79:709–714.
71. Wise PM, Weiland NG, Scarbrough K, Sortino MA, Cohen IR, Larson GH: Changing hypothalamopituitary function: Its role in aging of the female reproductive system. *Horm Res* 1989;31:39–44.
72. Finch CE, Felicio LS, Mobbs CV, Nelson JF: Ovarian and steroidal influences on neuroendocrine aging processes in female rodents. *Endocrine Rev* 1984;5:467–497.
73. Mobbs CV, Gee DM, Finch CE: Reproductive senescence in female C57BL/6J mice: Ovarian impairments and neuroendocrine impairments that are partially reversible and delayable by ovariectomy. *Endocrinology* 1984;115:1653–1662.
74. Swaab DF, Fisser B, Kamphorst W, Troost D: The human suprachiasmatic nucleus: Neuropeptide changes in senium and Alzheimer's disease. *Bas Appl Histochem* 1988;32:43–54.
75. Morimatsu M, Hirai S, Muramatsu A, Yoshikawa M: Senile degenerative brain lesions and dementia. *J Am Geriatr Soc* 1975;390–406.
76. Corso JF: *Aging sensory systems and perception.* New York, Praeger, 1981.
77. Lakatta EG: Diminished beta-adrenergic modulation of cardiovascular function in advanced age. *Cardiol Clin* 1986;4:185–200.
78. Lakatta EG: Hemodynamic adaptations to stress with advancing age. *Acta Med Scand Suppl* 1986;711:39–52.
79. Levitzky MG: Effects of aging on the respiratory system. *Physiologist* 1984;27:102–107.
80. Brandstetter RD, Kazemi H: Aging and the respiratory system. *Med Clin North Am* 1983;67:419–431.
81. Lindeman RD, Goldman R: Anatomic and physiologic age changes in the kidney. *Exp Gerontol* 1986;21:379–406.
82. Davies I: Ageing in the hypothalamo-neurohypophysial-renal system. *Compr Gerontol* 1987;1:12–23.
83. Meyer BR: Renal function in aging. *J Am Geriatr Soc* 1989;37:791–860.
84. Shock NW, Andres R, Norris AH, Tobin JD: Patterns of longitudinal changes in renal

function, in Orimo H, Shimada K, Iriki M, Maeda D (eds.), *Recent Advances in Gerontology.* Amsterdam, Excerpta Medica, 1979, pp 384–386.
85. Resnick NM, Yalla SV: Aging and its effect on the bladder. *Seminars Urol* 1987;5:82–86.
86. Smith DWE, Warner HR: Does genotypic sex have a direct effect on longevity? *Exp Gerontol* 1989;24:277–288.
87. Block E: Quantitative morphological investigations of the follicular system in women: Variations at different ages. *Acta Anat* 1952;14:108–123.

Chapter 4

Alterations of Host-Defense Mechanisms and the Susceptibility to Infections

Gurkamal Chatta, MD, and David C. Dale, MD

Immunosenescence is often accompanied by an increased incidence of neoplasia, autoimmune diseases, and infections. With the burgeoning geriatric population in the United States, there is heightened interest in the illnesses of the elderly and the economic implications thereof. Infectious diseases are among the most important problems; bacterial pneumonias and influenza rank as the fourth leading cause of death for persons over 65 years old.[1-4]

Although there has been much research into the effects of aging of the immune system, the data are somewhat conflicting and do not provide simple explanations for the kinds of infections seen. In addition to the immune defects, there are age-related decrements in organ structure and function, and an increased incidence of many diseases which independently effect host-defense mechanisms. Superimposed on this are environmental changes (ie, increasing institutionalization, social isolation, and neglect in the elderly). It is the interaction of all these factors which leads to the pattern of clinical illnesses seen.[5]

In this chapter, we will discuss: (1) the epidemiology of infectious diseases in the elderly; (2) normal host-defense mechanisms; (3) immune defects with aging; (4) age-related decrements in organ structure and function; (5) increased incidence of underlying diseases; (6) environmental factors; (7) specific infections in the elderly; and (8) prevention and treatment.

Epidemiology

Although only 12% of the U.S. population is over 65 years of age, 30% of acute-care beds and 90% of beds in chronic-care facilities are occupied by the elderly. In economic terms this translates into 35% of total health-care costs.[5-7] A significant proportion of this is accounted for by infectious diseases. In much of the existent aging research, it is impossible to differentiate between the effects of aging per se and the effects of accumulated insults and underlying chronic diseases. Nevertheless, there is ample clinical evidence for an age-related increase in certain infections, and a number of general statements can be made.

1. Regardless of setting, there is an increased incidence of bacterial pneumo-

Table 4.1 Pneumonia in the Elderly

	> 65 yr	< 65 yr
1. Hospitalization for acute pneumonia (per 1000 population/year)	11.5	2.0
2. Length of stay (days per 100 hospital discharges)	10.3	7.5
3. Mortality (deaths per 100 hospital discharges)	12.8	1.5

From the National Health Survey, 1981 (Ref. 9)

nias, associated bacteremias, and resultant morbidity in the elderly.[1] A study of pneumococcal bacteremia revealed that 75% of the patients were over 60 years old, 50% had an atypical presentation, and 60% had polymicrobial sputum cultures. Despite antibiotic treatment, there was 40% mortality and uniformly a protracted hospital course in the survivors.[8] A 1981 National Health Survey of cases with pneumonia (Table 4.1) clearly shows the increased morbidity and mortality in the elderly.[9]

2. Bacteremia, irrespective of source, occurs more often in the elderly. A retrospective study, of 500 patients with positive blood cultures, revealed that 60% of these occurred in the elderly. On multivariate analysis, age held up as an independent predictor for increased mortality.[10] The phenomena of afebrile bacteremia also occur almost exclusively in the elderly.[11]

3. Asymptomatic bacteriuria and symptomatic urinary tract infections are more prevalent in the elderly. Up to 15% of ambulant elderly women and 50% of the elderly in nursing homes are bacteriuric.[12] There is also an increased incidence of bacteremia following urinary tract infections. In one recent study of hospitalized women with nonobstructive pyelonephritis, 12 of 18 elderly women (median age 75 years) developed urosepsis as opposed to 0 of 7 young women (median age 27 years).[13]

4. Intraabdominal infections (ie, cholangitis, liver abscess, and diverticulitis) are more prevalent in the elderly with a uniformly poor prognosis.

5. Nosocomial infections of all types (ie, urinary tract infections, pneumonia, bacteremia, and wound infections) occur with a three- to fivefold increased frequency in the 70- to 90-year age group. One-third of all hospitalizations from a nursing home are also infection-related.[14-16]

6. The incidence of tuberculosis and the reactivation of the varicella-zoster virus is age-related and linked to a decline in cell-mediated immunity with aging.

7. Bacterial endocarditis is becoming primarily a geriatric disease, is invariably nonrheumatic in origin, and has an atypical presentation and a 20% to 50% mortality.

Another characteristic of infections in the elderly is the extreme variability in clinical presentation. Localizing symptoms and signs are often absent; and the only presenting features may be anorexia, malaise, dehydration, a change in mental status, or even frank delirium. A high index of suspicion is necessary to recognize serious infections of the elderly in a timely way. Not only is the

Table 4.2 Outcome of Fever in Adults Without Known Underlying Disease

	17–39 yr	40–59 yr	60–79 yr	>80 yr
Not hospitalized	79%	46%	23%	6%
Hospitalized but no life-threatening disease	20%	46%	60%	73%
Life-threatening disease	1%	7%	16%	16%
Mortality	0%	1%	1%	4%

From Keating et al.[19]

febrile response to infection blunted,[17] but also the usual neutrophilia in response to infection may be absent.[18] Thus there is often a delay in diagnosis and appropriate therapy, further compounding the already high morbidity and mortality to which the elderly are prone.

The absence of fever in response to infection in the elderly is ominous; however, even when it is present, it forebodes a serious illness. In a prospective study of 1202 ambulatory patients presenting with a temperature of 101°F or more, advancing age was significantly associated with more serious disease, a higher rate of hospitalization, and a poorer outcome (Table 4.2). In the study illustrated in Table 4.2,[19] a viral syndrome was thought responsible for the fever in 60% of the under-40-year-olds, 20% of the 40- to 60-years age group, and only 4% of over-60-year-olds. This again underscores the importance of a complete workup for a febrile illness in the elderly.[20]

Normal Host-Defense Mechanisms

Host-defense mechanisms[2,21] are often subdivided into *nonspecific* and *specific*. The nonspecific mechanisms provide defense against all types of microbes. The specific defenses reflect enhanced responsiveness due to previous exposure or immunization (Table 4.3).

To gain access to the body, an invading organism or foreign antigen has to breach the mucocutaneous barrier. The intact skin not only acts as a physical barrier, but also produces secretions which are microbicidal, and has a flora which prevents colonization by other microorganisms. The mucosal layer prevents microbial invasion by ciliary action, secretion of mucus and production of local immunoglobulin (IgA).

Having traversed the mucocutaneous barrier, the invading organism usually releases toxins which cause local tissue injury and increased vascular perme-

Table 4.3 Host Defenses

Nonspecific	Specific
Skin and mucosa	B-lymphocytes (humoral immunity)
Monocytes-macrophages	T-lymphocytes (cell-mediated immunity)
Polymorphonuclear leukocytes	Natural killer cells (NK cells)
Complement	

ability. Exudation of plasma proteins, including the complement proteins, follows. Complement is activated by interaction with many foreign surfaces and bacterial products. Complement components from this activation serve as chemoattractants for neutrophils and as opsonins to facilitate phagocytosis. Neutrophils are rapidly deployed to the site of insult, where they kill most common types of bacteria and limit infection. The involvement of tissue macrophages also aids the phagocytic process and results in elaboration of interleukin-1 (IL-1) and chemoattractants, which further augment the neutrophilic response.

As part of the acute inflammatory response, antigens are processed by phagocytes and presented to T-lymphocytes in association with the histocompatibility molecule (DR). The antigen-DR complex binds to the T-cell. Under the influence of IL-1, activation of T-cells takes place. The activated T-cells elaborate interleukin-2 and other lymphokines, which cause clonal expansion of T-cells and activation and differentiation of B-cells. The latter are transformed to plasma cells. The plasma cells then secrete antigen-specific antibodies, (ie, IgM, IgG, IgA, IgD, and IgE), which assist in host defense by fixing complement, opsonizing organisms, and neutralizing toxins. A primary antibody response (first exposure to antigen) involves secretion of IgM, and a secondary antibody response involves secretion of IgG. In a previously sensitized host, B-cells are involved in the immune response from the very outset by virtue of circulating memory B-cells.

T-cells constitute 80% of circulating lymphocytes and are the effectors of cell-mediated immunity. They kill intracellular organisms, mediate delayed hypersensitivity reactions, and modulate immune responses by means of T-helper and T-suppressor cells. The natural killer cells do not require prior exposure to reach their target and directly lyse cells.

It is important to understand that all the limbs of the immune network function in concert, many of the steps occurring simultaneously (Figure 4.1).

Lymphokines[1,5,22] are polypeptide products of activated lymphocytes that participate in a variety of cellular responses. They are produced by a variety of cells and have wide-ranging biological effects (Table 4.4).

Immune Defects with Aging

Aging has many important effects on the immune system, although in a number of areas the data tends to be conflicting. In part, this is a result of difficulties traditionally encountered with aging research. Not only is the aging process heterogeneous, but there is also the perennial difficulty of separating age per se from accumulated insults of acute and chronic illnesses. It is also recognized that different components of the immune system age at differential rates, adding complexity to understanding how aging influences this vital system.[4,5,23-29]

The effect of age on various components of the immune system is summarized below.

Neutrophils

Neutrophils constitute the first line of defense against invading microorganisms.[30] Neutrophils leave the circulation by adhering to endothelial cells via a complement receptor (CR3) and then make their way to the site of infection.

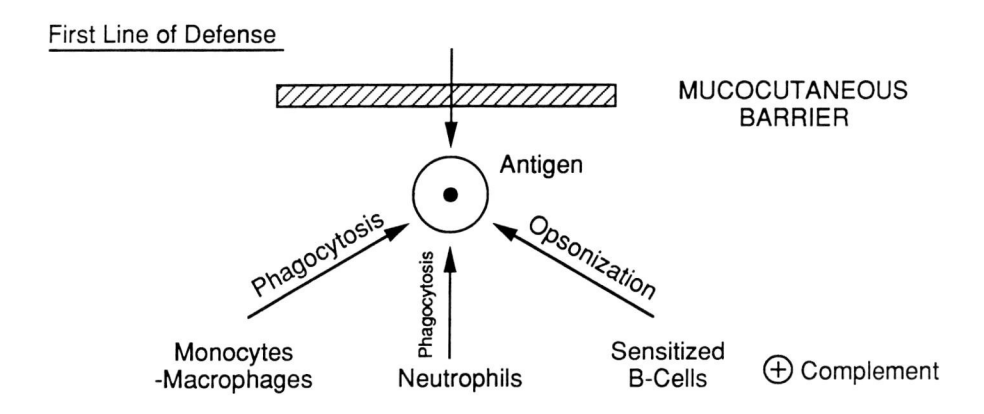

First Line of Defense

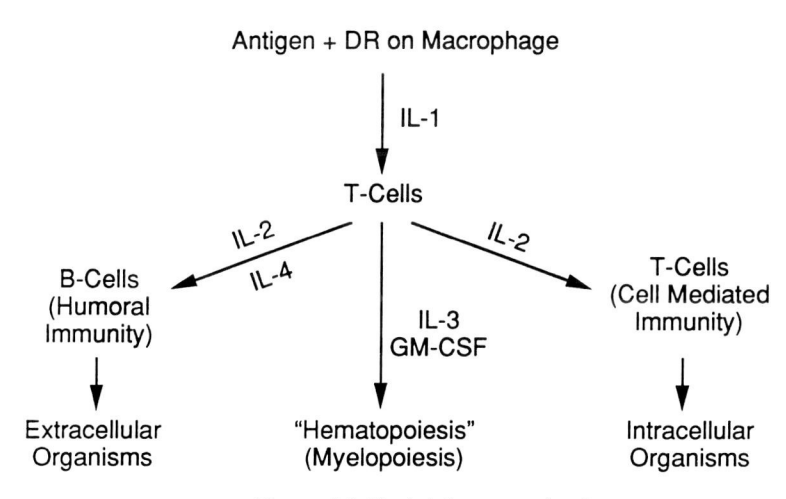

Figure 4.1 Host defense mechanisms.

They kill microorganisms by: (i) an oxidative pathway, involving the intracellular generation of hydrogen peroxide and superoxide; and (ii) a nonoxidative pathway, involving the intracellular release of neutrophil polypeptides (released by degranulation), which possess antimicrobial activity. There have been several studies which have evaluated different aspects of neutrophil function with aging (ie, adherence, chemotaxis, phagocytosis, and microbicidal capability). Although the data is somewhat conflicting, neutrophil function appears not to change significantly with aging.[31,32]

Despite preserved function of individual cells, the total supply of neutrophils available to fight infections may be reduced in the elderly.[33] Neutropenia, in the face of infection, occurs more often in the elderly and is associated uniformly with a poor outcome. The neutrophil response to infection is initiated by circulating cells and is sustained by the supply of neutrophils from bone marrow stores, which in turn is replenished from the hematopoietic stem cell pool. The suboptimal neutrophilic response to infection, which often occurs in the elderly,

Table 4.4 Major Lymphokines and Their Biologic Effects*

Lymphokine	Major biologic properties
Interleukin-1 (IL-1)	Activates resting T-cells; induces fever; activates endothelial cells and macrophages
IL-2	Growth factor for activated T-cells; synthesis of other lymphokines; activates cytotoxic lymphocytes
IL-3	Supports growth of multilineage bone-marrow stem cells
Granulocyte-macrophage colony stimulating factor (GM-CSF)	Promotes growth of neutrophilic, eosinophilic, and macrophagic cells
Granulocyte CSF (G-CSF)	Promotes growth of neutrophilic cells
Macrophage CSF (M-CSF)	Promotes growth of monocytes and macrophagic cells
IL-4	Growth factor for activated B-cells and mast cells
Alpha and beta interferon	Antiviral activity; induces class-I antigen expressions; augments NK cells
Gamma-interferon	Induces class-I, class-II (DR) antigens on the surface of cells; antiviral activity
Tumor necrosis factor	A cytotoxin; induces fever and acute phase responses; stimulates the synthesis of other lymphokines

* See Ref. 22.

raises the possibility of a defect in neutrophil production and/or regulation. Studies in both animals and humans suggest a diminution in precursor cells in the bone marrow, a decreased responsiveness of these cells to regulating cytokines, *or* decreased cytokine production.[34,35]

Monocytes and Macrophages

Monocytes are produced in the bone marrow. The circulating monocytes are transformed into tissue macrophages and are the principle cells for processing antigens. They elaborate interleukin-1 (IL-1) and other lymphokines. Their function is thought not to be affected by the aging process.[36] Although the elderly have a blunted febrile response to infection, the production of IL-1 (a mediator of fever) remains normal with aging. Currently, it is thought that there is a decreased responsiveness to IL-1 at the hypothalamic level.[37,38]

Complement

Complement is a complex of 20 or more proteins in the blood. Neither total complement levels nor its function is impaired by the aging process.[39]

T-cells

T-cells account for 80% of circulating lymphocytes in the blood and are effectors of cell-mediated immunity. Their precursor cells are bone-marrow-derived, and these in turn migrate to the thymus, undergo a process of maturation, and subsequently circulate in the blood as either T-helper cells (ie, the T4 subset) or T-suppressor cells (ie, the T8 subset). The specificity of T-cells is determined by clonotypic cell surface receptors (the T3-Ti complex).[40]

The increased predisposition to infections with intracellular organisms (ie, tuberculosis, listeria, legionella, and reactivation of varicella-zoster virus) suggests a decline in cell-mediated immunity with aging. The diminished ability in the elderly to mount cutaneous delayed hypersensitivity reactions to skin-test antigens also suggests a T-cell abnormality.[4,24,41] Extensive research has been done on the effects of aging on T-cell production, maturation, and regulation at the cellular and molecular levels. A synopsis of these studies follows.

Thymus and Thymic Hormones

Thymic involution commences at sexual maturity and is complete by age 50. There is also a concomitant decline in thymic hormone concentrations. There is decreased transit of immature cells from the bone marrow to the thymus, and also an increase in immature cells within the thymus.[4,24]

Animal models of immune reconstitution have revealed partial correction of T-cell defects with thymic extract in aged mice. Reconstitution in man is currently under study.[42]

Blood Lymphocyte Counts

These counts may be either normal or reduced with aging. Most studies showing reduced counts indicate that all T-cell subsets are affected equally.[43] According to one longitudinal study done over a 16-year period, a low blood lymphocyte count is an important marker for mortality within 3 years.[44] Flow cytometric analysis reveals an increase in circulating immature cells with aging. According to some studies, there is also a decrease in number and/or function of cytotoxic T-cells (CD8).

T-Cell Function

The consensus favors a decrease in T-cell proliferative responses with aging. Changes at the cellular level that contribute to this are: (a) decreased binding of ligand to the T3-Ti receptor on the surface of T-cells; and (b) defects in the activation of the protein kinase C system. Other studies of T-cell function reveal decreased production of IL-2, tumor necrosis factor, and gamma interferon. There also tends to be increased susceptibility to ultraviolet-radiation-induced damage, and a decrease in levels of DNA repair enzymes in the T-cells from older subjects.[4,24,29]

B-cells

Lymphocytes of the B-lineage are effectors of humoral immunity; they do this by elaborating antibodies to foreign antigens, microorganisms, or toxins. B-cells are bone-marrow-derived, and undergo their maturation there. The process of maturation involves acquiring surface immunoglobulin receptors. Antibody specificity to a wide variety of antigens is a result of immunoglobulin gene rearrangements. B-cell responses to a large measure are regulated by T-cell subsets and their lymphokines.[45] Derangements in B-cell-mediated immunity with aging are suggested by:

(i) Reduced antibody responses to T-cell-dependent and T-cell-independent antigens.[4,24]

(ii) Lower antibody levels with vaccination (ie, hepatitis B, influenza, and pneumococcal polysaccharide) in the elderly.[4,24,46]

(iii) Age-dependent decrease in isoagglutinins.

(iv) A rising incidence of autoantibodies and monoclonal proteinemias (3% over the age of 70) with aging. It is of note, however, that there is little or no age-related change in the levels of serum immunoglobulins,[47] and no study to date has incontrovertibly documented intrinsic B-cell defects. The low antibody response to vaccination is also thought to be partially circumventable with a higher challenge dose of the vaccine. It may reflect a T-cell rather than a B-cell effect of the aging process.[48]

NK Cells

Most studies report either decreased or no change in NK cell function. It is not known if alteration of NK cells may relate to the increased incidence of malignancies or infections in the elderly.

Age-Related Changes in Organ Structure and Function

Aging causes widespread changes in essentially all organ systems.[1,5] The changes which impact upon the body's ability to fight infection are briefly summarized below.

Skin

Aging affects all the layers (ie, epidermis, dermis, and subcutaneous tissue along with its organelles). Changes in collagen and elastic tissue can be attributed to aging per se and are characterized by progressive cross-linkaging of collagen and increased fragmentation of elastic tissue. The net result is a generalized thinning of the integument, an increased propensity to dehiscence, and reduced skin vascularity. Hence, the skin is easily breached, with an attendant risk of skin and soft-tissue infections. Furthermore, healing also tends to be delayed in the elderly and the strength of the healed skin is decreased.

Pulmonary System

Senescence of the respiratory tract results in (i) decreased mucociliary clearance of inhaled antigens and (ii) increasing collapse of the alveoli and reduction in vital capacity as a result of fragmentation of elastic tissue. These changes are further exacerbated by a decrease in respiratory muscle strength, reduced chest wall compliance, and smoke/dust-related insults. Thus, not only is pneumonia more likely to occur, but it also tends to be more often bronchopneumonic in distribution.

Gastrointestinal System

The two most significant age-related changes occur in the esophagus and the stomach. In the former, there is decreased peristalsis, reduced lower-esophageal sphincter tone, and thus increased likelihood of aspiration. Gastric acidity declines significantly, leading to survival of bacteria in ingested foods and more frequent bacterial colonization of the stomach and small intestines. In one study, 30% of people over 60 years of age were found to be achlorhydric, a change associated with increased respiratory infections with enteric organisms.

Genitourinary System

Both symptomatic and asymptomatic bacteriuria increase with aging. In the female, weakening of the pelvic floor leads to incomplete bladder emptying and resultant accumulation of residual urine. Atrophic vaginitis contributes to bladder infections from alterations in the surface bacterial flora and increased colonization by enteric organisms.

Increased Indicence of Underlying Diseases

The changes described in the preceding section are thought to be invariable concomitants of aging. The diseases mentioned in this section are more prevalent in the elderly. They are responsible for some of the defects in immune response, delayed wound healing, and the propensity to infection observed in a general population of older persons.[1,5]

Atherosclerosis is by far the most significant contributor to infection-related morbidity and mortality in the elderly. Its salient clinical expressions tend to be the following.

(i) *Peripheral vascular disease* predisposes to skin and soft-tissue infections, intractable ulcers, and occasionally osteomyelitis. It also contributes to delayed wound healing.
(ii) *Congestive heart failure* may contribute to the development of pneumonia and, because of poor tissue perfusion, slow healing of wounds.
(iii) *Cerebrovascular disease* is primarily a geriatric problem. The associated neurologic deficits often cause loss of mobility, falls, altered mental status, and aspiration pneumonias. Incontinence and urinary tract infections also occur frequently.

The prevalence of diabetes increases with aging, ie, 15% to 17% in the over-60-year-olds.[5] Also, it compounds the effects of atherosclerosis, causes neutrophil dysfunction, and contributes to delayed wound healing. Similarly, the age-related increase in chronic obstructive pulmonary disease and lung cancer causes an increased incidence of pulmonary infections.

Changes in Environment

It cannot be overemphasized that all aspects of care of the elderly have to be planned in the context of their biopsychosocial milieu. Old age is often associated with loneliness, economic deprivation, and social isolation. Multiple sensory deficits, immobility, malnutrition, and self-neglect also take their toll. All these factors contribute to both atypical presentations of infection as well as delay in care of the elderly.[1,5,49]

Twenty-five percent of persons over 65 years and 50% of those over 85 years of age require assistance with their activities of daily living. Five percent of persons over 65 years of age are in nursing homes and require frequent hospitalizations. These environmental changes (ie, immobility and institutionalization) are known to promote colonization with gram-negative organisms and to foster nosocomial infections.[50]

Nutrition in the elderly has been the focus of recent interest. Estimates of protein calorie malnutrition in the elderly range between 15% and 50%, with lower prevalence rates occurring in the ambulant elderly and higher prevalence rates in the institutionalized elderly.[51–53] Malnutrition is thought to impact adversely upon both lymphocyte and neutrophil function.

Specific Infections

Aging is associated with an increased incidence of certain infections, and the presentation for many of these illnesses often differs substantially in older versus younger adults. For instance, fever and the neutrophil response to infection may be absent. Bacteremic episodes (irrespective of source) and the resultant morbidity and mortality are also higher in the elderly. The more common infections are described below.

Pneumonias

Pneumonias[1,18,54,55] are predominantly bacterial in origin, and the etiologic organisms depend on the clinical setting (ie, community-acquired or nosocomial) (Table 4.5).

Pneumonia usually occurs because of aspiration of oropharyngeal bacteria. Aspiration is more likely in patients with strokes, dementia, and esophageal dysfunction. In many instances, bacterial pneumonia follows influenza, because this viral infection damages the bronchial mucosa and impairs ciliary function.

The treatment of patients with suspected pneumonia should be dictated by gram stain of the sputum. However, in the elderly, the sputum exam is often inconclusive because of a weak cough, dehydration, or other problems. In this situation, empiric treatment has to be instituted. In moderately ill patients, a single drug [eg, a "second generation" cephalosporin or ampicillin/sulbactam (Unisyn)] is usually adequate. Sicker patients and those with nosocomial infections require the addition of gram-negative coverage (ie, an aminoglycoside or aztreonam). Postinfluenzal pneumonia requires adequate coverage for *Staphylococcus aureus* (Table 4.6).

Table 4.5 Etiologic Organisms in Pneumonia*

Community		Hospital		Nursing home	
S. Pneumoniae	40–60%	Gram negatives	45%	Gram negatives	29%
Gram negatives	6–40%	S. Pneumoniae	10–20%	S. Pneumoniae	26%
H. influenzae	2–20%	Legionella	0–15%	H. influenzae	20%
S. aureus	2–10%	S. aureus	3–11%	S. aureus	8%
Legionella	0–20%				

* See Ref. 54.

Table 4.6 Common Infections, Etiologic Organisms, and Empiric Treatment*

Infection	Organisms	Antibiotics
Pneumonia		
Community-acquired†	*S. pneumoniae*, gram negative, *H. influenza*, *S. aureus*, *Legionella*	Cefazolin or cefoxitin or erythromycin
Nursing-home-acquired	Gram negative, *S. pneumoniae*, *H. influenza*, *S. aureus*	Cefoxitin and aminoglycoside‡ or aztreonam
Hospital-acquired	Gram negative, *S. pneumoniae*, *Legionella*, *S. aureus*	Cefoxitin and aminoglycoside or aztreonam or piperacillin
Postinfluenzal	*S. aureus*	Naficillin
Urinary tract		
Clinically stable	*E. coli*	Trimethoprin-sulfamethoxazole
Urosepsis	*Proteus, Klebsiella, Enterococcus, E. coli, Enterobacter*	Ampicillin§ and aminoglycoside
Cellulitis		
Uncomplicated	*S. aureus*, group A *streptococcus*	Naficillin
Complicated	Anaerobes and gram-negative rods	Clindamycin and aminoglycoside

* See Refs. 1, 12, 54, 57, 58.
† Intravenous erythromycin should be initiated at the outset in suspected *Legionella*.
‡ In general, for sicker patients, aminoglycosides should be used as initial therapy and discontinued if unneeded, based on culture results.
§ Ampicillin must be used to cover enteroccocus. In the event of penicillin allergy, vancomycin may be substituted.

Urinary Tract Infections

The prevalence of bacteriuria increases with aging and ranges anywhere between 10% and 40%. The sex differential of urinary tract infections also decreases considerably with aging.[12,13,56,57] The etiologic organisms include a variety of gram-negative organisms (eg, *Escherichia coli, Klebsiella, Enterobacter*) and enterococci. Organisms other than *E. coli* are more frequently encountered in the elderly. Urosepsis (particularly with enterococci) is always a concern.

Catheter-associated bacteriuria, which can be present in up to 80% of the nursing home elderly, is another major concern. Over 50% of nursing home subjects are incontinent, and more than half of them have catheters. The catheters are invariably colonized, and attempts to eradicate bacteriuria with antibiotics are not only futile but also select out resistant organisms. Treatment should only be instituted if there is a change in the clinical status of the patient, and that too only after appropriate cultures have been sent. It is usually best to change the patient's catheter before the sample for urine culture is sent. In the absence of chronic catheterization, chronic asymptomatic bacteriuria generally should not be treated unless there is a change in the patient's clinical status (Table 4.6).

Skin and Soft-Tissue Infections

The major problems associated with skin and soft-tissue infections[1,58,59] are cellulitis and infected decubitus ulcers. Cellulitis can either be uncomplicated or occur in the setting of venous insufficiency, peripheral vascular disease, and diabetes. If uncomplicated, the etiologic organism is usually either Group A streptococcus or *S. aureus*. With diabetes or vascular disease, it is usually a mixed infection with anaerobes and gram-negative rods.

Decubitus ulcers or "pressure sores" are invariably colonized and occasionally give rise to episodes of sepsis and/or osteomyelitis. Debridement of necrotic areas and the use of frequent wet to dry saline dressings to stimulate the growth of granulation tissue remain the mainstay of therapy. It is important to avoid occlusive dressings and topical agents which inhibit granulation. Systemic antibiotics should be instituted in the event of suspected sepsis (Table 4.6). In caring for the elderly, the single most important factor is keeping the pressure "off" susceptible areas (ie, the sacrococcyx, the greater trochanter, and the heels).

Tuberculosis

The elderly have become the single largest group of patients with active tuberculosis.[60–62] Although the majority of cases represent reactivation of past disease, in one study, 17% of newly diagnosed cases were due to primary infection.[61]

Pulmonary tuberculosis in the elderly is often characterized by a paucity of localizing symptoms, nonspecific manifestations, and cutaneous anergy in up to 30% of patients with active disease. Sputum for Ziel–Nielsen staining is often negative and the chest x-ray may be noncontributory, revealing only old apical fibrosis. In this setting, bronchial washings obtained at bronchoscopy may greatly increase diagnostic yield. In the presence of a pleural effusion, a pleural biopsy has an over 80% diagnostic yield. Epidemics of tuberculosis in nursing home patients are an emerging problem and miliary tuberculosis is also a predominantly geriatric problem. The latter, because of its insidious presentation, is often difficult to diagnose antemortem.

Pulmonary tuberculosis is usually treated with INH and rifampin for 9 to 12 months. Chemoprophylaxis in skin convertors only (ie, new responders to intermediate strength PPD with > 10 mm induration) is controversial for the elderly because of the potential risk of age-related INH hepatotoxicity. In selected individuals, however (ie, contacts with a positive tuberculin test), INH prophylaxis for a period of 12 months with regular monitoring of liver functions should be considered.

Intraabdominal Infections

Thirty percent of people in the eighth decade have gallstones and 50% have diverticulosis.[63,64] Not infrequently, complications like cholecystitis, diverticulitis, and even frank sepsis develop. At other times, the initial process is insidious and the only presenting features may be nonspecific gastrointestinal symptoms, including "failure to thrive." In this setting, a liver abscess must be suspected and diagnosis pursued aggressively. A CT scan with contrast is particularly helpful in this regard. When liver abscesses are present, they are often multiple. Drainage under CT guidance or ultrasound is the mainstay of treatment. Antibiotic treatment should adequately cover gram-negative rods and anaerobes. In the case of a biliary source, initial coverage should include enterococci as well (Table 4.7).

Table 4.7 Intraabdominal Infections: Common Organisms and Empiric Treatment*

Source	Aerobes	Anaerobes	Antibiotics
Biliary tract	*E. coli, Klebsiella, Enterococcus*	*Clostridium*	Ampicillin + clindamycin + aminoglycoside or ampicillin + cefoxitin
Colon (ie, severe diverticulitis)†	*E. coli, Proteus, Klebsiella*	*Bacteroides, Peptostreptococcus*	Aminoglycoside‡ + clindamycin or cefoxitin or metronidazole
Liver abscess	*E. coli, Streptococcus, Proteus, Klebsiella*	*Bacteroides, Peptostreptococcus, Fusobacterium, Clostridium*	Aminoglycoside + metronidazole or clindamycin or cefoperazone

* See Refs. 63 and 64.
† The efficacy of antimicrobial treatment in mild diverticulitis is not established.
‡ In general, for sicker patients, aminoglycosides should be used as initial therapy and discontinued if unneeded, based on culture results.

Infective Endocarditis

Over the last two decades, infective endocarditis has become a geriatric disease with over 50% of the cases occurring in patients over 60 years old.[65–67] Contributory factors include increased life expectancy, proliferation in use of endovascular devices, and the higher incidence of bacteremia in the elderly. Diagnosis requires a high index of suspicion and still depends primarily on positive blood cultures and, to some extent, on echocardiography. Mortality rates are between 20% and 50%. Staphylococcal endocarditis carries the worst prognosis. The organisms isolated most often are streptococci (ie, *S. viridans, S. bovis,* and *S. fecalis*) and staphylococci (ie, *S. aureus* and *S. epidermidis*). *Staphylococcus bovis* should prompt a search for an underlying colonic cancer, and *S. fecalis* usually emanates from the urinary tract. *Staphylococcus epidermidis* is most frequently associated with endovascular devices (ie, valves, shunts, and intravenous catheters). Less frequently, endocarditis (secondary to gram-negative organisms or candida) occurs (ie, invariably in a nosocomial setting).

In general, antimicrobial treatment should be given intravenously for 4 to 6 weeks. Streptococcal endocarditis is treated with high doses of penicillin G and an aminoglycoside (for the first 2 weeks) for synergism. For staphylococcal endocarditis, intravenous naficillin is used; vancomycin is required for *S. epidermidis* infections. Renal function should be monitored throughout and the dosage should be tailored appropriately. Refractory heart failure and persistently positive blood cultures are indications for proceeding to surgery with prosthetic valve endocarditis.

Herpes Zoster

Herpes zoster[68–70] represents a reactivation of the varicella-zoster virus which usually lies dormant in sensory ganglia following childhood chicken pox. The age-related decline in cell-mediated immunity correlates with the increasing incidence of herpes zoster. Immunosupression, either disease- or drug-induced, also causes a recrudescence of the virus.

Clinically, there is usually the sudden onset of burning or lancinating dermatomal pain (usually thoracic and invariably unilateral), followed 3 to 4 days later by a macular eruption in the same dermatomal distribution. Involvement of the trigeminal ganglion and facial nerve can cause keratitis and deafness. In the severely immunocompromised host, encephalitis, myelitis, and dissemination of the virus can occur. These complications are infrequent in the elderly in the absence of immunosuppressive drugs, hematologic malignancies, or other factors severely altering host-defense mechanisms. The most common complication in the elderly is postherpetic neuralgia, which can last for months.

The goals of treatment are symptomatic relief (ie, with wet compresses and analgesics) in the acute phase and prevention of postherpetic neuralgia. A short course of prednisone has been advocated for the prevention of neuralgia, although the issue is still controversial. In the severely immunocompromised host, a 7-day course of acyclovir is given during the acute stage to prevent dissemination of virus, but for others this is not indicated. A vaccine for the varicella zoster virus is currently under trial.

Prevention and Treatment

In this section, the general principles of treatment are stressed and the subject of prophylaxis examined in greater detail. Prevention of infection may be achieved either by immunoprophylaxis or chemoprophylaxis.

Immunoprophylaxis

In the elderly, vaccination is currently recommended for influenza, pneumococcus, and tetanus.

Influenza

Influenza and postinfluenzal pneumonia cause great morbidity and mortality in the geriatric population. During influenza epidemics, the attack rate in closed communities (ie, nursing homes) can approach 35%. Despite a suboptimal antibody response to vaccination in the elderly, overall vaccine efficacy is in the 70% range. In vaccinated populations, even if influenza occurs, it is less severe. In closed communities, vaccination also reduces morbidity in the nonvaccinated by inducing "herd immunity."[71,72] Yearly vaccination is recommended for people over 65 years of age, inmates of chronic-care facilities, patients with chronic cardiopulmonary problems, and patients with diabetes and chronic renal failure. The vaccine can be administered concurrently with pneumococcal vaccination, at a different site. Side effects are minimal and the only contraindication is an allergy to chicken eggs, which are used in preparing the vaccine.

Several studies have validated the effectiveness and the cost–benefit of the influenza vaccine.[73] During epidemics of influenza A, the drug Amantadine can be used for chemoprophylaxis of influenza A in nonvaccinated or recently vaccinated (ie, less than 2 weeks) subjects.

Table 4.8 Studies on the Efficacy of Pneumovax

Reference	Design	Comments
75	Prospective randomized*	Healthy, elderly subjects—77% efficacy
76	Prospective randomized*	Elderly with chronic illnesses—no efficacy
74	Retrospective case control	Elderly with chronic illness—no efficacy
78	Retrospective case control	Healthy, elderly—70% efficacy
77	Retrospective case control	Healthy, elderly—70% efficacy

* The 14 serotype vaccine was used in these studies.

Pneumococcus

Pneumococcal vaccination has been the subject of intense debate; the present vaccine contains 23 serotypes.[74-79] Recently, several studies have looked at its efficacy (Table 4.8). Despite methodologic differences and varying attack rates in these studies, it was concluded that the efficacy of the vaccine correlated directly with one's ability to mount an antibody response. Hence, it is felt by many, but not all experts, that all healthy elderly should receive the vaccine; additionally, asplenic individuals should be vaccinated. Side effects are mild.

Tetanus

Although low in incidence, tetanus now occurs primarily in the elderly (ie, 60% of new cases in the over-60-years age group).[80,81] Mortality is also disproportionately high in the elderly. Immunity to tetanus declines with aging and, in one study, 50% of the elderly had inadequate levels of circulating antitoxin. Current recommendations are for a booster of the adult tetanus–diptheria (Td) toxoid preparation every 10 years. In the absence of previous immunization, or an unclear history thereof, a primary series is recommended.

Chemoprophylaxis

In brief, any procedure in the presence of prosthetic heart valves, surgically constructed shunts, valvular heart disease, or a previous history of infective endocarditis is the basis for recommending chemoprophylaxis.[1,82,83] In particular, dental manipulations and gastrointestinal and genitourinary procedures have a high incidence of bacteremia. Antibiotic prophylaxis in these settings should cover the local microbial flora associated with these tissues.

Surgical prophylaxis in the absence of heart disease aims to prevent wound infections, infections at the operative site, and bacteremia. Chemoprophylaxis is currently recommended for colororectal surgery, vaginal hysterectomy, biliary tract surgery, cardiac surgery, hip operations, and urologic procedures. Antibiotics are usually administered in two doses (ie, pre-operatively and 24 to 48 hours postoperatively), and cover regional microbial flora and staphylococcus (in the case of bone surgery).

Summary

Aging is associated with an increased frequency and severity of many types of illness, including infectious diseases. Specific changes in host-defense mechanisms account for only part of this increased susceptibility to infections. Good health care for the elderly requires an appreciation for the more subtle presentation of infections (eg, a blunted febrile response, occult signs of inflammation) and more frequent nonspecific signs (eg, altered mental status, immobility, and anorexia). When fever is present or the suspicion for infection is high, antibiotic intervention should be prompt. It usually must be based on recognized patterns of infections in the elderly, since smears and cultures may be neither available nor helpful. Preventative measures—including vaccinations, chemoprophylaxis, as well as maintenance of nutritional status and physical stamina—are very important for prevention of infections in elderly individuals.

References

1. Yoshikawa TT, Norman DC: *Aging and Clinical Practice: Infectious Diseases, Diagnosis and Treatment.* New York, Igaku-Shoin, 1987.
2. Garibaldi RA, Nurse BA: Infections in the elderly. *Am J Med* 1986;81:53–58.
3. Berk SL, Smith JK: Infectious diseases in the elderly. *Med Clin North Am* 1983;67:273–293.
4. Saltzman RI, Peterson PK: Immunodeficiency of the elderly. *Rev Infect Dis* 1987;9:1127–1139.
5. Andres R, Bierman EL, Hazzard WR: *Principles of Geriatric Medicine.* New York, McGraw-Hill, 1985.
6. Fredman L, Haynes SG: An epidemiologic profile of the elderly, in Phillips HG, Gaylord SA (eds.): *Aging and Public Health.* New York, Springer, 1985, pp 1–41.
7. Hodgson TA, Kopstein AN: Health care expenditures for major diseases: Health and prevention profile, United States. Hyattsville, Maryland, USDHHS, Public Health Service, National Center for Health Statistics, 1983, pp 79–84.
8. Finklestein MS, Petkun WM, Freedman ML, et al: Pneumococcal bacteremia in adults: Age dependent difference in presentation and in outcome. *J Am Geriatr Soc* 1983;31:19–27.
9. Current estimates from the National Health Interview Survey: United States 1982. Data from the National Health Survey, series 10, no. 150 (DHHS publication no. PHS 85-1578), Hyattsville, Maryland, National Center for Health Statistics, 1985.
10. Weinstein MP, Murphy JR, Reller LB, et al: The clinical significance of positive blood cultures: A comprehensive analysis of 500 episodes of bacteremia and fungemia in adults. II. Clinical observations with special reference to factors influencing prognosis. *Rev Infect Dis* 1983;5:54–70.
11. Gleckman R, Hibert D: Afebrile bacteremia: A phenomenon in geriatric patients. *JAMA* 1981;248:1478–1481.
12. Yoshikawa TT: Unique aspects of urinary tract infection in the geriatric population. *Gerontology* 1984;30:339–344.
13. Gleckman RA, Bradley PJ, Roth RM, et al: Bacteremic urosepsis: A phenomenon unique to elderly women. *J Urology* 1985;133:174–175.
14. Setia U, Serventi I, Lorenz P: Bacteremia in a long-term care facility: Spectrum and mortality. *Arch Intern Med* 1984;144:1633–1635.
15. Finnegan TP, Austin TW, Cape RDT: A 12 month fever surveillance study in a veterans' long-stay institution. *J Am Geriatr Soc* 1985;30:590–594.
16. Irvine PW, Van Buren N, Krossley K: Causes for hospitalization of nursing home residents: The role of infection. *J Am Geriatr Soc* 1984;32:103–107.
17. Norman DC, Grahn D, Yoshikawa TT: Fever and aging. *J Am Geriatr Soc* 1985;33:859–863.

18. Murphy TF, Fine BC: Bacteremic pneumococcal pneumonia in the elderly. *Am J Med Sci* 1984;288:114–118.
19. Keating HJ III, Klimek JJ, Levine DS, et al: Aging and the clinical significance of fever in ambulatory adult patients. *J Am Geriatr Soc* 1984;32:282–287.
20. Finkelstein MS: Unusual features of infections in the aging. *Geriatrics* 1982;37:65–78.
21. Nossal GJV: The basic components of the immune system. *N Engl J Med* 1987; 316:1320–1325.
22. Dinarello CA, Mier JW: Current concepts: Lymphokines. *N Engl J Med* 1987;317:940–944.
23. Fox RA: The effect of aging on the immune response, in Fox RA (ed.): *Immunology and infection in the elderly*. New York, Churchill Livingstone, 1984, pp 289–309.
24. Weksler ME: Senescence of the immune system. *Med Clin North Am* 1983;67:263–272.
25. Charpentier B, Fournier C, Fries D, Mathieu D, Noury J, Bach JF: Immunological studies in human ageing: I. In vitro function of T cells and polymorphs. *J Clin Lab Immunol* 1981;5:87–93.
26. Weksler ME, Hutteroth TH: Impaired lymphocyte function in aged humans. *J Clin Invest* 1974;53:99–104.
27. Makinodan T, James SJ, Inamizu T, et al: Immunologic basis for susceptibility to infection in the aged. *Gerontology* 1984;30:279–289.
28. Delafuente JC: Immunosenescence: Clinical and pharmacologic considerations. *Med Clin North Am* 1985;69:475–486.
29. Makinodan T, Lubinski J, Fong TC: Cellular, biochemical and molecular basis of T-cell senescence. *Arch Pathol Lab Med* 1987;111:910–914.
30. Malech HL, Gallin JI: Current concepts: Immunology, neutrophils in human diseases. *N Engl J Med* 1987;317:687–692.
31. Nagel JE, Pyle PS, Chrest FJ, et al: Oxidative metabolism and bactericidal capacity of polymorphonuclear leukocytes from normal young and aged adults. *J Gerontol* 1982;37:529–534.
32. Corberand J, Ngyen F, Laharrague P, et al: Polymorphonuclear functions and aging in humans. *J Am Geriatr Soc* 1981;29:391–397.
33. Timaffy M: A comparative study of bone marrow function in young and old individuals. *Geront Clin* 1962;4:13–18.
34. Baldwin JG: Hematopoietic function in the elderly. *Arch Intern Med* 1988;148:2544–2546.
35. Lipschitz DA, Udupa RB, Milton RY, et al: Effect of age on hematopoiesis in man. *Blood* 1984;63:502–509.
36. Gardner ID, Lim STK, Lawton JWM: Monocyte function in aging humans. *Mech Ageing Dev* 1981;16:233–239.
37. Norman DC, Yamamura RH, Yoshikawa TT: Fever response in old and young mice after injection of interleukin 1. *J Gerontol* 1988;43:M80–M85.
38. Jones PG, Kauffman CA, Bergman AG, Hayes CM, Kluger MJ, Cannon JG: Fever in the elderly: Production of leukocytic pyrogen by monocytes from elderly persons. *Gerontology* 1984,30.182–187.
39. Nagaki K, Hiramatsu S, Inai S, et al: The effect of aging on complement protein levels. *J Clin Lab Immunol* 1980;45–50.
40. Royer HD, Reinherz EL: T lymphocytes: Ontogeny, function, and relevance to clinical disorders. *N Engl J Med* 1987;317:1136–1142.
41. Phair JP, Kauffman CA, Bjornson A, Gallagher J, Adams L, Hess EV: Host defenses in the aged: Evaluation of components of the inflammatory and immune responses. *J Infect Dis* 1978;138:67–73.
42. Gravenstein S, Duthie EH, Miller BA, Roecker E, Drinka P, Prathipati K, Ershler WB: Augmentation of influenza antibody response in elderly men by thymosin alpha one. A double-blind placebo-controlled clinical study. *J Am Geriat Soc* 1989;37:1–8.
43. Nagel JE, Chrest FJ, Adler WH: Enumeration of T lymphocyte subsets by monoclonal antibodies in young and aged humans. *J Immunol* 1981;127:2086–2088.

44. Bender BS, Nagel JE, Adler WH, Andres R: Absolute periphereal blood lymphocyte count and subsequent mortality of elderly men: The Baltimore longitudinal study of aging. *J Am Ger Soc* 1986;34:649–654.
45. Cooper MD: B lymphocytes: Normal development and function. *N Engl J Med* 1987;317:1452–1456.
46. Ammann AJ, Schiffman G, Austrian R. The antibody responses to pneumococcal capsular polysaccharides in aged individuals. *Proc Soc Exp Biol Med* 1980;164:312–316.
47. Buckley CE, Dorsey FC. The effect of aging on human serum immunoglobulin concentrations. *J Immunol* 1965;105:964–972.
48. Bender BS: B lymphocyte function in aging. *Rev Biol Research in Aging* 1985;2:143–154.
49. Katz S: Functional assessment. *J Am Geriatr Soc* 1983;31:721–726.
50. Garibaldi RA, Brodine S, Matsumiya S: Infections among patients in nursing homes. *N Engl J Med* 1981;305:731–735.
51. Chandra RK: Nutrition, immunity and infection: Present knowledge and future direction. *Lancet* 1983;1:688–691.
52. Corman LC: The relationship between nutrition, infection and immunity. *Med Clin North Am* 1985;69:519–531.
53. Morley JE: Nutritional status of the elderly. *Am J Med* 1986;81:679–695.
54. Bentley DW: Bacterial pneumonia in the elderly: Clinical features, diagnosis, etiology, and treatment. *Gerontology* 1984;30:297–307.
55. Verghese A, Berk SL: Bacterial pneumonia in the elderly. *Medicine* 1983;62:271–285.
56. Nordenstam GR, Brandberg CA, Oden AS, et al: Bacteriuria and mortality in an elderly population. *N Engl J Med* 1986;314:1152–1156.
57. Kunin CM: Duration of treatment of urinary tract infections. *Am J Med* 1981;71:849–854.
58. Hook EW III, Hooton TM, Horton CA, et al: Microbiologic evaluation of cutaneous cellulitis in adults. *Arch Intern Med* 1986;146:295–297.
59. Reuler JB, Cooney TG: The pressure sore: Pathophysiology and principles of management. *Ann Intern Med* 1981;94:661–666.
60. Nagami PH, Yoshikawa TT: Tuberculosis in the geriatric patient. *J Am Geriatr Soc* 1983;31:356–363.
61. Stead WW, Lofgren JP, Warren E, et al: Tuberculosis as an endemic and nosocomial infection among the elderly in nursing homes. *N Engl J Med* 1985;312:1483–1487.
62. Committee on Chemotherapy of Tuberculosis: Standard therapy for tuberculosis 1985. *Chest* 1985;87:117S–124S.
63. Nichols RL: Intraabdominal infections: An overview. *Rev Infect Dis* 1985;7(S):709–715.
64. Norman DC, Yoshikawa TT: Intraabdominal infection: Diagnosis and treatment in the elderly patient. *Gerontology* 1984;30:327–338.
65. Cantrell M, Yoshikawa TT: Aging and infective endocarditis. *J Am Geriatr Soc* 1983;31:216–222.
66. Wilson WR, Danielson GK, Guiliane ER, et al: Prosthetic valve endocarditis. *Mayo Clin Proc* 1982;57:155–161.
67. Mintz GS, Kotler MN: Clinical value and limitations of echocardiography: Its use in the study of patients with infective endocarditis. *Arch Intern Med* 1980;140:1022–1027.
68. Hope-Simpson RE: The nature of Herpes zoster: A long-term study and a new hypothesis. *Proc Roy Soc Med* 1965;58:9–13.
69. Burke BL, Steele RW, Beard DW, et al: Immune responses to varicella-zoster in the aged. *Arch Intern Med* 1982;142:291–293.
70. Weller TH: Varicella and herpes zoster: Changing concepts of the natural history, control, and importance of a not-so benign virus. *N Engl J Med* 1983;309:1363–1368.
71. Barker WH, Mullooly JP: Influenza vaccination of elderly persons: Reduction in pneumonia and influenza hospitalizations and deaths. *JAMA* 1980;244:2547–2549.

72. Patriarca PA, Weber PA, Parker RA, et al: Efficacy of influenza vaccine in nursing homes: Reduction in illness and complications during an influenza A epidemic. *JAMA* 1985;253:1136–1139.
73. Patriarca PA, Arden NH, Koplan JP, Goodman RA: Prevention and control of type A influenza infections in nursing homes. *Ann Intern Med* 1987;107:732–740.
74. Forrester HL, Jahnigen DW, LaForce FM: Inefficacy of pneumococcal vaccine in a high-risk population. *Am J Med* 1987;83:425–430.
75. Gaillat J, Zmirou D, Mallaret MR, et al: Essai clinique due vaccin antipneumococcique chez des personnes agées vivant en institution. *Rev Epidemol Sante Publique* 1985;33:437–444.
76. Simberkoff MS, Cross AP, Al-Ibrahim M, et al: Efficacy of pneumococcal vaccine in high risk patients. *N Engl J Med* 1986;315:1316–1327.
77. Sims RV, Steinmann WC, McConville JH, King LR, Zwick WC, Schwartz JS: The clinical effectiveness of the pneumococcal vaccine in the elderly. *Ann Intern Med* 1988;108:653–657.
78. Shapiro ED, Austrian R, Adair RK, Clemens JD: The protective efficacy of pneumococcal vaccine (abstract). *Clin Res* 1988;36:470A.
79. LaForce FM: Pneumococcal vaccine: An emerging consensus. *Ann Intern Med* 1988;108:757–759.
80. Weiss BP, Strassburg MA, Feeley JC: Tetanus and diphtheria immunity in an elderly population in Los Angeles County. *Am J Public Health* 1983;145:802–804.
81. Berk SL, Alvarez S: Vaccinating the elderly: Recommendations and rationale. *Geriatrics* 1986;41:79–87.
82. Guglielmo BJ, Hohn DC, Koo PJ, et al: Antibiotic prophylaxis in surgical procedures. *Arch Surg* 1983;118:943–955.
83. Shulman ST, Amren DP, Bisno AI, et al: Prevention of bacterial endocarditis: A statement for health professionals by the Committee on Rheumatic Fever and Infective Endocarditis of the Counsel on Cardiovascular Disease in the Young. *Circulation* 1984;70:1123A–1127A.

Chapter 5

Aging and Pharmacotherapeutics

G. Aagaard, MD

Chemistry and pharmacology have ushered physicians into an era of great promise. An endless stream of new drugs goes through the stages of development and clinical trials. Many are proved safe and effective and are added to the drug therapy armamentarium. The optimal use of this armamentarium in the prevention and treatment of illness in older women is an opportunity and a challenge to physicians.

The challenge of the safe and effective use of drugs in older patients exists for several reasons. First, older patients have more diseases. More diseases usually means that more drugs are prescribed. More drugs means the possibility of more adverse drug reactions as well as the greater chance of significant drug–drug interactions. Branch found that 15% of an elderly population took two or more prescription medications daily.[1] Law and Chalmers reported that 87% of patients 75 years of age and older were receiving drug therapy regularly, and that 34% of these took 3 or 4 drugs per day.[2]

Second, apart from the greater exposure to drugs associated with an increased burden of chronic disease, there may be an increased vulnerability to drugs, which is related to the aging process. A drug may be handled differently (pharmacokinetics) in older patients, or a drug may act differently (pharmacodynamics) in older patients.

Third, the aging process may cause changes which make it more difficult to obtain compliance from older patients. Hearing loss may make it difficult to understand spoken explanations or instructions. Visual changes may impair the ability to understand written instructions or to read the labels on drug containers. Loss of memory or confusion may make it difficult to comprehend or follow instructions regarding medications.

The considerations noted above explain why the idea prevails that drug therapy in elders should be approached with caution because elders are more vulnerable to adverse reactions. Certainly, it is true that elders are more likely to have postural hypotension even without drugs. Therefore, they are more likely to have a significant postural drop in blood pressure with any drug that may cause this important and dangerous response. However, elders show a wide range of responses to drugs, and this requires that physicians prescribe thoughtfully for the individual and follow closely.

Pharmacokinetic Effects of Aging

Drug Absorbtion

Since most prescribed drugs are given by mouth, this discussion will be limited to changes with aging in the gastrointestinal tract and their effect on the absorbtion of drugs. There are a number of aspects of gastrointestinal function that might change with aging, which could influence the absorbtion of a drug. These include: (1) gastric fluid pH; (2) gastric emptying time; (3) intestinal motility; (4) gastrointestinal fluid secretion (volume and composition); (5) gastrointestinal blood flow; and (6) gastrointestinal disease and the general health of the patient. However, there is little or no evidence that changes related to aging influence drug absorbtion significantly. Changes in the pH of the gastric fluid are offered as an example.

The pH of gastric fluid tends to increase with age and to a greater degree in women than in men. This could influence both the rate at which a drug goes into solution and the rate at which it is absorbed from the stomach. The dissolution rate of alkaline drugs could theoretically be impaired by achlorhydria or a significant decrease in gastric acidity. This would suggest that drugs might be prescribed in solution, instead of as pills, to avoid the process of dissolution in the stomach. Alkalinity of the gastric juice might also reduce the rate of absorbtion of alkaline drugs in the stomach. However, despite the changes in gastric acidity with age, which are well-established, there is not good evidence of reduced drug absorbtion.

Drug Distribution

When a drug is absorbed into the blood, it becomes available to all the tissues and organs to which blood circulates. The drug shifts from the blood to receptor sites, to storage depots, and to sites where it may be metabolized or excreted. The rate and extent of movement of a drug depends on the concentration of the drug, and the affinity of the drug for receptors and for storage tissues. Drugs tend to move from sites of higher concentration to sites of lower concentration.

Drugs in the plasma are present in two forms, free drug and plasma protein-bound drug. The amount of drug which is bound to plasma proteins is dependent on the affinity of the drug for plasma protein. Most protein-bound drug is bound to plasma albumen. In a sense, plasma protein-bound drug serves as a readily available store of drug, which is called upon when free drug is removed from plasma.

It is free drug which acts by binding to receptors. It is free drug which is also metabolized by liver cells, or excreted by the kidney. When free drug is removed from the plasma for any of these purposes, it is replaced by plasma protein-bound drug. If free drug is increased by the administration of a larger dose of drug, more drug will become bound to plasma protein but an additional amount of drug will be available at sites where it may be metabolized or excreted.

With aging, bodily changes occur which can influence the distribution of drugs. Total body water and blood volume tend to decrease. Lean body mass (muscle tissue) tends to decrease. There is a relative increase in body fat. Novak compared body fat in young adults with those 65 to 85 years of age.[3] Body fat increased from 18% to 36% of total body weight in men, and from 33% to 45%

in women. This means that drugs which are readily soluble in fat are more readily stored in older patients and to a greater extent in women than in men. Such a drug would have a greater volume of distribution, and when a single dose is administered would have a lower plasma concentration than would be attained if the drug were relatively insoluble in fat.

Drug Metabolism

Liver size decreases with age. Liver blood flow also decreases with age. It is logical to assume that drugs which are metabolized by the liver would have reduced clearance and a prolonged plasma half-life. However, studies to determine the site and rate of metabolism of a drug are difficult to design, conduct, and interpret.

O'Malley found that the plasma half-lives of antipyrine and phenylbutazone were increased 45% and 29%, respectively, in aged patients as compared to young adults.[4] The increase for the antipyrine half-life was even greater for women (78%).

In a large study, Vestal found that there was a great individual variation between subjects, and that only a small part of the reduced clearance could be ascribed to the influence of age alone.[5] Vestal and Wood also showed that smoking had less effect in inducing enzymatic metabolism in the aged.[6]

Renal Excretion

Kidney function decreases with age, with the result that drugs which are eliminated chiefly by the kidney show an increased plasma half-life and a decreased clearance rate. Beginning in the fourth decade of life, changes in renal blood flow, renal mass, glomerular filtration rate, and active tubular secretion and resorbtion occur.[7] The decrease in renal blood flow is greater than would be explained by the decrease in cardiac output which occurs with aging.

The reduced capacity to excrete drugs may not be adequately reflected by the serum creatinine concentration, which may be normal in an elderly patient while the creatinine clearance is definitely abnormal. The serum creatinine concentration may be in the normal range because of reduced production of creatinine due to a reduced muscle mass in the older patient. Therefore, it is best to use creatinine clearance to estimate renal function in prescribing a drug which is eliminated largely by excretion by the kidney.

Pharmacodynamics in Aging

Pharmacodynamics deals with the response that a drug elicits in a patient. Is that response greater or smaller than the "usual" response? The idea is widely held that the aged are more "sensitive" or more responsive to drugs than are younger adults. This is true in some instances, but it is not universally true. It takes significantly more isoproterenol to produce an increase of 25 beats per minute in aged subjects than is required in younger subjects.[8] The same study reported that the response to the β-adrenergic blocker, propranolol, was reduced in older patients. Vestal's findings suggest that the affinity of β receptors for both agonists and antagonists may decrease with age. Another explanation is that the sensitivity of aged patients to drugs which act on β receptors is decreased.

Increased sensitivity to drugs with aging is suggested by several studies. Reidenberg et al showed that the dose of diazepam, which caused depression, was inversely related to age.[9] In addition, the drug plasma level at which depression occurred was inversely related to age.

Increased sensitivity to a single 10 mg dose of nitrazepam was found in old as compared to young patients.[10] Older patients made more mistakes in a psychomotor test despite similar plasma concentrations and half-lives in the two groups.

Cook et al studied the response to intravenous diazepam in patients being prepared for dental or endoscopic procedures.[11] They found that patients 80 years of age required an average dose of 10 mg compared to 30 mg for patients age 20 years. The plasma levels required for sedation at age 20 were two to three times those required at age 80.

Older patients also appear to be more sensitive to warfarin. In both humans and rats, Shepard et al found that older subjects had a greater anticoagulant response even though they received a smaller weight-related dose.[12] They also found that at the same plasma level of warfarin there was a greater inhibition of vitamin K clotting factor synthesis in the older group. They found no significant differences in pharmacokinetics between the two age groups.

In summary, older patients may be more or less sensitive to drugs. The opiates, benzodiazepines, barbiturates, and anticoagulants may elicit an increased response. For other drugs, such as isoproterenol or β blockers, the response may be reduced. Drug treatment must be individualized, and the response of the patient must be closely followed.

Adverse Effects of Drugs

In prescribing any drug, a physician must consider and balance three major factors: (1) the natural history of the disease (What are the hazards to life and health if the disease is left untreated?); (2) the effectiveness of the drug in the disease as now presented in the patient; and (3) the hazards of the drug in a patient with a similar clinical picture. In a mild self-limited illness, it would be unwise to prescribe a drug that caused serious adverse effects in a significant number of patients. On the other hand, the possibility of adverse effects would not deter the use of a drug in a life-threatening illness.

In any discussion of adverse drug effects, it must be acknowledged that it may be difficult to reach agreement on a definition. Karch and Lasagna have suggested that an adverse drug reaction is "any response to a drug that is noxious and unintended and that occurs at doses used in man for prophylaxis, diagnosis, or therapy, excluding failure to accomplish the intended purpose."[13] Even with agreement on a definition, it may be difficult to get agreement of experienced clinicians on the classification of specific symptoms or signs in a patient. The differentiation between signs of adverse drug effects and the symptoms and signs of an illness may be challenging.

Many studies of adverse drug effects suffer from a lack of controls. Reidenberg and Lowenthal compared healthy students and hospital staff who were taking no medications with a group who were receiving medications.[14] They found that many symptoms commonly considered adverse drug effects were complained of by their healthy subjects. Prominent among these symptoms were fatigue, inability to concentrate, irritability, and insomnia.

Despite the difficulties mentioned above, there is good reason to suggest that adverse effects of drugs are more frequent and more severe in older patients. Seidl et al found an adverse drug reaction in 9.9% of patients 21 to 30 years of age and in 24% of patients 81 years of age and older.[15] Castleden and Pickles reviewed spontaneous reports of adverse drug reactions (ADR) received by the Committee on Safety of Medicines in the United Kingdom.[16] They found a correlation between the use of drugs and the number of ADR reports. This was true for two nonsteroidal antiinflammatory drugs (NSAID). They also found that the ADR was more likely to be serious or fatal in the elders. The most common ADRs caused by the two NSAIDs in the elderly affected the gastrointestinal and hemopoietic systems. The drug suspected of causing a gastrointestinal ADR was an NSAID in 75% of the reports, and 91% of fatal reports of gastrointestinal bleeds and perforations were in patients over 60 years of age.

Of equal importance to drugs as a cause of life-threatening ADRs is the unfavorable effect they may exert on the quality of life of patients. It is important to determine if a drug disturbs ability to function socially, decreases initiative, impairs memory, impairs sexual function, disturbs sleep patterns, or increases fatigue.

A host of drugs can cause psychiatric symptoms, ranging from mania and hallucinations to confusion, disorientation, and depression.[17] Mental confusion, especially in the elderly, has been reported with cimetidine.[18] In the days when sulfonamides were available but penicillin was not, pneumonia was often treated with a sulfonamide. Acute psychoses were reported, which would clear when the drug was discontinued. Lamy has estimated that 40 drugs or groups of drugs may cause delirium.

Cognitive impairment due to an ADR was found in 35 of 308 patients being evaluated for Alzheimer-type dementia. The drugs most often involved were minor tranquilizers, antihypertensives, and major tranquilizers.[19]

Sexual dysfunction may be an ADR from antihypertensive drugs. Central sympatholytics, β-adrenergic blockers, and α-adrenergic blockers are frequent offenders, although even the thiazide diuretics can cause trouble especially if hypokalemia is present.[20] Psychotropic drugs can also cause sexual dysfunction. The major tranquilizers, the antidepressants, and the benzodiazepines all have this potential.

Cimetidine and metoclopramide may both cause increased prolactin levels, which may be associated with decreased libido and later with impotence.

Anticholinergic drugs may also be associated with sexual dysfunction. These include atropine, some of the antispasmodics, the antiparkinson agents, the antihistamines, muscle relaxants, and antiarrhythmics. Not all of the drugs in these classes will cause sexual dysfunction, but the potential is present and should be ruled out in those patients who complain of an impairment.

In older patients a significant problem is drug-induced Parkinsonism (DIP).[21] Major tranquilizers, antiemetics, methyldopa, reserpine, and diazepam have all been implicated.

Many ADRs are dose-related: either the daily dose is too large or the drug is given for too long, with toxicity occurring over time. In some instances it may be possible to eliminate the ADR by reducing the dose or temporarily stopping the drug.

Drug–Drug Interactions as a Cause of Adverse Drug Reactions

Since older patients take more medications, they are more vulnerable to drug–drug interactions. A patient who is taking one or more different drugs has the potential for a drug–drug interaction if an additional drug is prescribed. Similarly, the patient who is taking two or more drugs could be at risk if one drug is discontinued.

Space does not permit a full discussion of this subject, but it is important to emphasize that drugs may influence the manner in which the body handles or responds to another drug. A drug may change the rate of absorbtion of another drug, or it may increase or decrease the rate of metabolism or the rate of excretion of another drug. If drug B reduces the rate of metabolism or the rate of excretion of drug A, it is possible that the plasma level of drug A will increase when drug B is prescribed. Cimetidine, for example, reduces the metabolism of diazepam. Hence, a dose of diazepam, which was well-tolerated previously, may become toxic after cimetidine is added to the patient's regimen. Similarly, a drug that competes very successfully for plasma protein-binding sites may displace another drug with a lesser affinity. For example, protein-bound warfarin may be displaced by a nonsteroidal antiinflammatory drug which is prescribed. The result could be a significant increase in the level of free warfarin in the plasma, and an increase in anticoagulant effect.

Because older patients take more drugs, they are theoretically at greater risk of drug–drug interactions. Fortunately, clinically significant adverse reactions are much less frequent than the theoretical possibilities. Nonetheless, it is important to look for a change in pharmacokinetics whenever a new drug is prescribed or a drug is discontinued.

Practical Suggestions for Optimal Drug Therapy in Older Women

1. Take a careful drug history, including all drugs currently being taken, both prescriptions and others. Ask the patient to bring all drugs currently being taken to the office for the first visit. What was the response to each drug? A prolonged response to a modest dose of diazepam given in preparation for a procedure suggests caution when considering the use of a benzodiazepine. Learn about past adverse effects. Have there been compliance problems? Why? Inquire about the use of cigarettes, alcohol, caffeine-containing beverages, laxatives, asperin, tylenol, antacids, and sleeping preparations.
2. Prescribe a drug only if there is a clear need and if the chances of benefit clearly outweigh the costs in adverse effects and dollars.
3. Enlist the patient's continuing participation in the drug-treatment program. Explain the need for, and the goals of, drug therapy. Describe how the medication should be administered. Ask for feedback on the response to the

drug, with emphasis on any adverse effects. Include a family member or other observer in the instructions and in the arrangements for feedback.

Request information regarding the time and degree of a favorable response. A prompt favorable response to a low dose or to a few doses suggests that the patient may develop toxicity to the drug over a relatively short time.

4. Evaluate the patient frequently and carefully for the desired response and for adverse effects. After any change in the drug-treatment program (any addition or deletion), follow the patient closely for any possible drug–drug interaction.
5. Always consider the drug-treatment program as a possible cause for any unfavorable change in the patient. If it is possible that a drug may be at fault, discontinue the drug and observe the patient closely.
6. Prescribe a low dose initially. If the dose must be increased, make the increments smaller and at longer intervals than you would use in younger patients. If the patient has any difficulty in swallowing tablets, try to obtain a liquid preparation.
7. Give the patient written instructions regarding medications. Keep instructions up to date. Make certain that the patient can read and understand the instructions. Review the instructions with the patient and have all the medications available.
8. Be certain that the patient can open the drug containers and can read the labels. Help the patient to identify each drug and to differentiate between tablets of similar appearance. Highlight those drugs which need special attention; for example, to be taken at least 1 hour before meals, or before bedtime.
9. Help the patient to develop or acquire a system that will help her to be confident that she has taken all of the drugs which have been advised. Insofar as possible, try to fit the drug-treatment program into the patient's daily schedule.
10. For a patient in the hospital, be certain that all drugs that will be taken after discharge are reviewed and that written instructions are given. If possible, have a family member present.
11. Ask the patient to bring all medications with her for each office visit. Review these at each visit to see if any might be discontinued.
12. When appropriate, use plasma drug levels for guidance in drug dosage and the interval between doses.

References

1. Branch LG: Understanding the health and social service needs of people over age 65. Washington, D.C., Department of HEW, 1977, p 77.
2. Law R, Chalmers C: Medicines and elderly people: A general practice survey. *Brit Med J* 1976;1:565.
3. Novak LP: Aging, total body potassium, fat-free mass and cell mass in males and females between age 18 and 85 years. *J Gerontology* 1972;27:438.
4. O'Malley K, et al: Effect of age and sex on human drug metabolism. *Brit Med J* 1971;3:607.

5. Vestal RE, et al: Antipyrine metabolism in man: Influence of age, alcohol, caffeine, and smoking. *Clin Pharm Thera* 1975;18:425.
6. Vestal RE, Wood AJJ: Influence of age and smoking on drug kinetics in man: Studies using model compounds. *Clin Pharmacokinetics* 1980;5:309.
7. Hollenberg NK, et al: Senescence and the renal vasculature in normal man. *Circ Res* 1974;34:309.
8. Vestal RE, et al: Reduced beta-adrenoreceptor sensitivity in the elderly. *Clin Pharm Thera* 1979;26:181.
9. Reidenberg MM, et al: The relationship between diazepam dose, plasma level, age and central nervous system depression in adults. *Clin Pharm Thera* 1978;23:371.
10. Castleden CM, et al: Increased sensitivity to nitrazepam in old age. *Brit Med J* 1977;1:10.
11. Cook PJ, Flanagan R, James IM: Diazepam tolerance: Effect of age, regular sedation and alcohol. *Brit Med J* 1984;289:351.
12. Shepard AMM, et al: Age as a determinant of sensitivity to warfarin. *Brit J Clin Pharm* 1977;4:315.
13. Karch FE, Lasagna L: Toward the operational identification of adverse drug reactions. *Clin Pharm Thera* 1977;21:247.
14. Reidenberg MM, Lowenthal DT: Adverse nondrug reactions. *N Engl J Med* 1968;279:678.
15. Seidl LG, et al: Studies on the epidemiology of adverse drug reactions: III. Reactions in patients on a general medical service. *Johns Hopkins Hosp Bull* 1966;119:299.
16. Castleden CM, Pickles H: Suspected adverse drug reactions in elderly patients reported to the Committee on Safety of Medicines. *Brit J Clin Pharm* 1988;26:347.
17. Drugs that cause psychiatric symptoms. *Medical Letter* 1984;26:75.
18. Cimetidine (Tagamet): Update on adverse effects. *Medical Letter* 1978;20:77.
19. Larson EB, et al: Adverse drug reactions associated with global cognitive impairment in elderly persons. *Ann Internal Med* 1987;107:169.
20. Drugs that Cause Sexual Dysfunction. *Medical Letter* 1983;25:73.
21. Wilson JA, Maclennan WJ: Review: Drug-induced Parkinsonism in elderly patients. *Age and Aging* 1989;18:208.

Chapter **6**

Preventive Health Care of Older Women

Wylie Burke, MD, PhD, and Wendy H. Raskind MD, PhD

In contrast to conventional medical treatment of active symptoms, the goal of preventive health care is to maintain or improve future health. This goal has three components: (1) the prevention of disease when possible; (2) the early identification of treatable conditions; and (3) the preservation of independence and useful function. All of these should be considerations during a routine visit to a physician. History-taking, physical examination, and screening tests each contribute to preventive health care. In addition, patient education is important. Patients vary in their awareness of preventive care and of current screening recommendations, and often need to have the rationale and benefits of these activities explained.

Disease prevention is possible only when modifiable precursors of disease can be recognized early. Frequently, such efforts require patients to undertake changes in their life-style. Helping the patient to understand the importance of such changes is a key part of preventive care. For example, smoking cessation significantly reduces the risk of chronic obstructive pulmonary disease, coronary artery disease, stroke, lung cancer, and other cancers. Most smokers find quitting to be extremely difficult. Furthermore, if the patient gives up smoking, no guarantee can be given that the diseases associated with smoking will be fully prevented. These realities complicate the task of helping a patient to stop smoking. Specific information on the value of a preventive measure helps a patient to undertake changes in long-standing habits. Similarly, the physician's counseling efforts are made easier when patients can be given concrete suggestions to follow. Approaches to counseling patients on smoking cessation and other preventive life-style changes are discussed in more detail below.

Other true preventive measures include immunizations, control of elevated blood pressure, and periodic dental cleaning. Some measures thought of as preventive in nature are actually measures aimed at identifying disease in early, treatable stages. These include screening for colon, cervical, and breast cancer. While not strictly preventive, such screening may make cure a possibility or significantly limit the morbidity of a disease process. Like life-style changes, effective screening often requires education of patients, so that they can understand both the purpose and the limitations of screening procedures.

The maintenance of useful function and independence involves a different kind of preventive care; in this area, potentially disabling conditions are identified in order to make interventions that preserve or improve an individual's functional state. For example, a hearing disorder may be ameliorated by use of a hearing aid, and an exercise program may offset some of the physical limitations imposed by arthritis.

A variety of screening techniques are available to aid in reaching the goals of preventive health care. Issues of cost, efficacy, and convenience are important in evaluating these techniques. The individual patient's needs must also be considered, since her risks will depend to some extent on her age, past medical history, family medical history, and risk-factor exposure.

Cardiovascular Disease

Coronary Artery Disease

The most common cardiovascular disease, and the one for which screening is most effective, is coronary artery disease (CAD). Risk factors for CAD are well-defined (see Table 6.1 and Ref. 1), and many of these can be modified to reduce risk through life-style changes and medical treatment.

A significant percentage of individuals affected with CAD will have either sudden death or a myocardial infarction as the first manifestation of their disease. For this reason, it is worthwhile to detect and, when possible, reduce risk factors in asymptomatic adults. It should be noted, however, that women have both lower rates and later onset for all manifestations of CAD compared to men. For example, a woman of 65 with moderately elevated blood pressure (eg, a systolic blood pressure of 165) has a 6% chance of developing coronary heart disease over the next 6 years, as compared to an 11% chance for a 65-year-old man with the same blood pressure.[1] This lower rate of CAD needs to be considered in choosing risk-reduction programs for women.

Stroke

Cerebrovascular disease is the second most common cardiovascular disease after CAD, and the third leading cause of death in the United States, after heart disease and cancer.[4] Hypertension, smoking, and diabetes are the leading risk factors for stroke.[5,6] The presence of CAD also reperesents a risk factor for stroke.[7,8] Thus, attention to risk factors for CAD contributes as well to stroke prevention.

Table 6.1 Risk Factors for Coronary Artery Disease*

Male sex
Age
Hypertension
Smoking habit
Hypercholesterolemia
Diabetes
Positive family history
Sedentary life-style

* See Refs. 1 to 3.

Hypertension

Although often considered a disease in itself, hypertension is usually asymptomatic. The cut-off point between normal and elevated blood pressure is a matter of arbitrary definition, since blood pressure is a continuous trait. In general, blood pressures up to 140/90 mm Hg are considered normal in adults over the age of 50, because it is only at blood pressures above this range that marked increases in cardiovascular disease occur. In the elderly, elevated blood pressure is the most important risk factor for CAD[1,9] and, for all ages, systolic blood pressures are more predictive of risk for CAD than diastolic blood pressures.[1] Blood pressure elevation is common, occurring in at least 15% to 20% of the adult American population.[10] Since in developed countries average blood pressure rises with age, the prevalence increases with each decade of life.[10,11] Isolated systolic hypertension is defined as a systolic pressure greater than 160 mm Hg and a diastolic pressure less than 90 mm Hg. The ranges for mild and severe diastolic hypertension are 90 to 104 mm Hg, and 115 mm Hg or greater, respectively, while the middle range of 105 to 114 mm Hg is moderate hypertension.[12] Blood pressures in the 140–159/85–89 range are considered borderline.

Many individuals have labile blood pressure, with measurements varying between normal and hypertensive levels. Labile blood pressure is presumed to increase the risk both for fixed hypertension and for the complications of hypertension. However, the risk of disease appears to be lower than that conferred by continuous hypertension.[10] Some individuals have normal blood pressure at home and elevated pressure when under circumstances of anxiety—for example, when in a doctor's office. Such individuals have lower risks of cardiovascular disease than would be expected from their high office blood-pressure readings.[13,14]

These patterns of variation in blood pressure underscore the importance of having several blood pressure measurements taken before a patient is diagnosed to be hypertensive. When an elevated reading is obtained, unless the level is dangerously high, the patient should be encouraged to have several readings taken outside the doctor's office. Community screening programs, fire stations, and some pharmacies provide this service. Patients should be informed of the importance of measuring blood pressure in a resting state (after at least 5 minutes of sitting).

Technique is also important. The cuff, appropriately sized for the patient's upper arm, should be inflated to at least 30 mm Hg above the systolic pressure determined by radial artery palpation. The cuff is deflated at a rate of 2 to 3 mm Hg/second to record the systolic pressure (point at which the first Korotkoff sound is heard) and diastolic pressure (point at which the Korotkoff sounds disappear). Change in tone is not a reliable measure of the diastolic pressure. Falsely elevated pressures can be obtained if the patient clenches her fist, the cuff is too small, or the arm is below the level of the right atrium. If the patient purchases a home blood-pressure apparatus, it should be calibrated against the office mercury sphygmomanometer. Office personnel responsible for blood-pressure measurements should review instructions for accurate measurement on a regular basis.[12]

Control of hypertension markedly reduces cerebrovascular mortality and morbidity.[15] The effect of blood-pressure lowering on CAD is less dramatic, possibly because some antihypertensive drugs introduce other risks for cardiac disease by lowering potassium or raising lipid levels.[15,16] These observations underline the importance of treating hypertension in the context of careful evaluation of other cardiac risk factors, and of minimizing the use of drug treatment when possible.

Treatment should usually be initiated with life-style changes. In general, patients with any degree of hypertension will benefit from dietary changes, relaxation techniques, and regular exercise.[17-20] In some patients, blood pressure may be reduced by as much as 10 to 20 mm Hg with reduction of salt in the diet. Not all individuals are salt-sensitive, and there is no simple objective method to identify those hypertensive individuals who will benefit from salt reduction. However, limiting salt intake to moderate levels (1.5 to 2.5 g of sodium per day) is safe, and should be recommended as an initial measure to all patients with elevated blood pressure.[12] Other dietary changes which may contribute to blood-pressure lowering include increased calcium, magnesium, and potassium intake, moderation in alcohol use,[12,18,21] increased fiber, and decreased saturated fat.[12,20,21] Increased dietary potassium is also associated with a lowered risk of stroke-associated death, independent of its effect on blood pressure.[22] These dietary changes are best accomplished through changes in the kinds of foods eaten, rather than through the use of pharmacologic supplements. Some specific guidelines for dietary counseling are discussed below under *Nutrition*.

Obesity is associated with an increased risk for hypertension. For patients who are obese, even a modest weight loss of 5 to 10 pounds may be associated with some blood-pressure lowering,[23] and hypertension may resolve in patients who reduce to their lean body mass. Weight loss should be undertaken by sensible alterations in diet and exercise patterns, since pounds lost during "crash" diets are almost always quickly regained. See further discussion of weight-loss programs under *Nutrition*.

Exercise and relaxation are both helpful in reducing blood pressure. Moderate exercise, such as brisk walking, reduces blood pressure and may prevent hypertension.[24] A program of regular, daily exercise is preferable to infrequent strenuous workouts. Rest in a quiet room, transcendental meditation, and biofeedback are among the relaxation techniques that may be helpful in the treatment of hypertension.[25] Patients generally benefit most from specific training in a particular technique by a skilled teacher.[26]

Patients whose blood pressures remain above 140/90 mm Hg despite hygienic measures may need pharmacologic treatment. The decision regarding the appropriate blood-pressure level at which to begin a drug is made on an individual basis and must take into account the existence of other cardiovascular risk factors. Drug therapy should be initiated cautiously, since untoward reactions are common if the blood pressure is reduced too rapidly. Decreased metabolism and delayed excretion of drugs are mechanisms that render the elderly particularly prone to develop orthostatic hypotension. The lowest dose available should be prescribed initially. Antihypertensive medications may cause many side effects.[27] These include hypokalemia, slowed heart rate, and elevated plasma low-density lipoprotein (LDL) or lowered plasma high-density lipoprotein (HDL) levels, and reduced kidney or liver function. Patients taking blood-pressure medicines have increased frequency of somatic complaints, including malaise and weakness, and may develop significant depression. The choice of medication for a patient also must be individualized, based on possible benefit for other existing conditions, drug interactions, and the likelihood that the patient will suffer side effects of the particular drug. The benefits of hypertension treatment occur only if the treatment is sustained. Noncompliance with medication is common, particularly if the cost is high; multiple daily doses are required, or side effects occur. Compliance may be improved by continuity of care with a single health-care provider.[28] Long-term therapy is usually required; therefore, cost of medication and frequency of dosing are important considerations.

Smoking

The cardiovascular health hazards of smoking are well-documented. Approximately 30% to 40% of deaths from CAD can be attributed to smoking,[29,30] and smokers have an almost twofold higher risk of heart disease than nonsmokers. Smoking is harmful to health in numerous other ways as well, and for this reason smoking cessation should be a first step in any program to reduce cardiac risks. Health effects of smoking and guidelines for helping smokers to quit are discussed below.

Hypercholesterolemia

Epidemiologic studies have demonstrated that the risk for CAD increases with serum cholesterol level in both men and women. Although the demarcation between "normal" and "abnormal" cholesterol levels is arbitrary, as it is with blood pressure, demonstrable increases in CAD rate can be shown for levels of cholesterol above 200 mg/dL, and levels above 300 mg/dL are associated with a marked increase in CAD rate (Figure 6.1).[1] When cholesterol is fractionated, the low-density lipoprotein (LDL) fraction is found to be most predictive of risk

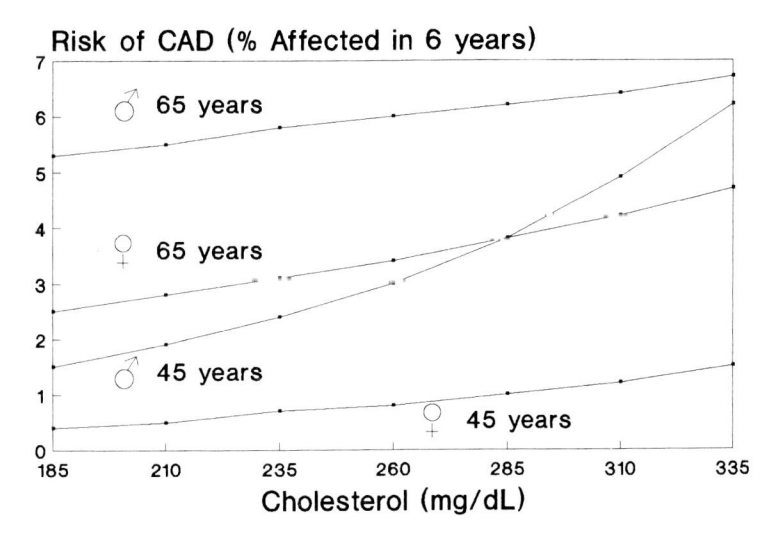

Figure 6.1 Risk of CAD as a function of cholesterol level. The percentage of asymptomatic individuals developing CAD over a 6-year period is shown for men and women who are either 45 or 65 years old at entry, and who are nonsmokers without hypertension, glucose intolerance, or left ventricular hypertrophy. Data from Gordon et al.[1]

of CAD.[31] The high-density lipoprotein (HDL) fraction exerts a protective effect. HDL levels are higher in postpubertal women than in men, and remain so even after menopause.[32] The protective effect of HDL may contribute to the overall lower risk of CAD seen in women as compared to men.

As shown in Figure 6.1, the risk of CAD related to cholesterol is dependent on both sex and age, and is lower in women at all ages. Several trials of cholesterol-lowering treatment in middle-aged men without previously identified CAD have demonstrated that mortality and morbidity from CAD can be reduced; the results of these trials have been widely cited as a rationale for aggressive screening and intervention programs.[33-35] However, the actual reduction in myocardial infarction or CAD death was small (1% to 2%) and the overall mortality was not reduced. Thus, the risk–benefit ratio for the use of lipid-lowering medications is not clear, particularly in women whose a priori risk for CAD is significantly lower than in men.[36-39]

Who, then, should be screened? Panels of health officials in Canada and the United States have set different guidelines, and these are likely to be modified in the future.[36,40,41] It is most important to screen individuals with other identified CAD risk factors. When a persistently elevated cholesterol level is found on screening, a full lipid profile should be obtained to determine LDL and HDL fractions. In contrast to total cholesterol, which is relatively unaffected by recent fat ingestion, HDL and LDL levels should be obtained after an overnight fast. The HDL assay is not well-standardized and is much less reproducible than the total serum cholesterol.[42] Unless the LDL level is extremely high (eg, over 180 mg/dL)[36,38] and the HDL level proportionately low (less than 35 mg/dL), pharmacologic treatment should be deferred until life-style measures have been tried.

As with hypertension, a number of life-style changes can improve the serum cholesterol level. The most important of these is reduction in dietary cholesterol and fat. Weight control and exercise also play a major role in control of cholesterol level. In the usual American diet, 36% or more of calories derive from fats, well above the 30% recommended for the general population by the American Heart Association. Much of the excess fat is contained in processed foods or in food preparation at restaurants, especially buffets or those serving "fast food." Older individuals, especiallly those living alone, may frequently eat in such restaurants, for reasons of budget and convenience, and may be unaware of the high fat and salt content of the food they are eating.

Diabetes

Diabetics are at increased risk for CAD and for other vascular diseases, including both stroke and peripheral vascular disease. A diabetic patient should receive regular supervision by a physician experienced in the management of this condition. Some patients will receive preventive health care from a physician other than the one who supervises their diabetes. This is particularly likely to be the case if routine preventive health care is provided by a gynecologist, while an internist or family practitioner manages the diabetes. Under these circumstances, it is prudent to remind the patient of the importance of regular physician visits for management of the diabetes, and of adhering to dietary restrictions.

Positive Family History

Family history of early coronary artery disease (age 55 or younger in men, age 60 or older in women) is the strongest single risk factor for CAD.[43,44] Certain rare lipid disorders (eg, familial hypercholesterolemia; familial combined hyperlipidemia) account for a small proportion of families in which early CAD occurs. These families are characterized by a pattern of autosomal dominant transmission, in which the increased risk of CAD is inherited vertically from one generation to the next; and in which each child of an affected individual is at 50% risk to inherit the lipid disorder and associated increased risk for CAD.[45] In the majority of families with early CAD, the increased risk for CAD is a polygenic trait, with the additive effect of several genes each contributing in a small way to the overall risk. Polygenic inheritance of blood pressure and cholesterol levels accounts for the increased incidence of early heart disease in some of these families.[43] Shared environmental factors, such as smoking or high-fat diets, may also contribute to the familial incidence of early heart disease. However, even when other known risk factors are taken into account, a family history of early CAD confers an increased risk of heart disease.[46,47]

When a patient has a positive family history for early heart disease, modification of other cardiac risk factors becomes more important. Explaining the significance of the positive family history to the patient may help to motivate life-style changes, including smoking cessation, reduced saturated fat in the diet, and increased exercise. Modification of other cardiac risk factors has been shown to reduce the incidence of CAD in individuals with a strong family history for heart disease.[48,49]

Sedentary Life-style

As part of a program to reduce the risk of CAD, all women should be advised to pursue a regular exercise program, unless they are physically unable to do so. While no studies have specifically assessed the cardiac benefits of exercise for older women, studies of male cohorts suggest that a sedentary life-style represents a risk factor of almost the same magnitude as cholesterol elevation for CAD.[50] Some studies have suggested that regular exercise may help to prevent the development of hypertension, diabetes, and obesity, as well as improve elevated blood-pressure and cholesterol levels. Benefits of exercise are discussed further under *Life style*.

Obesity

Obesity has been implicated as an independent risk factor for cardiovascular disease in some but not all studies addressing this issue.[51,52] Obesity is associated with other risk factors (notably, hypertension, diabetes, and a sedentary life-style), and it is difficult to determine the effect attributable to each separate factor. Recent data have suggested that a particular pattern of obesity—intraabdominal fat deposition, identified by a high waist-to-hip ratio—is associated with increased cardiovascular risk.[53,54] Intraabdominal fat deposition appears to be increased in smokers[55] and is also associated with lipid and insulin abnormalities,[56] so questions about the interrelationship of obesity and other risk factors remain. In any case, women with central obesity will benefit from im-

Table 6.2 Incidence of Cancer in American Women*

	Annual incidence[†]	Deaths[‡]	Lifetime risk[§]
Lung cancer	55,000	27	
Breast cancer	150,000	27	9.0
Colorectal cancer	79,000	17	5.7
Endometrial cancer	48,500		2.4
Ovarian cancer	20,500	8	
Melanoma	12,800		0.6
Leukemia/lymphoma	38,000		

* See Refs. 57 and 58.
[†] New cases/year.
[‡] Deaths/100,000/year.
[§] % likelihood of being affected.

provement in other cardiac risk factors, especially smoking, and may also benefit from weight loss.

Cancer

Many preventive health activities concern the early identification or prevention of cancer. Current practices reflect the fact that some cancers can be effectively screened for or prevented, while others cannot. For example, there is no accurate method of screening for early ovarian cancer, while early breast cancer can often be detected by mammography. The incidence of most cancers increases with age. Cancer screening is thus an important aspect of health maintenance for older women. The most common cancers affecting older women are lung, breast, and colon cancer (see Table 6.2). The life-time risk for each of these cancers is significant, and appropriate preventive measures should be pursued for all individuals. For other cancers, the value of preventive measures will depend partly on their convenience and efficacy, and partly on the specific characteristics of the patient being screened.

Lung Cancer

Lung cancer in women has increased dramaticaly from the mid-1960s to the present, and in some age groups now exceeds breast cancer as the most common cause of cancer death in women.[57–59] This increase is correlated with changes in smoking patterns for women. The percentage of women who smoked began to increase in the 1920s, and that increase is reflected in current lung cancer rates among women.[59] Smoking has declined during the last decade, but this decline has occurred more slowly in women than in men.[60] Of particular concern is a recent increase in smoking among young women.[60] These smoking trends suggest that lung cancer will continue to be frequent among women for some time to come.

Although lung cancer represents a significant health problem, unfortunately there is no effective screening method available. Several clinical trials have assessed the efficacy of annual chest x-rays, with and without periodic sputum cytologies, for identifying lung cancer in early, more treatable stages.[61–63] These trials were done with male smokers, who have an approximately threefold higher risk of lung cancer than female smokers.[64] Even in this high-risk group, no difference in mortality from lung cancer from regular screening could be demonstrated.[62-64] Small differences in stage of cancers detected and in 5-year mortality among those with lung cancer could be shown in some trials. However, the lack of a difference in overall mortality suggests that such differences derive primarily from false positive results in more intensively screened groups and from lead-time bias.[64] Lead-time bias is the effect of *apparent* increased length of survival seen when a cancer is identified at an earlier stage by screening than it would have been by clinical symptoms. Because there is no difference in ultimate mortality rate, it can be concluded that screening resulted in earlier diagnosis, without additional benefit to the patient with lung cancer.[64]

The lack of any benefit from trials of screening in high-risk patients indicates that routine screening for lung cancer should not be done, particularly in women, given their lower rate of lung cancer. One cautionary note should be made, however. In the trials of chest x-ray screening for lung cancer, even the control groups tended to have chest x-rays done relatively frequently as part of their regular health care. For example, in the Mayo Clinic Trial, one third of the lung cancers detected in the study were found in chest x-rays done for purposes other than screening.[62] Even when this effect is accounted for, there is no statistical evidence that chest x-ray screening identifies lung cancers at an early enough stage to change mortality outcome.[64] The finding does illustrate, however, that in a high-risk patient (ie, a smoker) the incidental finding of lung cancer is a possibility when a chest x-ray is taken for other reasons. With no effective method of screening for lung cancer, and limited success in treating it when it occurs, smoking cessation is the only preventive measure of proven value.

Breast Cancer

Breast cancer is one of the two most common cancers in American women. The average life-time risk of breast cancer for American women is 9%.[57] A number of risk factors have been identified for this cancer, and are listed in Table 6.3. Others, also listed in Table 6.3, are controversial. Many of the risk factors (eg, parity, age at menarche and menopause) relate to female hormone exposure,

Table 6.3* Risk Factors for Breast Cancer

Factors which increase risk of breast cancer
Early breast cancer in sister or mother
Nulliparity or late first pregnancy
Early menarche/late menopause
Previous breast, ovarian, or colon cancer
Family cancer syndrome
Factors which may increase risk of breast cancer
Hormone therapy
High-fat diet
Central obesity

* See Refs. 65 to 70.

and estrogen treatment may be a risk factor in some women 68 to 70. As with cardiovascular disease, the increased risk contributed by obesity appears to be specific to intraabdominal fat deposition,[67] and this "male pattern" of obesity may also be related to female hormone levels.

In contrast to lung cancer, two effective screening techniques exist for the detection of early, treatable breast cancer. These are breast self-exam and mammography. Breast self-exam is a simple procedure, readily learned by most women. Its benefit as a screening tool is probably small. However, it is a technique with no associated risk. There is some evidence to suggest that breast cancers detected by self-exam are on average found at an earlier stage than breast cancers found by physician exam or mammography.[71] All women should be questioned about their use of breast self-exam on a regular basis, and offered the opportunity to have the technique demonstrated.

Mammography provides the opportunity to identify cancer at an early stage, sometimes before a palpable lump is present. Concerns about radiation exposure were raised when this radiologic procedure was first introduced. However, current techniques result in only very limited radiation exposure, and the calculated risks from this exposure are minimal compared to the benefit of identifying early breast cancer.[72] Regular mammographic screening has been shown to result in reduced mortality from breast cancer in women 50 years of age and older. For this reason, annual mammography screening is uniformly recommended in this age group.[73-75]

Controversy exists regarding the use of mammography screening before the age of 50, in large part because the incidence of breast cancer is still relatively rare in this younger age group. Consequently, routine screening would result in a high rate of falsely positive findings.[72,73,76] For example, the incidence of breast cancer in women aged 40 to 44 years is only 1/1000, but 2% of women in this age group will have abnormalities on a mammography study.[72] Thus, most mammographic abnormalities in women between 40 and 50 are benign processes, and screening in this age group results in many unnecessary biopsy procedures.

Studies attempting to demonstrate reduced mortality from mammography screening in women under 50 have produced conflicting results.[76,77] While recognizing that definitive data are not available, several agencies and organizations have made recommendations regarding mammography screening in younger age groups. These recommendations fall into two groups. The American College of Physicians and the U. S. Preventive Health Task Force recommend no mammography screening of asymptomatic women before the age of 50, pending data that demonstrate an objective benefit from such screening.[73,78] The risk of false positive results is cited in arguing against routine screening in this age group,[73] and avoidance of unnecessary anxiety may also be a benefit of a policy against screening women in their forties.[79]

The American Cancer Society, the National Cancer Institute, and the American Medical Association recommend a baseline mammogram between the ages of 35 and 40, and mammography at 1- to 2-year intervals between the ages of 40 and 50.[74,75,80] With these recommendations, a call is made for additional data to resolve the degree of risk and benefit associated with mammography screening before the age of 50.[75]

There is, however, uniformity regarding the recommendation that mammography should be done at younger ages in patients whose family histories place them at increased risk for breast cancer. In assessing the importance of family history, several factors are taken into consideration: number of affected relatives; age at which relatives were affected; and bilateral versus unilateral disease. The greater the number of relatives affected, and the closer the biologic relationship of the affected relatives, the more significant the family history.[81,83] Early age of onset is also an indicator of higher genetic risk. For example, a woman whose mother and sister both developed breast cancer before age 50 has a 5- to 10-fold increased risk above average for breast cancer,[82] and is likely to benefit from annual mammography screening beginning as early as age 30. On the other hand, a woman with a family history of unilateral breast cancer in an aunt aged 65 has little, if any, increased risk for breast cancer above that of the general population. Women from families meeting the criteria for family cancer syndrome (see below) should also receive early and regular screening.

The actual use of mammography in the United States is low, even in the over-50 group. Surveys indicate that only 25% to 50% of women over age 50 have ever had a mammogram, and fewer have had mammography on an annual basis.[84] In one case-control study of older women, those with breast cancer were found to have a lower likelihood of metastatic disease if they had undergone screening, as would be expected; however, most surprisingly, only 6% of control women had ever had mammography.[85] These data underscore the importance of physician advice regarding the use of this screening technique in age groups where it has a proven benefit.

Colorectal Cancer

Colorectal cancer is the third most frequent cancer in women, after lung and breast cancer. The life-time risk for colorectal cancer among North American women is 5%.[57] It is believed that most colon cancers arise in the distal colon from adenomatous polyps.[86] Adenomatous polyps occur in as many as 10% to 25% of the population, and are readily visible on endoscopic examination of the colon. Not all adenomatous polyps will become cancerous[87,88]; the time course for development of cancer from a polyp has been estimated as 5 to 10 years.[88,89] Factors which increase the risk of colorectal cancer are shown in Table 6.4.

Two methods of screening for colorectal cancer are available. These are testing of stool for occult blood (which may be caused by polyps or cancer, or other benign conditions) and lower endoscopy (sigmoidoscopy or colonoscopy), which permits direct visualization of a polyp or cancer. Controversy exists regarding the cost and efficacy of each method.

Table 6.4 Risk Factors for Colorectal Cancer

Factors which increase risk:
    First-degree relative with colon cancer
    History of colorectal, breast, endometrial, or ovarian cancer
    History of adenomatous polyp(s)
    Ulcerative colitis
Highest-risk group:
    Two or more first-degree relatives with colorectal cancer
    Family cancer syndrome
    Family history of polyposis coli

The American Cancer Society currently recommends testing of stool for occult blood on an annual basis, beginning at age 50.[90] Not all polyps and cancers will bleed, and this method may fail to detect 50% of colon cancers.[91] However, it offers the opportunity to detect early cancer or a precancerous polyp through use of a simple, noninvasive test.[90,91]

The U.S. Preventive Services Task Force recommends testing of stool for occult blood only for those individuals with risk factors which increase the likelihood of colon cancer, as listed in Table 6.4.[78] The primary argument against the routine use of this test is the high false-positive rate; only 5% to 10% of occult blood reactions are due to cancer or precancerous lesions, and the majority are due to benign conditions, such as hemorrhoids and diverticulosis.[92] Bowel workups resulting from stool testing (usually a flexible sigmoidoscopy and a barium enema) involve a small risk of significant complications, including hemorrhage and bowel perforation.[93] In addition, testing for occult blood in stool has not been proven to improve survival,[92,94] and a negative test may engender a false sense of security.[92]

Nevertheless, testing for occult blood in stool permits the identification of individuals at increased risk of colon cancer, with a test that is both inexpensive and noninvasive.[91] Given the high life-time risk of colon cancer in our society, and the absence of better screening methods, it is our opinion that routine stool testing is appropriate in adults 50 years of age and older.

As with stool testing, there are differing recommendations regarding the use of endoscopy procedures for colon cancer screening. The American Cancer Society recommends routine use of flexible sigmoidoscopy screening for all adults, beginning at age 50. Two sequential annual examinations are recommended, with repeat testing every 3 years thereafter.[90] The U.S. Preventive Services Task Force recommends this procedure only for individuals at increased risk for colon cancer.[78]

The rationale for sigmoidoscopy screening is straightforward.[95,96] The flexible sigmoidoscope permits visualization of the colon to 60 cm. In addition to cancerous lesions, polyps can be located and biopsied. Colonoscopy is performed on any individuals found to have adenomatous polyps on sigmoidoscopy, to permit visualization of the entire colon and to remove the adenomatous polyp(s). Theoretically, actual prevention of cancer can be accomplished. However, reduced mortality from colorectal cancer as a result of this screening process has not yet been shown.[97] Initial trials of sigmoidoscopic screening were for the most part uncontrolled, so that an accurate assessment of the effect of screening on morbidity and mortality of the screened population could not be obtained.[97] A controlled study from Kaiser Permanente used rigid sigmoidoscopic screening, and showed only a marginal reduction in mortality.[98] The flexible sigmoidoscope allows examination of two to four times more colon than the rigid sigmoidoscope, and has been shown to be more effective in identifying polyps.[96] Screening by flexible sigmoidoscopy is thus expected to provide a greater benefit than could be obtained from the rigid sigmoidoscope, but this has not yet been proven.

As with other cancer screening measures, there is concern regarding false-positive results and procedure risks from flexible sigmoidoscopy screening, as well as the significant cost attached to routine screening of all adults 50 and over. Hyperplastic polyps, which are benign and not associated with colorectal cancer, are more common than adenomatous polyps, and their presence may lead to additional workup and procedure risk. A negative flexible sigmoidoscopy examination may also create a sense of false security, as proximal polyps and cancers are not ruled out.

The uncertainties and controversy concerning sigmoidoscopy screening measures make it impossible to argue for a specific approach at this time. It may be prudent to inform patients of the range of recommendations proposed by expert panels regarding colorectal cancer screening, and to help patients to decide which screening program is most appropriate for them, taking into account the average life-time risk of colorectal cancer, and the uncertainty, cost, and risk intrinsic to the screening procedures.

It is generally agreed that patients with high-risk family histories should be routinely screened (see Table 6.4). These include individuals with a family history of polyposis coli, two or more first-degree relatives with colorectal cancer, or a history otherwise compatible with the family cancer syndrome (see below). Others at increased risk include individuals with ulcerative colitis, a past history of colon polyps, or a past history of colon, endometrial, ovarian, or breast cancer.

Family Cancer Syndrome

The term *family cancer syndrome* is used to define familial clustering of cancer. The most common cancers involved are colorectal, breast, ovarian, and endometrial cancer. If two or more first-degree relatives are affected with cancer of these types, this syndrome should be suspected.[99–101] Typically, early onset of cancer and multiple primary tumors in one or more of the affected individuals are also seen. There is no specific laboratory test to identify affected individuals from such families, and careful cancer screening is the only measure that can be offered. For all individuals with these high-risk family histories, colorectal cancer screening with both stool testing and endoscopy is recommended.[90,102] The U.S. Preventive Services Task Force and most experts recommend colonoscopy, rather than sigmoidoscopy, for screening in these high-risk individuals.[78] Other preventive measures for individuals with a family history suggestive of family cancer syndrome include mammography, beginning in the early 30s, and annual pelvic exams at all ages. Women from these families may benefit from ultrasound screening of the ovaries, although this is a screening measure with too low a sensitivity to be of value in average-risk women.[103]

Skin Cancer

Melanoma

The incidence of melanoma has doubled every 10 to 15 years since the 1930s. The life-time risk of melanoma for the average American is currently 0.6%, and is estimated to rise to 1% by the year 2000.[104,105] Factors which increase the risk for melanoma include fair skin and hair color, positive family history for melanoma, large congenital nevi, and the presence of pigmented lesions meeting the criteria for dysplastic nevi.[106,107] A history of severe sunburn or blistering also appears to increase the risk for melanoma.[108,109] For example, after controlling for other known risk factors, patients with 6 or more severe sunburns (pain lasting more than 48 hours) were found to have a 2.4-fold increased risk of melanoma compared to those without a history of sunburns.[109]

Congenital nevi of greater than 20 cm diameter have a 5% to 20% risk of degenerating into melanoma.[107] These are readily identified, and treatment of the nevus is often sought for cosmetic reasons. The risk from smaller congenital nevi has not been well quantified, but is assumed to be above that of the general population.[107] Acquired nevi rarely exceed 5 mm or 6 mm, so that nevi larger than this merit careful review. Dysplastic nevi occur in 2% to 8% of the population, and are defined by four characteristics: (1) macular and papular components, (2) irregular borders, (3) variegated pigmentation within the same lesion, and (4) diameter of 5 mm to 12 mm. Congenital nevi or nevi with dysplastic characteristics can be biopsied; specific pathologic findings confirm that a nevus is dysplastic.[107] When lesions with dysplastic characteristics are 1 cm or larger, or show progressive increase in size or asymmetric growth, melanoma should be suspected.[107]

An annual full-skin examination is recommended for patients with dysplastic nevi, large congenital nevi, or a positive family history of melanoma. Melanomas may occur de novo, without a prior suspicious nevus. A high index of suspicion toward new or changed pigmented lesions will help to prevent diagnostic delay.[110] Patients with both dysplastic nevi and a positive family history are at particularly increased risk. The life-time risk of melanoma is estimated to be 100% when an individual has dysplastic nevi *and* two first-degree relatives (parents, siblings, or children) with melanoma.[111] Such individuals should be referred to a dermatologist for careful surveillance.

Other Skin Cancers

Sun exposure (both sunburn and accumulated life-time exposure) is the major risk factor for other skin cancers.[112] Fair-haired and fair-skinned individuals are at greatest risk, and should be advised to use sun-protective skin preparations when exposed to bright sunlight. The most common skin cancer is the *basal cell* cancer. This is identifiable as a pearly papule often displaying prominent associated telangiectasia. As basal cell cancers grow, they may develop a central ulceration. Surgical removal is generally curative. *Squamous cell* cancers arise from areas of *actinic keratosis*. The latter are erythematous lesions 0.5 mm to 5 mm in size, with irregular adherent scale. On pathologic examination they consist of dyplastic squamous cells confined to the epidermal layer of the skin. They can be readily treated with liquid nitrogen cryotherapy. As the dysplastic tissue extends into the dermal layer, the lesions increase in size and become indurated. Surgery is required at this stage to remove the cancerous process and, as with basal cell cancers, is curative.

Infectious Diseases

Immunizations

Tetanus and Diphtheria

Although tetanus and diptheria are rare diseases, with only 70 to 100 cases and 1 to 5 cases reported per year, respectively, they occur almost exclusively in adults who have not been adequately immunized.[113,114] Since immunity wanes over time, risks of infection and mortality increase with age. Diphtheria and tetanus toxoids are at least 95% effective in reducing both the risk and clinical severity of disease; and the immunization schedule recommended is very inexpensive.

The primary immunizing series of three doses of combined toxoids (the pediatric mixture also contains pertussis toxoid, which is not given to adults) and two booster doses is usually complete at age five. Adults who did not receive primary immunization or whose immunization status is unknown should be given the full primary series. All adults should be vaccinated with booster doses every 10 years at mid-decade.

Polio

Routine primary or booster immunizations of adults in this country is not deemed necessary and is recommended only for travel to endemic areas.[115] However, adults who have not been previously immunized or whose specific immunity to polio virus may have waned have a small risk of developing paralytic polio from the stool of a child who has recently received the live oral polio vaccine (OPV). Therefore, persons who have close contact with very young children (parents, grandparents, day-care workers) should be given a booster immunization if previously immunized or a three-dose primary immunization if never vaccinated (see Table 6.5). The Immunization Practices Advisory Committee (ACIP) recommends the more immunogenic live OPV for children. However, vaccine-associated polio, although rare, is more common in adults.[116] Therefore, an enhanced-potency (e) inactivated polio virus vaccine (IPV), available since the spring of 1988, is suggested for this population. The e-IPV is produced in cultured human diploid cells and may contain trace amounts of streptomycin and neomycin. Adults with a history of anaphylactic reactions to these antibiotics should not receive IPV.[117]

Measles (Rubeola)

The vaccination program for measles has been extremely successful, and this often very severe disease is now rare. Prior to development of the MMR vaccine most individuals will have had clinical or subclinical measles and have developed natural antibodies. Therefore, it is not necessary to vaccinate persons born before 1957. Patients who can reliably document a history of measles also need not be vaccinated. Patients who do not fall into these categories and who have never been immunized against measles or who are planning foreign travel should be given a primary series or booster dose of live, attenuated virus vaccine.[118] Measles vaccine is derived from chick embryo cell culture and may contain

Table 6.5 ACIP Recommendations for Adult Immunization

Immunization	Administration	When to be administered
Influenza	IM, SC	Autumn, for persons 65 and over *and* high-risk groups (see text)
DT	IM	q 10 years—mid-decade
Polio (e-IPV)	SC	1 dose, if previously immunized; 2 additional doses, at 4–8 weeks and 6–12 months, if never immunized
Pneumovax	IM or SC	Once
Measles	SC	See text

traces of neomycin. A history of anaphylactic reaction to neomycin or eggs is a contraindication to administration of live measles vaccine.

Influenza

"Flu" results from infection with one of the antigenically and immunologically distinct myxovirus influenza groups. Epidemics are caused mostly by type-A viruses, whose surface antigen composition undergoes frequent mutational change—the so-called antigenic drift. Since the immune response to these viruses is mounted against the antigen phenotype, past infection or vaccination with one strain may not confer adequate protection against another strain with an altered antigenic profile. For this reason, to prevent or attenuate the severity of disease, it is necessary to vaccinate at-risk persons each year with a vaccine that includes the viral strains predicted to be prevalent. The most important complication of influenza is bacterial pneumonia, which can occur concurrently or as a secondary infection. Between 1972 and 1981, an average of 20,000 excess deaths occurred in association with yearly influenza epidemics.[119] In the 1988 to 1989 influenza season, 78% of the pneumonia or influenza deaths reported occurred in persons at or older than 65 years of age.[120] Although influenza vaccination is less effective in elderly populations than in young, healthy adults, 75% reduction in mortality was seen in nursing home residents who had been vaccinated compared with those who had not.[121] Routine vaccination of persons 65 years and older has been shown to be cost-effective[122] and should be performed each year in the autumn. Persons with any chronic disease—such as cardiovascular, pulmonary, or renal impairment, diabetes, severe anemia, or depressed immunocompetence—should be vaccinated as well. It is also recommended that health-care personnel and household contacts of high-risk persons be immunized to prevent spread of influenza to the people who are most likely to develop complications. Vaccines should not be given during a febrile illness because an inadequate immune response may occur. A history of egg allergy is a contraindication to vaccination, since the vaccine contains traces of egg protein.

To reduce the risk of developing influenza A, high-risk patients who fail to receive influenza immunization may be given amantadine (200 mg/day for persons under 65 years of age and 100 mg/day for the elderly) for the duration of an outbreak (reviewed in Ref. 123). Rimantadine, a drug with less toxicity than amantadine, may soon be approved. Vaccination remains the best strategy for prevention since postexposure prophylaxis with either of these drugs may not be effective,[124] and no drug is yet available for prophylaxis or amelioration of influenza B. The primary usefulness of amantadine is in the reduction of severity and duration of influenza A illness. For this purpose, the recommended dose of 200 mg/day is begun within 48 hours of onset of symptoms.

Pneumococcal Vaccine

Pneumococcus is a common cause of pneumonia, with 150,000 to 570,000 cases per year, accounting for 10% to 25% of all pneumonias.[125,126] The overall mortality, even in the antibiotic era, is 5%, and subsets of infected individuals have substantially higher likelihood of poor outcome.[127] Those with higher mortality risk include individuals older than 55, alcoholics, and those with underlying chronic disease and impaired immunity, especially asplenia. Associated bacteremia carries a 15% to 40% mortality, and intensive-care support has had no impact on this figure.[128] Whereas there is general agreement regarding the immunization schedules discussed above, a controversy surrounds the topic of pneumococcal vaccine utility. Previous enthusiastic support for routine immunization[129] was dampened by a raft of negative reports. The vaccine does not protect against all of the more than 85 serotypes, is not 100% effective, and is even less effective in the chronically ill or immunoincompetent population segment most likely to benefit from immunization. However, although studies on low-risk populations (including that of otherwise healthy but aging women, in which attack rates are low) may fail to show a benefit from vaccination, the risk and cost of giving the vaccine is small.

The current vaccine formulation, licensed in the United States in 1983, contains polysaccharide components of 23 pneumococcal subtypes, responsible for almost 90% of bacteremic pneumococcal illness. Most healthy adults, including the elderly, do have a significant long-term elevation in type-specific antibody in response to vaccination.[130,131] In one study of immunocompetent persons aged 55 or older, the clinical effectiveness of pneumococcal vaccine in reducing the incidence of pneumococcal infection was estimated to be 70%.[132] Currently, the ACIP recommends that all people 65 years or older receive the pneumococcal vaccine.[133] Although response to immunization is lower in patients with chronic illness or compromised immune systems, the risk of mortality due to pneumococcal infections is so great in these individuals that they should be vaccinated. Pneumococcal vaccination should not be repeated, even if the previous immunization was with the older 14-valent preparation, since severe local reactions can occur.[134,135]

Travel Immunizations

People traveling outside the United States may require additional immunizations for diseases, such as typhus, which are still frequent in some countries. Other prophylaxis may also be needed; for example, malaria prophylaxis is required when traveling to endemic regions in Central America, Africa, and the Far East. Patients contemplating travel to areas other than Canada or Western Europe should be advised to consult a Travel Clinic, if one is available, for the most up-to-date information on potential exposures and immunization recommendations. If there is no facility providing this information, guidelines can be obtained from the Center for Disease Control or the U.S. Department of Health and Human Services (eg, see Ref. 118).

Musculoskeletal Disease

Osteoarthritis

Osteoarthritis, often called degenerative joint disease (DJD), is the most frequent cause of disability in the elderly. In fact, autopsy studies have shown that even as early as 40 years of age some pathologic abnormalities can be detected in weight-bearing joints of almost all individuals.[136] By age 75, there is radiographic evidence for degenerative joint changes in 85% of patients[137] and, in contrast to osteoporosis, the disease occurs with similar frequency in all ethnic groups. The most frequently involved regions are the distal and proximal interphalangeal joints, knees, hips, and lower lumbar and cervical vertebrae.[138] The pattern of joint involvement suggests a genetic component. Although osteoarthritis often develops in joints previously damaged by trauma or affected by inflammatory arthritis, it also occurs without identified precipitating cause. With the exception of knee involvement, there is conflicting opinion regarding the role of obesity in etiology or exacerbation of DJD.[139,140]

The main symptom is pain, which is aching in nature and usually of moderate severity. Except with advanced disease, the pain is commonly increased with activity and relieved by rest. Although brief morning stiffness is frequently present, DJD usually is not characterized by the prolonged postrest stiffness seen in inflammatory arthritis. Muscle spasms may contribute to the discomfort. Physical exam can reveal enlargement of joints, without the boggy synovial swelling of the inflammatory arthritides, pain on palpation, and crepitus with movement. Osteophyte growth and cartilage irregularities can result in limitation of movement, which can be disabling in severe cases with hip and knee involvement. Radiographic studies often show the specific changes of osteoarthritis, and the diagnosis is usually made without difficulty.

Treatment should be conservative, as long as it is possible, since the disease is chronic, slowly progressive, and rarely crippling. The patient should be reassured that the natural history of DJD usually does not necessitate aggressive intervention and that benign therapies often provide relief. It is reasonable to suggest a plan of weight reduction for the obese patient, especially those with involvement of weight-bearing joints. Warm baths or moist heat packs can decrease muscle spasm and joint stiffness. Physical therapy can maintain or improve range of motion and strengthen supporting musculature, but care must be taken to avoid repetitious movements that may accelerate joint degeneration. The provision of walking aids and large-handled appliances can simplify and improve the activities of daily living. The nonsteroidal antiinflammatory drugs (NSAID) have become a mainstay of therapy for DJD. These drugs decrease the mild synovitis that may be present and provide good pain relief. Enteric-coated aspirin is usually well-tolerated, but the drug of choice for an individual patient is chosen empirically on the basis of patient compliance, frequency of dosing, side effects, and cost. It must be remembered that a major morbidity of aspirin and NSAIDs is upper gastrointestinal bleeding, especially in the elderly. In addition, NSAIDs may result in fluid retention and renal dysfunction. Narcotics should be avoided; the disease is long-term, not "curable," and other pain-reducing measures are available. Narcotics have some very undesirable side effects for the geriatric population, including constipation and central nervous system depression. Surgical procedures are usually reserved for patients with intractable pain or progressive functional disability.

Osteoporosis

Osteoporosis results from a decrease in bone density, caused by increased bone resorption relative to bone formation. The maximum bone density in young adulthood varies, at least in part due to genetic factors. For instance, black women have a greater maximum bone density than do white or Asian women.[141] These and other risk factors for osteoporosis are shown in Table 6.6. Beginning

Table 6.6 Risk Factors for the Development of Osteoporosis*

Sex (female > male)
Age
Positive family history
Race: White or Asian
Endocrine: hyperthyroidism, hyperparathyroidism
Prolonged use of glucocorticoids
Cigarette smoking
Alcohol abuse
Early oophorectomy
History of lactose intolerance
Sedentary life-style/immobilization
Body habitus: small, lean
Low calcium intake

* See Refs. 141 to 147.

in the fourth decade of life, there is a continuous slow decrease in bone density. However, in women, the decade immediately postmenopause is marked by a more rapid loss.[142]

Increased incidences of Colles' and vertebral fractures are seen soon after menopause, whereas hip fractures occur later in life.[148] As the density of bone decreases, the severity of the trauma sufficient to cause a fracture also decreases. To compound the situation, falls occur more frequently as people age, in part due to decreased vision, neurologic impairment, dementia, arthritis, and medications. By some estimates, one fifth of all women over 65 years of age have vertebral fractures and one third of all women who reach very old age (>85 years) will have suffered a fractured hip.[148] The morbidity of hip fracture is extremely high—as many as 20% of patients die within 1 year of complications directly related to this event, and approximately half of the survivors are no longer able to live independently. Although sometimes characterized by immediate severe local back pain, vertebral fractures are often asymptomatic, detected only as loss of height or kyphosis. These fractures may also be diagnosed by chest x-ray ordered for another purpose.

Standard radiographs are not a good screen for osteopenia, since at least 30% of bone density must be lost before it is seen on x-ray.[141] Currently available techniques for quantitation of vertebral and other bone density[149] are expensive and show overlap between the groups with and without osteoporosis.[147,150] Although low bone density is the strongest known risk factor for osteoporotic fractures, most women have some degree of osteoporosis by the age at which hip fractures occur, and not all elderly women with decreased bone density suffer fractures.[151] The value of screening depends on whether the findings would influence a physician's or patient's decision regarding therapy. Since the evidence favors preventive estrogen therapy in many peri- and postmenopausal women, it is not felt that screening should be performed in large scale at this time.[150,152] Rather, bone-density assays should be reserved for patients with symptoms and those in the high-risk groups who are reluctant to begin estrogen or who have relative contraindications to it.

Several therapies have benefits in preventing or ameliorating osteoporosis. A fall in vitamin D levels leads to a decrease in calcium absorption, especially after age 70. The average intake of calcium is less than two thirds the recommended daily allowance, currently set at 800 mg/day, substantially less than the 1200 to 1500 mg/day that may be needed to restore a positive calcium balance after menopause.[141] If dietary calcium is low, and there is no history of nephrolithiasis or hypercalcemia, supplementation at least up to the RDA should be attempted using low-cost calcium carbonate tablets (each standard calcium carbonate tablet provides 200 mg of elemental calcium).

Calcium supplementation may have some beneficial effect on bone density, but postmenopausal estrogen replacement actually decreases the frequency of fractures.[153,154] The most significant factor in the development of osteoporosis in women is the estrogen deficiency that accompanies menopause. The benefit of estrogen replacement therapy (ERT) has been supported by many studies. Estrogen replacement has been shown to be most effective if started within 5 to 6 years of menopause, during the period of greatest bone loss.[141,155] Since estrogen therapy is not entirely benign, the risk–benefit ratio must be considered when advising widespread use of these medications. There is general agreement that high-risk patients, especially those with surgically induced early menopause, should be strongly advised to use replacement therapy. One study found that postmenopausal bone loss can be prevented by low-dose estrogen (0.3 mg/day) and calcium supplements,[156] but the usual recommended dose is 0.625 mg/day. Long-term use of conjugated estrogens is associated with a persistent three- to fourfold increased risk of endometrial cancer.[157] However, this relatively common cancer is not a leading cause of cancer deaths,[158] since it is often diagnosed at an early stage when cure is still possible. The addition of a progestin (and reinstitution of cycling) for patients who have not had a hysterectomy probably decreases the risk of endometrial cancer,[159] but patients may be reluctant to accept this therapy.[160] New regimens that combine low-dose continuous progestin with estrogen may prevent endometrial hypertrophy (and dysplastic changes) and decrease the incidence of withdrawal bleeding.[161,162]

Progestin therapy, however, may also be associated with negative side effects, including breast tenderness, depression, irritability, and decreased cardioprotective high-density lipoprotein levels.[163,167] Estrogens, on the other hand, cause increases in HDL levels. There is conflicting evidence regarding the cardiovascular benefit of ERT to women who have undergone natural menopause,[164,165] but a positive effect is seen in those patients who have had surgically induced menopause.[166] Since cardiovascular disease is so prevalent, even a small reduction in individual risk might be of benefit to the population. It is unclear whether the alteration in lipoprotein ratios that results from low-dose progestins will negate the beneficial effect of estrogens on cardiovascular disease. It should be noted that several studies have shown that exogenous estrogen use is associated with a lower all-cause mortality even in patients who have not undergone hysterectomy.[167] A 1988 consensus panel[168] recommended that ERT should be instituted immediately after the onset of menopause to women at high risk who do not have the absolute contraindications of acute or chronic liver disease, acute vascular thrombosis, or breast cancer. Recent studies have raised questions about hormone replacement as a risk factor for breast cancer. Conflicting data have been obtained, and an apparent association may reflect problems in study design.[68–70] This issue is likely to be resolved by future studies. Decisions regarding ERT in patients with one of the relative contraindications—including gallbladder disease, migraine headaches, chronic thrombophlebitis, hypertension, or a history of endometriosis—must be made on an individual basis. For a more complete discussion of hormone replacement refer to Chapter 12.

Peak premenopausal bone mass is related to the level of physical activity.[169] Exercise not only slows the rate of bone loss, but can result in some bone gain.[169-171] For this and other reasons discussed herein, increased physical activity should be encouraged and, of course, patients should be counseled to discontinue smoking. Decreased bone loss is one benefit of obesity.[144] Studies of fluoridation of the water supply give conflicting results, and the role of fluoride supplementation in the prevention and therapy of this disease is still unclear.[172] A recent study suggests that risk of fracture may in fact be increased by fluoride supplementation since it results in the deposition of cancellous rather than cortical bone.[173] Other medical therapies of moderate and severe osteoporosis are being evaluated in research settings; patients with complex problems should be referred to specialists for management.

Vision and Hearing

Impairments of visual and auditory senses are common occurrences during aging that may reduce the quality of life and contribute to social isolation. Patients may assume that decreased senses are normal consequences of aging and, therefore, may not volunteer that they have a problem. Primary care providers should specifically inquire about changes in vision and hearing so that appropriate referrals can be made. The frequency of significant eye disease (including presbyopia, glaucoma, and cataracts) is low in the population under 40 years of age, but thereafter increases steadily.[174]

Glaucoma is a condition of increased intraocular pressure that results from a decrease in drainage of the aqueous humor from the eye. If untreated, the increased pressure leads to cupping and then atrophy of the optic disc, and eventually to decreased visual fields and visual acuity.[175] Rare in childhood and early adulthood, glaucoma rises in prevalence with each decade over age 40. Approximately 0.4% to 1.6% of individuals older than 40 have some degree of visual impairment secondary to glaucoma.[176] As is the case for many conditions, patients with a positive family history of glaucoma are at increased risk to develop this condition. Timely intervention usually prevents loss of vision. Unfortunately, most patients with early glaucoma are asymptomatic; a significant loss of peripheral vision can occur before a patient is aware that there is a problem. The presence of glaucoma also places the patient at increased risk to develop cataracts.

A cataract is defined as an opacity in the lens. Congenital cataracts are stable defects, whereas presenile (occurring in late childhood and early adulthood) and senile cataracts (usually appearing after age 30 to 40) usually progress and may cause severe visual impairment.[177] Cataract formation is a physiologic change of aging so that, although they are "abnormal," some evidence of lens opacification can be detected by slit lamp examination in over 96% of people older than 60 years.[178] These common senile cataracts are usually characterized by very slow progression. Most never reach a size that causes significant visual deterioration. However, since the prevalence is so high, cataract formation is one of the most common causes of serious loss of vision, accounting for approximately 15% to 20% of cases of blindness.

There are factors besides aging that increase the likelihood that a person will develop cataracts. Many drugs, including ergotamines and systemic or ophthalmic corticosteroids, are toxic to the lens. Prolonged use may result in cataracts.[178] Diabetics tend to develop typical senile cataracts at an earlier age, and these cataracts enlarge more quickly than those occurring in the nondiabetic population. More rarely, diabetics may develop specific "diabetic cataracts," characterized by increased sorbitol, fructose, and glucose content in the lens.[178] Genetic factors are involved in the predisposition to cataracts. In some families, acquired cataract formation is transmitted as an autosomal dominant trait.[179] Finally, cataracts may form following trauma to the lens. Regardless of etiology, removal of the cataract is the only way to restore lost vision.

With aging, the nearest point at which an object can be brought into clear focus becomes more remote. This disturbance in accommodation for near vision is called presbyopia—literally, "aged vision"—and results from decreases in lens elasticity and contractibility of ciliary muscles.[180] The latter change reduces the ability of the eyes to converge, and physical hardening of the lens prevents it from assuming a rounded shape—movements that are both necessary for close vision. The maximum degree of accommodation decreases with age from childhood to approximately age 75, with onset of clinically significant presbyopia at about 45 years. Presbyopia interferes most with reading, but convex reading glasses can substitute for the loss of accommodative power.

Since most eye impairments are remediable and if untreated may lead to substantial deterioration in quality of life, it is important to identify those persons who might benefit from an ocular evaluation. In general, persons who complain of visual disturbances should be promptly referred to an ophthalmologist. Decreased visual acuity, blurred vision, impaired night vision, and eye pain are examples of symptoms that may indicate serious eye pathology. Frequent routine screening eye examinations are no longer recommended for all asymptomatic individuals, since abnormalities are rarely found and the cost–benefit ratio is unfavorable. The American Academy of Ophthalmology recommends that asymptomatic individuals aged 40 and older have ophthalmologic evaluations every 5 years, primarily for the detection of presbyopia. More intensive surveillance should be reserved for people who are at increased risk for eye diseases, such as those with diabetes, hypertension, or a family history of glaucoma or progressive blindness.

Hearing loss is a common finding in otherwise healthy people. Two major factors in hearing loss are noise exposure and aging. The most common effect of presbycusis ("aged hearing") is progressive bilateral loss of the ability to detect high-frequency tones.[181] The decrease in range of tone sensitivity is usually quite insidious, and the associated symptom of tinnitus may be the first hearing abnormality noticed by the patient. Approximately 5.2% of people aged 18 to 44 have some degree of hearing impairment, but the prevalence increases steadily to 13.6% at 45 to 64 years, 24.4% at 65 to 74 years, and 37.8% at or above age 75.[182] Although only a proportion of these people will have hearing losses severe enough to warrant intervention, screening is worthwhile, since inexpensive and easy-to-perform tests are available. The "gold standard" hearing test is the pure-tone audiogram to identify the frequencies at which a signal is not heard. Recently, a portable otoscope containing an audiometer has become available. This instrument emits tones at four frequencies and three intensities, and is appropriate for use by primary care physicians.[183,184] For purposes of screening, however, the most important parameter to study is the ability to discern normal spoken conversation, since this determines the degree to which the hearing impairment is a problem in daily life. For example, the patient may communicate without difficulty in a quiet examining room, but not by telephone or in the presence of background noise.

Two maneuvers that are fairly sensitive in detecting hearing impairment are whispered voice for speech discrimination and finger-rub tests.[185] The first test is performed by whispering a series of common one- or two-syllable words beginning at a distances of 6 inches from the test ear and gradually moving away. The distance at which the patient cannot correctly repeat at least 50% of the words is noted. Appropriate vocabulary lists are published.[186] Alternatively, after first positioning his hand close to the patient's ear, the examiner rubs his thumb and index finger together and slowly withdraws his hand until the patient can no longer hear the signal. Whispered voice should be correctly discerned to approximately 19 cm, and finger rub should be heard at 8 cm from the external auditory canal.[185]

A simple 15-question self-administered test developed by the American Academy of Otolaryngology—Head and Neck Surgery (AAO-HNS)[187] can be given to the patient to score at home (Figure 6.2). A score of 10 or above indicates that the patient is significantly hearing-impaired, and audiological evaluation by an ENT specialist should be urged. Scored between 6 and 9 suggest that the patient is at risk to develop future significant impairment. ENT evaluation can be recommended at this stage. Copies of this test can be purchased from the AAO-HNS.

One easily remedied contributory factor to impaired hearing at any age is cerumen impaction. There is a tendency for cerumen in older individuals to be dry and to inspissate. Once the external canal is cleared by gentle irrigation or wax-dissolving drops, recurrent impaction can be avoided by weekly instillation of a few drops of baby oil.

Mouth

All patients should be encouraged to have a yearly dental examination as part of an optimal health-maintenance program. However, some patients may see their dentists infrequently, especially if they lack insurance coverage for such care. Physicians who provide primary care to geriatric patients should be aware of the relatively common oral conditions that occur in this population.[188] Periodontal disease is the most common cause of tooth loss in the elderly. Areas of dentin normally protected by a covering of gum become susceptible to development of caries that also contribute to loss of teeth. Good oral hygiene practices, including daily brushing and flossing can prevent these dental problems. Oral examination can also reveal precursors to oral cancer that are most often the result of tobacco and alcohol exposure, but also occur in the presence of chronic irritation, such as might result from ill-fitting dentures. In contrast to candida (thrush), the white patches of leukoplakia are painless and cannot be scraped off. Most of these lesions are benign, but as many as 10% contain regions of dysplasia or carcinoma in situ. Erythroplakia are red lesions of mucosa that are much more frequently dysplastic or frankly malignant. Since early diagnosis increases the likelihood of curative surgery,[189] visual examination of

	5 Minute Hearing Test © 1989, American Academy of Otolaryngology–Head and Neck Surgery	Almost always	Half the time	Occasionally	Never
1.	I have a problem hearing over the telephone.				
2.	I have trouble following the conversation when two or more people are talking at the same time.				
3.	People complain that I turn the TV volume too high.				
4.	I have to strain to understand conversations.				
5.	I miss hearing some common sounds like the phone or doorbell ringing.				
6.	I have trouble hearing conversations in a noisy background such as a party.				
7.	I get confused about where sounds come from.				
8.	I misunderstand some words in a sentence and need to ask people to repeat themselves.				
9.	I especially have trouble understanding the speech of women and children.				
10.	I have worked in noisy environments (assembly lines, jackhammers, jet engines, etc.).				
11.	Many people I talk to seem to mumble (or don't speak clearly).				
12.	People get annoyed because I misunderstand what they say.				
13.	I misunderstand what others are saying and make inappropriate responses.				
14.	I avoid social activities because I cannot hear well and fear I'll reply improperly.				
	To be answered by a family member or friend: 15. Do you think this person has a hearing loss?				

Scoring

To calculate your score, give yourself 3 points for every time you checked the "Almost always" column, 2 for every "Half the time," 1 for every "Occasionally," and 0 for every "Never." If you have a blood relative who has a hearing loss, add another 3 points. Then total your points.

- 0 to 5 — Your hearing is fine. No action is recommended.
- 6 to 9 — Ask your doctor about a hearing test.
- 10 and above — strongly recommend a hearing test.

Figure 6.2 Five-Minute Hearing Test (From American Academy of Otolaryngology—Head and Neck Surgery: Five Minute Hearing Test. Washington, D.C., 1989.)

the oral mucosa and tongue is reasonable in patients who are at higher than normal risk to develop oral squamous cell carcinoma, especially those patients who do not regularly receive dental checkups.

Depression and Dementia

Depression is a common disorder in later life.[190] Because no biological parameter is useful clinically to diagnose depression, recognition of this treatable disorder depends upon a careful history. Diagnostic criteria for depression are listed in Table 6.7.[191] It is important to keep in mind that elderly patients may deny saddened moods even when depression is present. Instead, they may complain of somatic symptoms (eg, abdominal pain, headache) for which no anatomic or physiologic explanation is apparent. The recent onset of such hypochrondriacal behavior should prompt a careful search for the signs and symptoms of depression listed in the table.

Later life is a time of changes in life-style, and is marked by the deaths of friends and relatives. Prolonged grief is not normal. If mourning lasts longer than is appropriate for a person's sociocultural peer group, the diagnosis of depression should be considered. Talking with a family member may help in making this judgment. The presence of an apparent environmental precipitant does not influence response to antidepressant medication.

Dementia is a syndrome of acquired deficits of memory and other cognitive abilities sufficiently severe to impair social or occupational functions.[191] In our aging society, dementia is a health problem of truly staggering proportion. Population studies suggest that approximately 5% of persons over age 65 and 20% of persons over age 80 have the dementia syndrome.[192] Although dementia is common, these studies demonstrate that such impairment is not a normal concomitant of the aging process and imply that the term "senility" should be abandoned. Dementia of the Alzheimer's type (DAT), which is usually a relentlessly progressive disease, is by far the most common cause of dementia in the elderly, accounting for at least 70% of cases.[193] After DAT, the most frequent cause of dementia is multiple cerebral infarction (multiinfarct dementia), accounting for approximately 15% of cases. This dementing process potentially

Table 6.7 Criteria for the Diagnosis of Depression

1. Persistently sad mood or inability to experience pleasure for at least 2 weeks
2. At least four of the following signs and symptoms:
    a. Sleep disturbance
    b. Change of appetite
    c. Fatigue or lethargy
    d. Loss of interest in usual activities
    e. Impaired subjective ability to think or concentrate
    f. Decreased self-esteem or inappropriate guilt
    g. Psychomotor retardation or agitation
    h. Thoughts of death or suicide

From *Diagnostic and Statistical Manual of Mental Disorders*, 3rd ed.[191]

can be prevented by control of hypertension, but no treatment for the dementia itself is available. Ethanol is directly toxic to brain tissue and, with or without thiamine deficiency, can lead to alcoholic dementia,[194] comprising 5% of dementias in later life. This disorder often has a reversible component if the patient can be kept free of alcohol. Another 5% of dementias result from Parkinson's disease.[195] Among the causes of the remaining 5% of cases of dementia in later life are brain structural abnormalities (such as tumors, subdural hematomas, and normal pressure hydrocephalus), inherited and neurodegenerative diseases, metabolic derangements, and infectious processes [including tertiary syphilis, encephalitides, Creutzfeldt-Jacob disease, and, ever more commonly, acquired immune deficiency syndrome (AIDS)]. Although the dementias that result from metabolic abnormalities are theoretically curable, by the time recognizable mental dysfunction is present, intervention rarely produces complete resolution of the impairment.[196,197] Therefore, it may be reasonable to screen asymptomatic older persons for the more common of these diseases, including hypothyroidism and B12 deficiency, usually the result of pernicious anemia. Thyroid function tests and CBC with indices and smear evaluation will usually be sufficient to detect these disorders, although cognitive dysfunction has been reported in pernicious anemia before the development of anemia.[198]

Depression can mimic dementia. However, the apparent cognitive deficits in depression are more the result of poor concentration and motivation than of actual memory loss. Careful observation and interview should distinguish between the two diagnoses. For either depression or dementia a detailed drug history should be obtained. Sleeping pills, alcohol, β blockers, antihistamines, and muscle relaxants are among the medications that can significantly affect mood and intellectual function.

If dementia is suspected, a detailed neurologic exam seeking localizing signs is important. The Mini Mental State Exam (MMSE) is a 10-minute comprehensive and reliable instrument that evaluates memory, language, and praxis.[199] As part of the workup of dementia, a VDRL test for syphilis is often obtained. However, tertiary syphilis is now a rare disease in women, and screening VDRL in the absence of dementia and with no history of syphilis exposure is not indicated.

Aging women will often have aging husbands who are also at risk to develop dementia. The simple question, "How is your husband?" may elicit the patient's worries regarding the cognitive functions of her spouse. The patient should then be advised to have her spouse evaluated. Although, in this case, the patient is not the one with the "disease," the burden of caring for a demented person is significant, physically, psychologically, and financially. Unfortunately, there are currently no effective medical therapies for DAT or, as previously mentioned, for many of the other etiologies of dementia. Physicians should be aware of community resources, such as the Alzheimer's Association, a nationwide organization that can provide invaluable peer support.

Life-style

A major component of preventive health care is the promotion of a healthy lifestyle. For most Americans, this requires a conscious effort to improve eating patterns and increase levels of exercise. Smoking or excessive alcohol intake may also be issues. Patients should be reminded to use seat belts. The importance of life-style changes should not be underestimated. Time spent helping a patient to quit smoking or start an exercise program may provide greater benefit than more conventional medical care, such as prescribing antihypertensive medications. Because the education and emotional support required by a patient who is making drastic changes in her life-style is time-consuming, it may be appropriate to refer the patient to a program or provider specializing in this area. However, advice from a physician carries special weight. Patients should always be told in simple, unambiguous terms of the health benefits derived from life-style changes.

Smoking

Smoking is responsible for 11% of deaths among women.[60] It is a causative factor in CAD, stroke, peripheral vascular disease, chronic obstructive pulmonary disease, and several cancers (see Table 6.8). Public awareness of the health consequences of smoking is increasing,[60] but many still fail to appreciate the broad deleterious effects of smoking. Quitting should be a goal for all smokers.

The risk of disease has been shown to diminish when smoking has been discontinued. Persistent smokers have a 2.2-fold greater risk of dying from coronary heart disease and a 1.6-fold greater death rate than individuals who quit smoking.[205] A former smoker who remains without evidence of cardiovascular disease for 10 years after quitting will subsequently have minimal if any increased risk of heart disease compared to a nonsmoker,[206] and significant reduction in the risk of myocardial infarction is seen within 2 to 3 years.[207,208] The residual risk for cancer diminishes more slowly—over about a 15- to 20-year period—but, as with cardiovascular disease, the risks of disease are lower for quitters than they are for those who continue smoking.[29]

Even patients who have already developed smoking-related conditions benefit from quitting. Reduced reinfarction rates and slowed progression of COPD, for example, can be documented when patients with CAD or COPD stop smoking.[29,60] Abstention from smoking has been shown to improve cerebral perfusion in elderly patients[209] and is associated with improvement in symptoms from peripheral vascular disease.[29]

The physician plays an important role in motivating the smoker to quit. Brief

Table 6.8 Representative Disease Risks of Smoking*

Disease process	Relative risk[†]	Attributable risk[‡] (%)
Coronary artery disease	1.7	30
Stroke	1.2–1.5	18
Subarachnoid hemorrhage	5.7	
Lung cancer	7.3	87
Oral, laryngeal, and esophageal cancer	2–27	62
Bladder cancer	2–3	31
Chronic obstructive pulmonary disease	30	82

* See Refs. 200 to 205.
[†] Relative risk of death for smokers compared to nonsmokers.
[‡] Percent of deaths attributable to smoking.

physician counseling may result in quitting rates of 3% to 20%,[210,211] and repetitive counseling is likely to increase this rate. Key steps in helping a patient to quit include the following[29,210–213]:

1. Identify smoking as a medical problem for the patient.
2. Inform the patient of the risks of smoking and the benefits of quitting. The more specific and personalized the health advice is, the more likely it will have an effect.
3. Help the patient to formulate a concrete plan for quitting. This includes identifying alternatives to smoking (eg, exercise, social activities, chewing gum).
4. Discuss the benefit of changing the social environment. For example, it may help the patient to socialize with friends who are nonsmokers, or to coordinate her quitting efforts with those of friends. If the spouse is a smoker, cessation is much more likely to succeed if he tries to quit as well.
5. Provide continued follow-up. Ask the patient about progress on smoking each time she is seen.

When a patient is shown that she has smoking-related changes in pulmonary function and carbon monoxide levels, she is more likely to quit smoking.[214]

Additional interventions that may help a patient to quit smoking include the use of nicotine-containing gum and hypnosis.[211] It is not necessary for the primary physician to be actively involved in all aspects of the effort. Referral to other providers for an active smoking-cessation program should always be considered. However, the interest of the primary provider in the patient's progress helps maintain the motivation to quit.

Exercise

A regular exercise program should be recommended to all women unless a specific medical or physical condition prevents it.[215,216] Sedentary individuals benefit from even modest increases in regular physical activity. Health benefits include a reduced risk of heart disease and hypertension, easier weight control, maintenance of muscle strength, improved glucose control in diabetics, and decreased risk of depression.[216] In a study of ambulatory elderly individuals, regular physical activity was associated with a lower overall risk of bone fracture.[217] Moderate exercise programs have been shown to contribute to prolonged longevity as well as improved health.[2,218]

Nevertheless, surveys suggest that less than 10% of individuals 65 and older exercise on a regular basis,[215,219] despite data indicating that even modest levels of exercise provide health benefits.[2] An increased level of exercise has been identified as an important national health goal,[215,219] and represents a method for improving health that is simple and accessible for most patients.

It is important to advise the patient to advance slowly above her usual level of physical activity. A patient who has been almost entirely sedentary will benefit from brief walks of a few minutes, and should not attempt vigorous exercise.[216] For patients who are able to do so, the goal should be a program of moderate aerobic exercise (such as brisk walking, swimming, or the use of an exercise bicycle for 30 minutes three or more times a week).[216,220] It may take several months to achieve this goal, especially for patients who are not currently exercising. Although significant cardiovascular conditioning can be maintained by exercising three times a week,[216] additional benefits are obtained if exercise is accomplished daily. Patients who are trying to lose weight, for example, will benefit from daily exercise. It may be easier for a patient to maintain a daily exercise program if she includes different activities: walking, swimming, exercise bicycle. On busy days, even a brief walk is beneficial.

Nutrition

Most patients will benefit from some modifications in diet. Based on average patterns of food consumption in the United States,[221,222] the following guidelines should be provided.

Fats and Cholesterol

Saturated fats and cholesterol should comprise 30% or less of total calorie intake. In the current average American diet, calories from fat make up 36% to 43%[221,222] of the daily calorie intake, so that for most people, some reduction in fat-containing foods is required to reach this goal. Food preparation methods that add fat (eg, frying) should be avoided.

Fiber

All individuals should be encouraged to increase intake of fiber and complex carbohydrates. Ideally, fiber-containing foods and whole grain or cereal products should be eaten at each meal.

Sodium

There is no evidence that high-salt diets are harmful to individuals with normal blood pressure. Conversely, there is no benefit to a diet high in salt. The Surgeon General has recommended reduced salt intake as a nutritional goal for the general population.[223] This can be accomplished by avoidance of foods high in salt (eg, potato chips, canned soup) and by limiting the use of salt in food preparation. For individuals without hypertension, an appropriate goal for sodium intake is 5 to 6 g per day.[224] For individuals with hypertension, a more limited intake of 1.5 to 2.5 g is recommended.

Calcium

The National Research Council's recommended calcium intake for women over age 24 is 800 mg per day, while the actual intake is on average only 500 to 600 mg per day.[225] Some experts recommend higher calcium intake (eg, 1000 mg before menopause and 1500 mg after menopause.[222,226] Calcium deficiency is an important contributor to the development of osteoporosis in postmenopausal women (see *Osteoporosis*). The best way to achieve adequate calcium intake is through consumption of calcium-rich foods, specifically dairy products. An 8-ounce glass of milk provides 250 to 300 mg of calcium, irrespective of the fat content of the milk.[226] Other foods rich in calcium include spinach, broccoli, sardines, salmon, and tofu.[224,227,228] Comparative calcium contents for these foods are shown in Table 6.9.

Patients unable or unwilling to obtain adequate calcium from foods in their

Table 6.9 Calcium Content of Foods*

	Calcium content (mg)
Skim milk, 1 cup	303
Sardines, 8 medium	354
Salmon, 3 oz. canned	167
Broccoli, 1 medium spear	205
Spinach, 1 cup cooked	245
Tofu, 1 piece (1″ × 2.5″ × 2.75″)	108

* See Refs. 227 and 228.

diet can use calcium supplements. Absorption of calcium from supplements is low, averaging only about 30% and decreasing with age.[226] The most common side effects of calcium supplements are gastrointestinal discomfort and constipation. Different calcium salts do not appear to differ significantly in the production of side effects or in absorption.[222,226] Calcium supplements may interfere with iron absorption or cause depletion of phosphate, and intake of amounts higher than 3 to 4 g of elemental calcium per day causes hypercalcemia.[226] Calcium supplements are contraindicated in individuals with a history of calcium-containing urinary tract stones.

Potassium

Potassium contributes to blood-pressure control in hypertensive individuals and is protective against stroke mortality. A diet providing approximately 75 mEq of potassium daily is optimal.[224] This can be accomplished by consuming the recommended five or more servings of a combination of fruits and vegetables per day, including green and yellow vegetables and citrus fruits. (A serving equals a one-half cup portion or a medium-sized piece of fruit.) Dietary supplements are not recommended for the general population.[224]

Vitamins

Many elderly individuals are in the habit of consuming vitamin supplements, in the mistaken belief that they will provide "energy" and make up for waning appetites.[229] In fact, vitamin supplements are not required by individuals who eat a well-balanced diet[224] and represent a needless expense for many elderly individuals on fixed incomes. Further, overuse of vitamin pills may result in overdosing of fat-soluble vitamins (vitamins A, D, and E in particular) because these are not readily excreted.

Obesity and Weight Loss

In general, weight rises with age. For women, this may be due in part to reduced metabolism related to the cessation of menses; reduced physical activity is often a factor as well. Standard weight tables do not reflect this age-related increase, and underestimate the "ideal" body weight for older people.[230] As shown in Figure 6.3, a weight gain of as much as 1 pound per year, or 10 pounds per decade, is acceptable and without an associated increase in mortality.

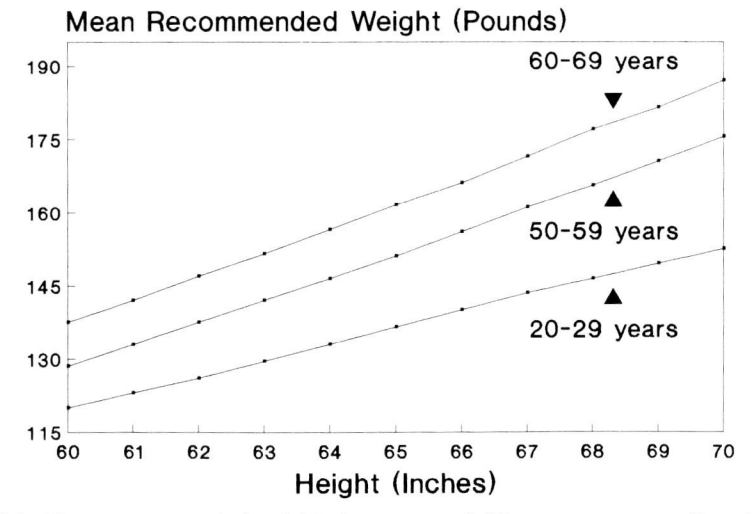

Figure 6.3 Mean recommended weights for women of different age groups. Based on the analysis of Andres.[230]

Women who are at or above 115% of ideal body weight, however, may experience excess morbidity and mortality, and appropriate counseling regarding weight loss should be offered. Similarly, central obesity is associated with increased risks for cardiovascular disease and breast cancer, as discussed above, and women with this pattern of weight gain may benefit from weight loss. Women with hypertension and diabetes may also benefit from weight loss, even with mild degrees of obesity.

Weight measurements should be taken on a regular basis, because rapid losses or gains may be significant. An involuntary weight loss of 10 pounds or greater over a year may be due to occult cancer, gastrointestinal or thyroid disease, diabetes, or depression, and an appropriate workup should be considered. Similarly, rapid weight gain may be an indicator of hypothyroidism, or, if an organic cause can be ruled out, suggests the need for counseling regarding food intake and exercise.

Diet Counseling

Safe and effective dieting can be accomplished by following simple guidelines. Most individuals who lose weight while dieting, however, will regain the weight subsequently, and patients should be encouraged to diet only when a specific medical indication is present.

When plans to diet are made, the patient should be counseled as follows.

1. Weight loss should be slow and steady. The goal should rarely exceed 2 to 4 pounds a month.
2. Regular, fully balanced meals should be eaten, with calorie reduction accomplished primarily by an increase in fruit and vegetable intake, and a decrease in foods containing fat and sugar.
3. A patient who is dieting should be encouraged to pursue moderate exercise on a daily basis.

4. Patients should not avoid their favorite foods, even those of a relatively high caloric content. Portions should be reduced. The diet should be one that can be tolerated for long periods of time.
5. It is often necessary for a patient who is dieting to be seen on a regular basis—weekly or monthly—by a dietitian or other counselor, to discuss meal plans and check weight. Community-based programs may serve this purpose, and additionally provide the patient with valuable social support.

Bowel Function

Constipation is a common complaint in older patients. Sometimes this complaint derives from the mistaken idea that normal bowel function requires daily evacuation; for some people, it may be normal to have a bowel movement every 2 to 3 days. Constipation implies the difficult evacuation of stool that is firm and hard. Patients will sometimes complain of having small "pellets" of stool. This is usually due to poor eating habits and lack of exercise. Laxative abuse may also be a factor. While there should always be concern for the possibility of a pathologic cause, particularly if the constipation represents a distinct change in bowel habit, most patients will benefit from a trial of increased fluid and fiber intake, and increased exercise. Medications which may contribute to constipation include codeine and other narcotics, calcium supplements, diuretics, antihistamines, and antidepressants. Patients who have used laxatives frequently may require the use of periodic enemas over a several-week period while a new bowel program is being established.

Fiber and Fluid

Ideally, fiber-rich foods or supplements should be taken with each meal. Bran is an excellent source of fiber; a quarter to a half a cup of bran can be added to cereal, salad, or other food each day. Bran muffins and bread are also helpful, but provide smaller quantities of bran. Other important sources of fiber are vegetables, fruit, beans, and whole-grain bread. Large portions should be encouraged. If adequate fiber cannot be derived from diet, the patient should be advised to use psyllium, 1 teaspoon to 1 tablespoon, up to three times a day.

A fluid intake of 6 to 8 glasses (48 to 64 oz.) a day is recommended. Older patients will sometimes avoid fluid intake for social reasons, as, for example, to prevent stress incontinence or nocturia. When a bowel program is begun, the patient should be encouraged to keep a diary of fluid intake for several days, to encourage adequate intake.

Gastrocolic Reflex

Bowel evacuation is more likely to occur after a meal, as a result of the gastrocolic reflex. Patients should be advised to arrange their day so that they have time and adequate facilities for bowel evacuation, after at least one of their daily meals. This may be particularly important while traveling. Arranging meals so they they occur at around the same time every day is also helpful.

Use of Medications

Older patients often use many medications, including both prescription and over-the-counter preparations. A full list of all medications being used should be obtained on an annual basis. The physician should be alert to medications as a cause of otherwise unexplained symptoms. Interactions between different medications may occur. As discussed in Chapter 5, older patients may experience an increased incidence of side effects from medications. A few examples of specific problems related to over-the-counter medications are noted below.

Antihistamines and Decongestants

Most over-the-counter cold preparations are combinations of antihistamines and decongestants. Antihistamines can cause drowsiness and anticholinergic side effects, including dry mouth, urinary retention, and, in the extreme, confusion. Decongestants, the most common of which is pseudoephedrine, typically cause symptoms related to sympathetic stimulation, including irritability, increased pulse rate and blood pressure, and sleeplessness. The combination of these two medications in a single preparation can, understandably, cause a mixture of side effects. Patients may experience fewer side effects if combined preparations are avoided. For example, pseudoephedrine may be taken during the day, and an antihistamine at nighttime, for control of nasal congestion. Doses lower than those recommended by the manufacturer are often sufficient to provide relief of symptoms.

Nose Drops

Many effective nasal preparations for nasal congestion contain sympathomimetics, such as oxymatazoline. They are effective in resolving congestion, but should not be used for longer than 3 days. With prolonged use, patients experience reactive congestion on withdrawal of the medication.

Sedatives

Sedative use is common. The active ingredient in most over-the-counter sleeping medications is an antihistamine (eg, diphenhydramine) with side effects as noted above.

Aspirin

Many individuals take aspirin on a regular basis, for headache, fever, or musculoskeletal pain. It may sometimes be prescribed for arthritis or to prevent stroke or myocardial infarction. Patients using aspirin should be informed about the potential for gastrointestinal side effects (bleeding, peptic symptoms) and the medication's effect on coagulation; elderly women, in particular, may be susceptible to the anticoagulant effect of aspirin, and should be instructed to report any easy bruising associated with use of the drug.

Nonsteroidal Antiinflammatory Drugs

Over-the-counter availability of nonsteroidals has benefitted patients because of the lower cost of these medications, which aid in the management of arthritis, other musculoskeletal pain, menstrual pain, and headache. In spite of labeling, however, patients are not always aware of side effects. These include esophageal reflux, gastrointestinal bleeding, and fluid retention.[231] These medications may also impair renal function; in patients using high doses of these medications chronically, renal function should be monitored on a regular basis.

Acetaminophen

Chronic use of acetaminophen may also have an adverse effect on renal function.[232] This medication is frequently used for headache, musculoskeletal pain, and fever. It is often recommended for patients who have had adverse gastrointestinal side effects from aspirin or NSAIDs, as a safer drug. Patients may thus underestimate the potential for side effects and may not report the regular use of this medication unless asked.

Screening Laboratory Tests

The development of automated instruments capable of simultaneously measuring blood levels of many components has dramatically altered many physicians' approaches to routine screening. Rather than requesting the measurement of one specific element, a panel of 6, 8, 12, or even 20 items is obtained. This is a situation in which more is not necessarily better than less. Each blood level is a continuous variable; there is no absolute demarcation between normal and abnormal. Therefore, the normal range cited for each variable is usually the mean value plus or minus 2 standard deviations calculated from a population of presumably normal individuals. By definition, for each test 5% of normal individuals will have values that fall outside the "normal" range—2.5% below and 2.5% above. As the size of the panel increases, the proportion of normal individuals having completely normal results decreases. A population of 8651 randomly selected patients attending a routine health-evaluation program were screened for 20 laboratory abnormalities. Whereas 74.1% of these patients had normal results for a subset panel of 8 components, only 45.1% had completely normal results for the entire set of 20 tests,[233] even in this population at low risk to have the illnesses suggested by the abnormal values. These results are consistent with the theoretical predictions of false-positive rates for panels of varying sizes.[234] Another observation of this study was that items found to be abnormal on the initial screen often reverted to normal on retesting.

One underlying premise of routine periodic screening is that earlier diagnosis of disease, before symptoms are recognized, will result in reduced morbidity or mortality. Unfortunately, for many illnesses detectable by such screening, early diagnosis usually does not change outcome. Another consideration of screening is that it should be cost-effective in terms of both economic and human terms. Again, for multi-item biochemical screening, this criterion is not met. The use of large batteries of tests increases the frequency of abnormal results, decreases the tests' practical significance, and leads to additional testing, additional office visits, and additional patient anxiety. A disease label may result in increased cost of or inability to obtain life or health insurance. After considering these and other factors, Canadian and American medical commissions recommended against the use of biochemical profiles as screening tools in asymptomatic individuals.[235,236] However, it is our opinion that screening tests for individual biochemical components are justified in some cases, depending on the physician's pretest level of suspicion that an abnormality might be found.

An abnormal test should always be repeated to ensure that the abnormality persists and is not the result of day-to-day variation. For each biochemical abnormality detected in a multiphasic profile, there is a list of conditions that could be etiologic. However, most of these conditions are uncommon and rarely present without symptoms or clinical signs. The less common the condition being considered, the more likely an abnormal value is a false-positive. Markedly abnormal values are more likely to represent a disease process than are marginal abnormalities. The ordering of some specific laboratory tests should be considered when there is even a limited suspicion that the patient may have one of the more common diseases discussed below.

Diabetes Mellitus

Diabetes mellitus is a heterogeneous group of diseases, characterized by an inability to process glucose properly. Insulin-dependent diabetes (type I) results from a destruction of the pancreatic islet cells that produce insulin. Although the usual age of onset is in childhood to young adulthood, some patients develop this form of diabetes much later in life. Noninsulin-dependent diabetes (type II) in most cases is a disease of older adults, affecting approximately 3% of the U.S. population.[237] The mechanism by which type-II diabetes arises is not entirely understood. There is relative insulin and glucose insensitivity, impaired but not absent insulin release, and a relationship to obesity, such that increased weight increases the risk to develop the disease.[238] Genetic factors are important for development of both forms of the disease.[239] A substantial portion of overt diabetics will develop complications including cardiovascular disease, renal failure, neuropathy, and blindness. Many patients with either form of diabetes will complain of polyuria, polydipsia, and polyphagia, making the diagnosis in these patients relatively straightforward. However, older people with diabetes often do not develop this classic symptom triad. The most common presentation of diabetes in the elderly is insidious weight loss and fatigue; diabetes should always be considered in the differential diagnosis of these nonspecific complaints. Some patients with abnormal glucose metabolism are entirely without symptoms. Routine periodic testing for diabetes in the asymptomatic population became part of the standard health-maintenance program when it was thought that initiation of treatment in the presymptomatic stage of diabetes was more effective than treatment begun at the onset of symptoms. As yet, studies have failed to document a benefit from early diagnosis (reviewed in Refs. 240 and 241), and overdiagnosis and therapy can be dangerous. It seems reasonable to limit screening to patients at higher-than-average risk to develop diabetes; that is, obese individuals, especially those with a family history of diabetes, and women with a history of gestational diabetes.[242] Although there may be no need to begin medications prior to development of symptoms, an overweight patient might be spurred to alter her diet and lose weight as an alternative to the prospect of medical therapy.

What test for glycemia should be employed? Urine testing, although simple and noninvasive, is insensitive. The renal threshold for glucose excretion in general is above 160 mg/dL, and varies both among patients and for a single patient over time.[243] The glucose tolerance test (GTT) will result in overdiagnosis of diabetes in the aging population, since there is a gradual increase in both fasting and postprandial glucose levels with age. Even with conservative standards set for the aged, nearly 50% of people over 60 years of age will have an abnormal GTT. The 2-hour postprandial glucose level normally rises by 5 to 10 mg/dL per decade over 50, whereas the fasting level changes much more modestly (1 to 2 mg/dL per decade over 50).[244] Therefore, the fasting plasma glucose measurement is a better screening tool for older persons. Both the National Diabetes Data Group[242] and the World Health Organization[245] would make a diagnosis of diabetes if the fasting plasma glucose concentration is at least 140 mg/dL on more than one occasion. A random plasma glucose level repeated 200 mg/dL or higher has also been accepted by consensus as diagnostic of diabetes.[242,245] The glycosylated hemoglobin level (HbA1C) provides a measure of the degree of hyperglycemia in the preceding 1 to 3 months.[246] Although HbA1C can be used to screen for diabetes,[247,248] more commonly it is used to assess the effectiveness of therapy.

One important caveat is that the majority of people with mild, asymptomatic glucose intolerance will not develop frank diabetes[249,250]; some revert to normal glycemia and others remain in the borderline range. Once a diagnosis of glucose intolerance is made, however, surveillance should be continued so that intervention can be started promptly once symptoms occur.

Thyroid Disease

Thyroid function does not naturally diminish with aging; thyroxine (T4) and thyroid stimulating hormone (TSH) levels remain normal. However, hypothyroidism is much more frequently seen in older than in younger populations. Most affected individuals present after age 50. Symptoms and signs of this condition include lethargy, constipation, dry skin, alopecia, memory impairment, and depression—complaints that may be attributed to the aging process and may not be investigated further. Some elderly patients may have none of the classic symptoms besides lethargy and weakness. Since untreated hypothyroidism can lead to irreversible dementia, physicians should be alert to symptoms that indicate this diagnostic possibility. In one study, 4% of patients at least 60 years old who were evaluated at the time of hospital admission were found to have previously unrecognized hypothyroidism.[251] In the healthy, nonhospitalized elderly population, the prevalence of hypothyroidism has been estimated to be as high as 5%.[252]

There is no consensus on whether to screen routinely for hypothyroidism in the healthy, asymptomatic elderly patient. Some argue that such screening is not cost-effective, since the yield is low. On the other hand, the consequences of untreated hypothyroidism in the elderly can be severe,[253] and include dementia. Certainly, those patients at increased risk should be tested, including those with a history of neck irradiation or hyperthyroidism. Hypothyroidism can be a long-term complication of hyperthyroidism, especially when the patient has received radioactive iodine. Given the benign nature and low cost of thyroid testing, it may be reasonable to screen all older patients every 1 to 2 years. An elevated TSH level reflects the response of the hypothalamic-pituitary axis to decreased thyroid hormone levels, and is sufficient as a screening test for thyroid gland failure.[254]

Unlike hypothyroidism, the elderly comprise only about 20% of patients affected by hyperthyroidism. Symptoms of hyperthroidism include decreased energy, weight loss, and muscle weakness. Again, however, symptoms are more common in young patients than in older patients and mimic "normal" aging. Hyperthyroidism should be suspected in a patient who appears more nervous and agitated than normal, especially when tachycardia is present. The elderly patient may present with atrial fibrillation or congestive heart failure, complications of hyperthyroidism that are unusual in younger people.[255,256] The etiology of hyperthyroidism in the elderly is often nodular goiter and rarely Grave's disease, so ophthalmopathy is usually not seen. One subset of older hyperthyroid patients has depressed activity and mental functioning and may appear to be hypothyroid. The term "apathetic hyperthyroidism" has been applied to this condition.[257] Although TSH levels are suppressed in hyperthyroid states, an elevated free-T4 index (FTI), calculated from T4 and triiodotyronine resin uptake (T3RU), is sufficient for the diagnosis to be made in otherwise healthy patients.

Hyperparathyroidism

Primary hyperparathyroidism is characterized by excessive parathormone secretion, usually the result of parathyroid adenomas, which leads to elevated plasma calcium levels. Symptoms include fatigue, weaknes, depression, bone and abdominal pain, and renal stones. Bone mineral loss can be significant, adding to the morbidity of osteoporosis that frequently coexists. Perhaps the most striking effect of multichannel autoanalyzers has been the dramatic increase in the diagnosis of primary hyperparathyroidism.[258] Once assumed to be a very rare disease, diagnosed only after onset of symptoms, primary hyperparathyroidism is now estimated to occur in 25 per 100,000 in the general population. The incidence of this disease is greater in women than in men and rises with age, so that approximately 188 per 100,000 women over age 60 are affected.[259]

There are several caveats to remember when interpreting an elevated random screening calcium. (1) As discussed, 2.5% of the normal population will have an elevated calcium on any one occasion—13 times the frequency of hyperparathyroidism in the segment of the population at highest risk. Therefore, an elevated calcium determination should be documented on at least three occasions prior to referral to a specialist. (2) The unbound ionized calcium fraction, upon which diagnosis rests, is dependent on the amount of binding to serum proteins. For this reason, the measured total calcium concentration obtained in a screening battery must be adjusted for the albumin level simultaneously obtained. For every 0.1 g/dL albumin above 4.0, 0.1 mg/dL should be subtracted from the calcium level. If the albumin level is below 4.0 g/dL, the correction factor is added to the calcium level. (3) Ionized calcium levels will rise in acidosis, such as might occur in blood pooling distal to a tourniquet. Repeat calcium determinations should be obtained with care to keep the tourniquet time to a minimum.

Laboratory tests that support the diagnosis of hyperparathyroidism include elevated plasma parathormone and urinary cyclic AMP levels, both of which increase with age.[260] There is an unresolved controversy regarding the appropriate therapy, medical versus surgical, during the asymptomatic stage, especially in the geriatric population.[261-263] If the diagnosis of hyperparathyroidism is seriously entertained, the patient should be referred to an endocrinologist for further evaluation.

Renal Disease

Even in the absence of diseases that directly affect the kidney, renal function changes dramatically in the process of normal aging. Beginning in young adulthood, renal plasma flow deceases by 10% each decade, so that by 80 years of age there has been a 50% reduction.[264] In addition, gradual loss in the number of nephrons leads to a decline in glomerular filtration rate (GFR).[265,266] These factors contribute to a fall in creatinine clearance which begins to be detectable at about age 35. A reciprocal rise in serum creatinine is not seen, however, since creatinine clearance depends on muscle mass, which also decreases with age.[265] The lower muscle mass of women results in approximately 20% lower creatinine clearance values than those in men. A creatinine value above 1.5 mg/dL is unlikely to be solely the result of normal aging, and indicates that renal disease may be present. When prescribing drugs that are renally excreted, it should be remembered that the serum creatinine overestimates the GFR in older people, and some measure of creatinine clearance should be obtained. A 24-hour urine collection for direct measurement of the creatinine excreted may be difficult for an older women to provide. A useful estimate can be calculated from the patient's serum creatinine, age, and weight as follows:

$$\frac{(140 - \text{Age}) \times \text{Weight in kg}}{72 \times \text{Creatinine}}$$

Aside from diminished creatinine clearance, other renal changes with aging include decreased concentrating and sodium-conserving abilities.[267] However, maximal renal capacity far exceeds what is needed; so, although renal function is markedly diminished with aging, under normal circumstances extracellular volume and osmolality are adequately regulated. Situations that perturb water and solute balance may overwhelm older kidneys, and significant volume depletion may result. Examples of such stresses are febrile illnesses, strenuous exercise, and decreased fluid intake while on diuretics. Even in the absence of heart disease, volume overload may result from increased intake of solute and water, either orally or in the form of radiologic contrast. Abnormal serum sodium concentrations, reflecting water excess or deficit, may also result in these situations.

Creatinine and BUN levels should be measured periodically in patients taking drugs that might have adverse effects on kidney function, such as NSAIDs and tylenol, antihypertensive medications, and diuretics. Patients with diseases that might result in renal dysfunction, including hypertension and diabetes, should have these blood tests as well.

Complete Blood Count

The complete blood count (CBC) is a common component of screening batteries performed on asymptomatic ambulatory patients. However, there is evidence to suggest that this screening test rarely detects a serious underlying disorder and often leads to further, more expensive testing.[268,269] Patients with significant anemia almost always have symptoms—fatigue being the most common complaint. Although mild anemia is common in otherwise healthy elderly persons, most studies have not found this to be of clinical consequence unless it is associated with an underlying illness. Certainly, a patient who has complaints suggestive of upper- or lower-gastrointestinal tract bleeding or unexplained fatigue deserves a hematocrit or hemoglobin measurement as part of the evaluation. There may also be merit in obtaining a screening hematocrit in women who have heavy menstrual bleeding, since the diet may not contain an adequate supply of iron, and iron supplementation may prevent the development of severe, symptomatic anemia. Red cell indices are helpful in the diagnosis of pernicious anemia, but the disease is not common, and permanent complications in the absence of symptoms are extremely rare. The white cell count and differential are only helpful in the evaluation of suspected illnesses, such as infections or malignancies. The values fluctuate too widely from day to day, and abnormalities are too nonspecific to be of utility in screening.[269,270]

Urinalysis

Dipstick evaluation of urine samples is easy to perform and relatively inexpensive. Chemically impregnated strips are able to detect several urine components, including hemoglobin, protein, and the white cell enzyme leukocyte esterase.[271] As with other screening tests, there is a controversy regarding the utility of this practice,[272] since it is not clear that identification of minor abnormalities or diagnosis of urinary tract diseases in the presymptomatic phase is of benefit. Some researchers, who oppose the ordering of urinalyses (UAs) in the absence of clear indications, argue that a change in therapy is rarely made on the basis of urine results, even when an abnormality is present.[273] This does not seem to be a valid reason for discontinuing the screening process, but rather indicates that additional studies are necessary to define the long-term outcome of patients whose urine abnormalities went untreated.

The frequency of abnormalities found on urinalyses in any population is very high; in 6000 women included in one study of mass screening of asymptomatic working adults, at least one abnormality was detected in 12%. The most frequent abnormal finding was hematuria, present in 8% of samples.[274] In contrast to gross hematuria, which requires full urologic workup, asymptomatic microhematuria rarely implies serious pathology. No neoplasms were identified in females ascertained with asymptomatic microhematuria who were followed prospectively for 10 years.[275] After thorough evaluation of patients whose urinalysis was abnormal, hematuria was most often attributed to trigonitis or a related condition. However, hematuria may indicate the presence of renal calculi which, if untreated, can lead to decreased renal function. Papillary necrosis, often the result of analgesic abuse, may also cause microscopic hematuria. Use of offending medications should be discontinued to prevent progression of renal disease.

Pyuria, detected by a positive leukocyte esterase reaction on dipstick testing, may indicate bacterial cystitis or bladder colonization. Although silent bacteriuria is associated with increased mortality in elderly people, there is no evidence to support a benefit from antibiotic treatment in this circumstance.[276,277] On the other hand, symptomatic urinary tract infection should be treated with appropriate antibiotics. Sterile pyuria, once the hallmark of renal tuberculosis, is now most frequently the result of interstitial nephritis, such as might result from analgesic abuse.

Proteinuria may reflect hematuria, urinary tract infection, or intrinsic renal disease, such as idiopathic nephrotic syndrome. However, protein may be excreted in the urine following strenuous exercise, fever, exposure to cold, or emotional stress.[278] If proteinuria is consistently present on a qualitative test, a measure of total daily protein excretion should be obtained accurately by 24-hour urine collection, if possible, or estimated from a single voided specimen.[279]

Published guidelines for periodic health examinations do not include urinalyses for asymptomatic persons.[280] Therefore, no firm recommendations can be made regarding the frequency with which UAs should be obtained. Instances in which UA is indicated include hypertension, diabetes, history of chronic use of potentially renal toxic medications, and, of course, symptoms attributable to the urinary system. As with other laboratory tests, abnormalities found initially on UA often become normal on retesting. Only if the abnormality persists should the more labor-intensive microscopic evaluation be performed. Patients with confirmed abnormal findings for which a benign explanation is not readily apparent should be referred to a nephrologist.

EKG and Chest X-Ray

Both EKG and chest x-ray have been used as routine screening tests in the past. Analyses of their effectiveness suggest that they are not useful as screening tests in asymptomatic individuals.[64,281,282]

Planning for the Future

As part of the preventive care practice, it is appropriate to counsel patients regarding certain specific issues for the future. One of these is the patient's wishes regarding the medical care she would want to have in the event that terminal debilitating medical illness interfered with her ability to make decisions for herself. Most states have "Living Will" legislation, permitting individuals to write directions concerning the level of support they would want if devastating illness should occur.[283] However, few physicians discuss these issues with patients.[284] This is a subject which must be approached delicately, to avoid creating unnecessary anxiety; patients may wonder, for example, whether the physician who raises issues of terminal care may be implying that the patient's health is failing.[285] A reassuring opening statement—for example, "It is my practice to discuss these matters with my patients well in advance, at a time when they are healthy"—may make it clear to the patient that no "hidden message" is being communicated.

Patients vary widely in their wishes regarding terminal care, but most prefer the opportunity to discuss the matter with their physicians.[284,285] A nondirective discussion, facilitating the patient's efforts to clarify her own wishes, is most helpful. The content of the discussion should be documented in the medical record.

Women are more likely than men to survive a spouse or become caretakers of an ailing spouse. Planning for the future should include a discussion of the need to prepare for such contingencies. Women whose husbands have been diagnosed to have heart disease may benefit from instruction in CPR.[286,287] Pa-

Health History

Have YOU had any of the following?

YES	NO		YES	NO	
___	___	Asthma	___	___	Cancer
___	___	Heart murmur	___	___	Liver disease, yellow
___	___	High blood pressure			jaundice, hepatitis
___	___	Mental breakdown or emotional problem	___	___	Pneumonia
___	___	Rheumatic fever	___	___	Serious injury or accident
___	___	Sugar diabetes	___	___	Thyroid gland trouble
___	___	Tuberculosis (TB)	___	___	Uncontrolled bleeding
___	___	Sexually transmitted disease (STD)	___	___	Exposure to asbestos
			___	___	Exposure to excessive sun

Obstetric History

Age periods began _____
Age periods stopped _____
Number of pregnancies _____
Number of miscarriages or lost pregnancies _____

Have you had a hysterectomy? Yes____ No____

Please list any allergies: _____

_____

Have you ever had a bad reaction to a drug? Yes____ No____

If yes, please list medication and type of reaction: _____

_____

Date of last immunization _____

Check each of the following diseases for which you have received immunization at any time in the past:

Polio ___ Tetanus ___ Diphtheria ___ Measles ___ Mumps ___ Pneumonia ___ Flu ___

Family Health History   **Hospitalizations**

Family Member	Birth Year	Health (if living)	Cause of death (if deceased)	Date	Location	Reason for hospitalization
Mother						
Father						
Brothers/sisters (Please List)						
Children (Please List)						

Habits:

	Now	Ever
Smoking Cigarettes	___	___
Other (Cigars etc)	___	___

Number of years smoked _____
Daily amount smoked _____

Alcohol (Please circle)
Beer   Wine   Other Liquors   None

Amount per week _____

Figure 6.4 Form for initial health history.

Annual Health Questionnaire

1. Do you have any of the following symptoms?

	Yes	No
Changes in eyesight	—	—
Trouble with hearing	—	—
Cough	—	—
Shortness of breath	—	—
Chest Pain	—	—
Frequent Indigestion	—	—
Fequent nausea	—	—
Bowel habit change	—	—
Vaginal bleeding	—	—
Other bleeding	—	—
Skin problem	—	—
Lack of energy	—	—
Memory trouble	—	—

2. Do you have any of the following problems?

	Yes	No
Heart disease	—	—
Diabetes	—	—
High blood pressure	—	—
Cancer	—	—
Asthma or breathing problem	—	—

Other _____

3. Current medications:

    _____   _____
    _____   _____

4. Have you been hospitalized in the past year? yes___ no___
   If yes, state reason_____

5. Immunizations:

Date of your last tetanus (DT) shot _____

Have you had a flu shot?   Yes___   No___

    If yes, date _____

Have you had a pnuemovax shot (immunization against pneumonia)?

    Yes___   No___

    If yes, date _____

Have you had any bad reactions to medications in the past year?

    Yes___   No___

If yes, please give details:_____

Figure 6.5 Form for annual updating of health history.

Table 6.10 Summary of Recommendations

Average-risk patient

Under age 40
  Annual:
    Blood pressure, weight, and pulse measurements
    Updating of medical history
    Review of symptoms and immunization status
    Immunizations as indicated
  Additional recommendations:
    PAP testing*

Age 40-49
  Annual:
    Blood pressure, weight, and pulse measurements
    Updating of medical history
    Review of symptoms and immunization status
    Immunizations as indicated
  Additional recommendations:
    PAP testing*
    Eye examination every 5 years
  Controversial:
    Mammography[†]

Age 50-64
  Annual:
    Blood pressure, weight, and pulse measurements
    Updating of medical history
    Review of symptoms and immunization status
    Immunizations as indicated
    Hearing testing as indicated
    Mammography
    Occult blood testing of stool
    Laboratory: TSH and UA; creatinine if taking medications
  Additional recommendations
    PAP testing*
    Eye examination every 5 years
  Controversial:
    Flexible sidmoidoscopy screening[‡]

Age 65 and Over
  Annual:
    Blood pressure, weight, and pulse measurements
    Updating of medical history
    Review of symptoms and immunization status
    Flu vaccine; other immunizations as indicated
    Hearing testing as indicated
    Mammography
    Occult blood testing of stool
    Laboratory: TSH and UA; creatinine if taking medications
  Additional recommendations:
    PAP testing*
    Eye examination every 5 years
  Controversial:
    Flexible sigmoidoscopy screening[‡]

Table 6.10 (*continued*)

Risk factor	Patient at increased risk See discussion under
Smoking	*Life-style (Smoking)*
Excessive sun exposure	*Skin Cancer*
Gestational diabetes	*Diabetes Mellitus*
Obesity	*Cardiovascular Disease; Breast Cancer; Life-style (Nutrition); Diabetes Mellitus*
Family history of:	
Early heart disease	*Cardiovascular Disease*
Cancer	*Breast and Colon Cancer; Family Cancer Syndrome*
Osteoporosis	*Osteoporosis*
Diabetes	*Diabetes Mellitus*

* See Chapter 11.
† See discussion under *Breast Cancer*.
‡ See discussion under *Colon Cancer*.

tients should be aided in identifying support groups which will help them to cope with the stresses of their husband's illness.[288] A patient with an ailing spouse should be urged to obtain periodic relief from the role of caretaker.

Summary Guide to Preventive Health Care of Older Women

Recommendations for routine screening in different age groups are summarized in Table 6.10. Forms such as those shown in Figures 6.4 and 6.5 can be helpful in obtaining initial medical history at a patient's first visit, and in annual updating. Areas of controversy are noted, with references to discussions in the text of this chapter. Discussions of specific high-risk groups and of counseling for life-style changes are also referenced.

References

1. Gordon T, Sorlie P, Kannel WB: Coronary heart disease, atherothrombotic brain infarction, intermittent claudication—A multivariate analysis of some factors related to their incidence: Framingham study, 16-year follow-up. Washington, D.C., Section 27, U.S. Government Printing Office, 1971.
2. Blair SN, Kohl HW, Paffenbarger RS, Clark DG, Cooper KH, Gibbons LW: Physical fitness and all-cause mortality. *JAMA* 1989;262:2395–2401.
3. Beard CM, Kottke TE, Annegers JF, Ballard DJ: The Rochester coronary heart disease project. *Mayo Clin Proc* 1989;64:1471–1480.
4. Chronic disease reports: Mortality trends 1979–1986. *MMWR* 1989;38:189–193.
5. Ostfeld AM: A review of stroke epidemiology. *Epidem Rev* 1980;2:136–152.
6. Roehmholdt ME, Palumbo PJ, Whisnant JP, Elveback LR: Transient ischemic attack and stroke in a community-based diabetic cohort. *Mayo Clin Proc* 1983;58:56–58.
7. Friedman GP, Loveland DB, Ehrlich SP: Relationship of stroke to other cardiovascular disease. *Circulation* 1968;38:533–541.

8. Herman B, Schmitz PIM, Leyton ACM, et al: Multivariate logistic analysis of risk factors for stroke in Tilburg, the Netherlands. *Am J Epid* 1983;118:514–525.
9. Applegate WB: Hypertension in elderly patients. *Ann Intern Med* 1989;110:901–915.
10. Epstein FH: The epidemiology of hypertension, in Robertson, JLS (ed.): *Handbook of Hypertension*. New York, Elsevier, 1983.
11. Rowland M, Roberts J: Blood pressure levels and hypertension in persons aged 6–74: United States 1976–1980. Washington, D.C., U.S. Department of Health and Human Services, publication PHS 82-1250.
12. The 1988 report of the joint national committee in detection, evaluation, and treatment of high blood pressure. *Arch Intern Med* 1988;148:1023–1038.
13. Perloff D, Sokolow M, Cowan R: The prognostic value of ambulatory blood pressures. *JAMA* 1983;249:1792–1798.
14. Floras JS, Hassan MO, Sever PS, Jones JV, Osikowska B, Sleight P: Cuff and ambulatory blood pressures in subjects with essential hypertension. *Lancet* 1981;2:107–109.
15. Hebert PR, Fiebach NH, Eberlein KA, Taylor JO, Hennekens CH: The community-based randomized trials of pharmacologic treatment of mild-to-moderate hypertension. *Am J Epidemiol* 1988;127:581–590.
16. Hennekens CH: Benefits of treatment of mild to moderate hypertension. *J Gen Intern Med* 1987;2:438–441.
17. MacGregor GA, Markanda ND, Sagnella GA, Singer DRJ, Capupuccio FP: Double blind study of the sodium intakes and long-term effects of sodium restriction in essential hypertension. *Lancet* 1989;2:1244–1247.
18. Pickering TG, Harshfield GA, Kleinert HD, Blank S, Laragh JH: Blood pressure during normal daily activities, sleep and exercise. *JAMA* 1982;247:992–996.
19. Porter G: Chronology of the sodium hypothesis and hypertension. *Ann Intern Med* 1983;98:720–723.
20. Kaplan NM: Maximally reducing cardiovascular risk in the treatment of hypertension. *Ann Intern Med* 1988;109:36–40.
21. Gruchow HW, Sobocinski KA, Barboriak JJ: Alcohol, nutrient intake, and hypertension in U.S. adults. *JAMA* 1985;253:1567–1570.
22. Kahw K-T, Barrett-Connor E: Dietary potassium and stroke-associated mortality. *N Engl J Med* 1987;316:235–240.
23. Tuck ML, Sowers J, Dornfield L, Kledzik G, Maxwell M: The effect of weight reduction on blood pressure, plasma activity, and plasma aldosterone levels in obese patients. *N Engl J Med* 1981;304:930–933.
24. Blair SN, Goodyear NN, Gibbons LW, Cooper KH: Physical fitness and incidence of hypertension in healthy normotensive men and women. *JAMA* 1984;252:487–490.
25. Benson H: Systemic hypertension and the relaxation response. *N Engl J Med* 1977;296:1152–1156.
26. Agras WS: Relaxation therapy in hypertension. *Hosp Pract* 1983;May:129–137.
27. Curb JD, Borhari NO, Blaszkowski TP, Zimbaldi N, Fotiu S, Williams W: Long-term surveillance for adverse effects of antihypertensive drugs. *JAMA* 1985;253:3263–3268.
28. McClellan WM, Hall WD, Brogan D, Miles C, Wilber JA: Continuity of care in hypertension. *Arch Intern Med* 1988;48:525–528.
29. Fielding JE: Smoking: Health effects and control. *N Engl J Med* 1985;313:491–498.
30. Petitti D, Wingerd J: Use of oral contraceptives, cigarette smoking, and risk of subarachnoid hemorrhage. *Lancet* 1978;2:234–235.
31. Abbott RD, Wilson PWF, Kannel WB, Castelli WP: High density lipoprotein cholesterol, total cholesterol screening and myocardial infarction: The Framingham study. *Arteriosclerosis* 1988;8;207–211.
32. Rifkind BM, Segal P: Lipid Research Clinics Program reference values for hyperlipidemia and hypolipidemia. *JAMA* 1983;250:1869–1872.

33. Lipid Research Clinics Program. The lipid research clinics coronary primary prevention trials result: I. Reduction in the incidence of coronary heart disease. *JAMA* 1984;251:351–364.
34. Frick MH, et al: Helsinki heart study: primary prevention trial with gemfibrizol in middle-aged men with dyslipidemia. *N Engl J Med* 1987;317:1237–1245.
35. Canner PL, et al: Fifteen year mortality in the coronary drug project: Long term benefits with niacin. *J Am Coll Cardiol* 1986;8:1245–1255.
36. Garber AM, Sox HC, Littenberg B: Screening asymptomatic adults for cardiac risk factors: The serum cholesterol level. *Ann Intern Med* 1989;110:622–639.
37. Garber AM: Where to draw the line against cholesterol. *Ann Intern Med* 1989;3:625–627.
38. Brett AS: Treating hypercholesterolemia: How should practicing physicians interpret the published data for patients? *N Engl J Med* 1989;321:676–680.
39. Leaf A: Management of hypercholesterolemia: Are preventive interventions advisable? *N Engl J Med* 1989;321:680–684.
40. Report of the National Cholesterol Education Expert Panel on detection, evaluation, and treatment of high blood cholesterol in adults. *Arch Intern Med* 1988;148:36–69.
41. Basinski A, Frank JW, Naylor CD, Rachlis MM: Detection and management of asymptomatic hypercholesterolemia: A policy document by the Toronto Working Group on Cholesterol Policy. Toronto, Ontario Ministry of Health, 1989.
42. College of American Pathologists: Comprehensive Chemistry 1987 Survey. College of American Psychologists, Skokie, Illinois, 1987.
43. Motulsky AG: Genetic research in coronary heart disease, in *Genetic Epidemiology of Coronary Heart Disease: Past, Present and Future.* New York, Alan R. Liss, 1984, pp 541–548.
44. Nora JS, Lortscher RH, Spangler RD, Nora AH, Kimberling JH: Genetic-epidemiologic study of early onset schenic heart disease. *Circulation* 1980;61:503–508.
45. Goldstein JL, Brown MS: Familial hypercholesterolemia, in Stanbury JB et al (eds.): *The Metabolic Basis of Inherited Disease.* New York, McGraw-Hill, 1983.
46. Tenkate LP, Boman H, Daiger SP, Motulsky AM: Familial aggregation of coronary heart disease and its relation to known genetic risk factors. *Am J Cardiol* 1982;50:945–953.
47. Snowden CB, McNamara PM, Garrison RJ, Feinleib M, Kannell WB, Epstein FH: Predicting coronary heart disease in siblings: A multivariate assessment. *Am J Epidemiol* 1982;115:217–222.
48. Hopkins PN, Williams RR, Hunt SC: Magnified risks from cigarette smoking for coronary prone families in Utah. *West J Med* 1984;141:196–202.
49. Khaw K-T, Barrett-Connor E: Family history of heart attack: A modifiable risk factor? *Circulation* 1986;74:239–244.
50. Harris, Caspersen CJ, DeFriese GH, Estes EH: Physical activity counseling for healthy adults as a primary preventive intervention in the clinical setting. *JAMA* 1989;261:3590–3598.
51. Hubert HB, Feinleib M, McNamara PM, Castelli WP: Obesity as an independent risk factor for cardiovascular disease: A 26-year follow-up of participants in the Framingham Heart Study. *Circulation* 1983;67:968–977.
52. Barrett-Connor EL: Obesity, atherosclerosis, and coronary artery disease. *Ann Intern Med* 1985;103:1010–1019.
53. Bray GA, Bouchard C: Role of fat distribution during growth and its relationship to health. *Am J Clin Nutrition* 1988;47:551–552.
54. Lapidus L, Bengtsson C, Larsson B, Pennert K, Rybo E, Sjostrom L: Distribution of adipose tissue and risk of cardiovascular disease and death: A 12 year follow-up of participants in the population study of women in Gothenburg, Sweden. *Br J Med* 1984;289:1257–1261.
55. Barrett-Connor E, Khaw K-T: Cigarette smoking and increased central obesity. *Ann Intern Med* 1989;111:783–787.

56. Peiris AN, Sothmann MS, Hoffmann RG, et al: Adiposity, fat distribution, and cardiovascular risk. *Ann Intern Med* 1989;110:867–872.
57. Silverberg E, Boring CC, Squires TS: Cancer statistics, 1990. *CA: A Cancer Journal for Clinicians* 1990;40:9–26.
58. Sondik E (ed.): *Annual Cancer Statistics Review 1988*. Washington, D.C., Division of Cancer Prevention and Control, National Cancer Institute, 1989.
59. Fielding JE: Smoking and women: Tragedy of the majority. *N Engl J Med* 1987;317:1343–1345.
60. Surgeon General's 1989 Report on Reducing the Health Consequences of Smoking: 25 Years of Progress; Executive Summary. *MMWR* 1989;38(Suppl S2):1–32.
61. Fontana RS, Sanderson DR, Woolner LB, Taylor WF, Miller WE, Muhm JR: Lung cancer screening: The Mayo program. *J Occup Med* 1986;28:746–750.
62. Melamed MR, Flehinger BJ, Zaman MB, Heelan RT, Perchick WA, Nartini N: Survival and mortality from lung cancer in a screened population: The Johns Hopkins study. *Chest* 1984;86:44–53.
63. Tockman MS: Survival and mortality from lung cancer in a screened population: The Johns Hopkins study. *Chest* 1986;89(Suppl):3245–3255.
64. Eddy DM: Screening for lung cancer. *Ann Intern Med* 1989;111:232–237.
65. Paffenbarger RS, Kampert JB, Chang H: Characteristics that predict risk of breast cancer before and after the menopause. *Am J Epidem* 1980;112:258–268.
66. Choi NW, Howe GR, Miller AB, et al: An epidemiologic study of breast cancer. *Am J Epidem* 1978;107:510–521.
67. Schapira DV, Kumar NB, Lyman GH, Cox CE: Abdominal obesity and breast cancer risk. *Ann Intern Med* 1990;112:182–186.
68. Mills PK, et al: Prospective study of exogenous hormone use and breast cancer in Seventh-Day Adventists. *Cancer* 1989;64:591–597.
69. Bergkvist L, Adami H-O, Persson I, Hoover R, Schairer C: The risk of breast cancer after estrogen and estrogen-progestin replacement. *N Engl J Med* 1989;321:293–297.
70. Breast cancer and estrogen replacement (letters to the editor). *N Engl J Med* 1990;322:201–203.
71. Foster RS, Lang SP, Costanza MC, Worden JK, Haines CR, Yates JW: Breast self-examination practices and breast cancer stage. *N Engl J Med* 1978;299:265–270.
72. Eddy DM: Screening for breast cancer. *Ann Intern Med* 1989;111:389–399.
73. McGuire LB: Screening for breast cancer. *Ann Intern Med* 1989;111:858–859.
74. Mammography guidelines 1983. *CA: A Cancer Journal for Clinicians* 1983;33:255.
75. Council on Scientific Affairs: Mammographic screening in asymptomatic women aged 40 years and older. *JAMA* 1989;261:2535–2542.
76. Eddy DM, Hasselblad V, McGivney W, Hendee W: The value of mammography screening in women under age 50 years. *JAMA* 1988;259:1512–1519.
77. Chu KC, Smart CR, Tarone RE: Analysis of breast cancer and stage distribution by age for the Health Insurance Plan clerical trial. *J Natl Cancer Inst* 1988;80:1125–1132.
78. U.S. Preventive Health Task Force: Draft statement: Preventive health care recommendations, 1989.
79. Devitt JE: False alarms of breast cancer. *Lancet* 1989;2:1257–1258.
80. National Cancer Institute: *Working Guidelines for Early Cancer Detection: Rationale and Supporting Evidence to Decrease Mortality*. Bethesda, Maryland, NIH, 1987.
81. Sattin RW, Rubin GL, Webster LA, et al: Family history and the risk of breast cancer. *JAMA* 1985;253:1908–1913.
82. Anderson DE: Some characteristics of familial breast cancer. *Cancer* 1971;28:1500–1504.
83. Ottman R, King M-C, Pike M, Henderson BE: Practical guide for estimating risk for familial breast cancer. *Lancet* 1983;2:556–558.
84. Heath CW, Fink DJ: Trends in screening mammograms for women 50 years and older. *MMWR* 1989;38:137–140.

85. Brown JT, Hulka BS: Screening mammography in the elderly: A case-control study. *J Gen Int Med* 1988;3:126–131.
86. Muto T, Bussey HJR, Morson BC: The evolution of cancer of the colon and rectum. *Cancer* 1975;36:2251–2270.
87. Lipshutz GR, Katon RM, McCool MF, et al: Flexible sigmoidoscopy as a screening procedure for neoplasia of the colon. *Surg Gynecol Obstet* 1979;148:19–22.
88. Gottlieb LS, Winawer SJ, Stwernbery S, et al: National polyps study: The diminutive colonic polyp. *Gastrointest Endosc* 1984;30:143.
89. Burt RW: Polyps: An approach to large bowel cancer detection and prevention. *Can Detec Prev* 1985;8:393–398.
90. American Cancer Society: ACS report on the cancer-related health check-up. *CA* 1980;30:208–215.
91. Allison JE, Feldman R, Tekawa IS: Hemoccult screening in detecting colorectal neoplasm: Sensitivity, specificity, and predictive value. *Ann Int Med* 1990;112:328–333.
92. Simon JB: Occult blood screening for colorectal carcinoma: A critical review. *Gastroenterology* 1985;88:820–837.
93. Eddy DM: The economics of cancer detection and prevention: Getting more for less. *Cancer* 1981;47:1200–1209.
94. Brodie DR (ed.): Screening and early detection of colorectal cancer. Washington D.C., U.S. Department of Health, Education, and Welfare, NIH publication No. 80-2075, 1979, pp 1–2.
95. Crespi M, Weissman GS, Gilbertsen VA, Winawer SJ, Sherlock P: The role of proctosigmoidoscopy in screening for colorectal neoplasia. *Cancer* 1984;34:159–165.
96. Yarborough GW, Waisbren BA: The benefits of systematic fiberoptic flexible sigmoidoscopy. *Arch Intern Med* 1985;145:95–96.
97. Ow CL, Lemar HJ, Weaver MJ: Does screening proctosigmoidoscopy result in reduced mortality from colorectal cancer? *J Gen Int Med* 1989;4:209–215.
98. Friedman GD, Collen MF, Fireman BH: Multiphasic health checkup evaluation: A 16-year follow-up. *J Chron Dis* 1986;39:453–463.
99. Family history information enables physicians to recognize genetically "at-risk" patients. *JAMA* 1980;243:19–20.
100. Li FP, Fraumeni JF: Prospective study of a family cancer syndrome. *JAMA* 1982;247:2692–2694.
101. Lynch HT, Follett KL, Lynch PM, Albano WA, Mailliard JL, Pierson RL: Family history in an oncology clinic. *JAMA* 1979;242:1268–1272.
102. Winawer SJ, Miller DG, Sherlock P: Risk and screening for colorectal cancer. *Adv Int Med* 1984;30:471–496.
103. Campbell S, Bhan V, Royston P, Whitehead MJ, Collins WP: Transabdominal ultrasound screening for early ovarian cancer. *BMJ* 1989;299:1363–1367.
104. Kopf AW, Rigel DS, Friedman RJ: The rising incidence and mortality rate of malignant melanoma. *J Dermatol Surg Onc* 1982;8:760–761.
105. Lee JAH: The rising incidence of cutaneous malignant melanoma. *Am J Dermatopath* 1985;7(Supp):35–39.
106. Elwood JM, Gallagher RP, Hill GB, Spinelli JJ, Pearson JCG, Threlfall N: Pigmentation and skin reaction to sun as risk factors for cutaneous melanoma: Western Canada melanoma study. *Brit Med J* 1984;288:99–102.
107. National Institutes of Health Consensus Development Conference Statement: Precursors to malignant melanoma. *J Am Acad Derm* 1984;10:683–688.
108. Lew RA, Sober AJ, Cook N, Marvell R, Fitzpatrick TB: Sun exposure habits in patients with cutaneous melanoma. *J Dermat Surg Onc* 1983;9:981–986.
109. Green A, Siskind V, Bain C, Alexander J: Sunburn and malignant melanoma. *Br J Cancer* 1985;41:393–397.
110. Cassileth BR, Temostok L, Frederick BE, et al: Patient and physician delay in melanoma diagnosis. *J Am Acad Derm* 1988;18:591–598.

111. Greene MH, Clark WH, Tucker MA, Kraemer KH, Elder DE, Fraser MC: High risk of melanoma in melanoma-prone families with dysplastic nevi. *Ann Intern Med* 1985;102:458–465.
112. Fitzpatrick TB, Sober AJ: Sunlight and skin cancer. *N Engl J Med* 1985;313:818–819.
113. Center for Disease Control: Tetanus—United States, 1985–1986. *MMWR* 1987;36:477–481.
114. Center for Disease Control: Tetanus—United States, 1987 and 1988. *MMWR* 1990;39:37–41.
115. U.S. Department of Health and Human Services: *Health Information for International Travel 1989*. Washington, D.C., Public Health Service Centers for Disease Control, HHS publication no. (CDC) 89-8280, 1989, pp 110–112.
116. Nkowane BM, Wassilak SGF, Orenstein WA, et al: Vaccine-associated paralytic poliomyelitis—United States: 1973 through 1984. *JAMA* 1987;257:1335–1340.
117. Immunization Practices Advisory Committee (ACIP): Poliomyelitis prevention: Enhanced-potency inactivated poliomyelitis vaccine—Supplementary statement. *MMWR* 1988;36:795–798.
118. U.S. Department of Health and Human Services: *Health Information for International Travel 1989*. Washington, D.C., Public Health Service Centers for Disease Control, HHS publication no. (CDC) 89-8280, 1989, pp 103–105.
119. Lui KJ, Kendal AP: Impact of influenza epidemics on mortality in the United States from October 1972 to May 1985. *Am J Public Health* 1987;77:712–716.
120. Center for Disease Control: Pneumonia and influenza mortality—United States, 1988–89 season. *MMWR* 1989;38:97.
121. Patriarca PA, Weber JA, Parker RA, et al: Efficacy of influenza vaccine in nursing homes: Reduction in illness and complications during an influenza A(H3N2) epidemic. *JAMA* 1985;253:1136–1139.
122. Riddiough MA, Sisk JE, Bell JC: Influenza vaccination: Cost-effectiveness and public policy. *JAMA* 1983;249:3189–3195.
123. Douglas RD: Prophylaxis and treatment of influenza. *N Engl J Med* 1990;322:443–450.
124. Hayden FG, Belshe RB, Clover RD, Hay AJ, Oakes MG, Soo W: Emergence and apparent transmission of rimantadine-resistant influenza A virus in families. *N Engl J Med* 1989;321:1696–1702.
125. Immunization Practices Advisory Committee: Update: Pneumococcal polysaccharide vaccine usage—United States. *MMWR* 1984;33:273–276, 281.
126. Williams WW, Hickson MA, Kane MA, Kendal AP, Spika JS, Hinman AR: Immunization policies and vaccine coverage among adults: The risk for missed opportunities. *Ann Intern Med* 1988;108:616–625.
127. Burman LA, Norrby R, Trollfors B: Invasive pneumococcal infections: Incidence, predisposing factors and prognosis. *Reviews of Infectious Diseases* 1985;7:133–142.
128. Hook EW III, Horton CA, Schaberg DR: Failure of intensive care unit support to influence mortality from pneumococcal bacteremia. *JAMA* 1983;249:1055–1057.
129. LaForce FM, Eickhoff TC: Pneumococcal vaccine: The evidence mounts. *Ann Intern Med* 1986;104:110–112.
130. Mufson MA, Krause HE, Schiffman G: Long-term persistence of antibody following immunization with pneumococcal polysaccharide vaccine. *Proc Soc Exp Biol Med* 1983;173:270–275.
131. Mufson MA, Krause HE, Schiffman G, Hughey DF: Pneumococcal antibody levels one decade after immunization of healthy adults. *Am J Med Sci* 1987;193:279–284.
132. Sims RV, Steinmann WC, McConville JH, King LR, Zwick WC, Schwartz JS: The cost-effectiveness of pneumococcal vaccine in the elderly. *Ann Intern Med* 1988;108:653–657.
133. Immunization Practices Advisory Committee: Pneumococcal polysaccharide vaccine. *MMWR* 1989;38:64–68,73–76.

134. Kaplan J, Sarnaik S, Schiffman G: Revaccination with polyvalent pneumococcal vaccine in children with sickle cell anemia. *Am J Pediatr Hematol Oncol* 1986;8:80–82.
135. Lawrence EM, Edwards KM, Schiffman G, Thompson JM, Vaughn WK, Wright PF: Pneumococcal vaccine in normal children. *Am J Dis Child* 1983;137:846–850.
136. Lowman EW: Osteoarthritis. *JAMA* 1955;157:487–488.
137. Roberts J, Burch TA: Prevalence of osteoarthritis in adults by age, sex, race, and geographic area, United States—1960–1962. National Center for Health Statistics: Vital and health statistics: data from the national health survey. U.S. Public Health Service, document no. 1000, Series 11, no. 15. Washington, D.C., U.S. Government Printing Office, 1966.
138. Moskowitz RW: Primary osteoarthritis: Epidemiology, clinical aspects, and general management. *Am J Med* 1987;83(Suppl 5A):5–10.
139. Goldin RH, McAdam L, Louie JS, Gold R, Bluestone R: Clinical and radiological survey of the incidence of osteoarthritis among obese patients. *Ann Rheum Dis* 1976;35:349–353.
140. Leach RE, Baumgard SS, Broom J: Obesity: Its relationship to osteoarthritis of the knee. *Clin Orthop* 1973;93:271–273.
141. Consensus Conference: Osteoporosis. *JAMA* 1984;252:799–802.
142. Mazess RB: On aging bone loss. *Clin Orthop* 1982;165:239–252.
143. Williams AR, Weiss NS, Ure CL, Ballard J, Daling JR: Effect of weight, smoking, and estrogen use on the risk of hip and forearm fractures in postmenopausal women. *Obstet Gynecol* 1982;60:695–699.
144. Daniell HW: Osteoporosis of the slender smoker: Vertebral compression fractures and loss of metacarpal cortex in relation to postmenopausal cigarette smoking and lack of obesity. *Arch Intern Med* 1976;136:298–304.
145. Bickle DD, Genant HK, Cann C, Recker RR, Halloran BP, Strewler GJ: Bone disease in alcohol abuse. *Ann Intern Med* 1985;103:42–48.
146. Richelson LS, Wabner HW, Melton LJ III, Riggs BL: Relative contributions of aging and estrogen deficiency to postmenopausal bone loss. *N Engl J Med* 1984;311:1273–1275.
147. Newcomer AD, Hodgson SF, McGill DB, Thomas PJ: Lactase deficiency: Prevalence in osteoporosis. *Ann Intern Med* 1978;89:218–220.
148. Riggs BL, Melton LJ III: Involutional osteoporosis. *N Engl J Med* 1986;314:1676–1686.
149. Mazess RB: The noninvasive measurement of skeletal mass, in Peck WA (ed.): *Bone and Mineral Research Annual*, vol. 1. Amsterdam, Excerpta Medica, 1983, pp 223–279.
150. Hall FM, Davis MA, Baran DT: Bone mineral screening for osteoporosis. *N Engl J Med* 1987;316:212–214.
151. Cummings SR: Are patients with hip fracture more osteoporotic? *Am J Med* 1985;78:487–494.
152. Cummings SR, Black D: Should perimenopausal women be screened for osteoporosis? *Ann Intern Med* 1986;104:817–823.
153. Ettinger B, Genant HK, Cann CE: Long-term estrogen replacement therapy prevents bone loss and fractures. *Ann Intern Med* 1985;102:319–324.
154. Nordic BEC, Horsman A, Crilly RG, Marshall DH, Simpson M: Treatment of spinal osteoporosis in postmenopausal women. *Br Med J* 1980;280:451–454.
155. Goldbloom R, Battista RN: The periodic health examination: 1. Introduction. *Can Med Assoc J* 1988;138:617–618.
156. Ettinger B, Genant HK, Cann CE: Postmenopausal bone loss is prevented by treatment with low-dosage estrogen with calcium. *Ann Intern Med* 1987;106:40–45.
157. Shapiro S, Kelly JP, Rosenberg L, et al: Risk of localized and widespread endometrial cancer in relation to recent and discontinued use of conjugated estrogens. *N Engl J Med* 1985;313:969–972.
158. Pritchard KI: Screening for endometrial cancer: Is it effective? *Ann Intern Med* 1989;110:177–178.

159. Luciano AA, Turksoy RN, Carleo J: Clinical and metabolic responses of menopausal women to sequential vs. continuous estrogen and progestin therapy. *Obstet Gynecol* 1988;71:39–43.
160. Ferguson KJ, Hoegh C, Johnson S: Estrogen replacement therapy: A survey of women's knowledge and attitudes. *Arch Intern Med* 1989;149:133–136.
161. Magos AL, Brincal M, Studd JWW, Wardle P, Schlesinger P, O'Dowd T: Amenorrhea and endometrial atrophy with continuous oral estrogen and progestin therapy in postmenopausal women. *Obstet Gynecol* 1985;65:496–499.
162. Weinstein L: Efficacy of a continuous estrogen-progestin regimen in the menopausal patient. *Obstet Gynecol* 1987;69:929–932.
163. Hirvonen E, Malkonen M, Manninen V: Effects of different progestogens on lipoproteins during postmenopausal replacement therapy. *N Engl J Med* 1981;304:560–563.
164. Ross RK, Paganini-Hill A, Mack TM, Arthur M, Henderson BE: Menopausal estrogen therapy and protection from death from ischaemic heart disease. *Lancet* 1981;1:858–860.
165. Sullivan JM, Zwaag RV, Lemp GF, et al: Postmenopausal estrogen use and coronary atherosclerosis. *Ann Intern Med* 1988;108:358–363.
166. Colditz GA, Willett WC, Stampfer MJ, Rosner B, Speitzer FE, Hennekens CH: Menopause and the risk of coronary heart disease in women. *N Engl J Med* 1987;316:1105–1110.
167. Bush TL, Cowan LD, Barrett-Connor E, et al: Estrogen use and all-cause mortality: Preliminary results from the lipid research clinics program follow-up study. *JAMA* 1983;249:903–906.
168. Lufkin EG: Estrogen replacement therapy: Current recommendations. *Mayo Clin Proc* 1988;63:453–460.
169. Aloia JF, Vaswani AN, Yeh JK, Cohn SH: Premenopausal bone mass is related to physical activity. *Arch Intern Med* 1988;148:121–123.
170. Krolne B, Toft B, Nielsen PS, Tondevold E: Physical exercise as prophylaxis against involutional vertebral bone loss: A controlled trial. *Clin Sci* 1983;64:541–546.
171. Dalsky GP, Stocke KS, Ehsani AA, Slatopolsky E, Lee WC, Birge SJ: Weight-bearing exercise training and lumbar bone mineral content in postmenopausal women. *Ann Intern Med* 1988;108:824–828.
172. Simonen O, Laitinen O: Does fluoridation of drinking water prevent bone fragility and osteoporosis? *Lancet* 1985;2:432–433.
173. Riggs BL, Hodgson SE, O'Fallon WM, et al: Effect of fluoride treatment on the fracture rate in postmenopausal women with osteoporosis. *N Engl J Med* 1990;322:802–809.
174. National Society to Prevent Blindness: Vision problems in the U.S. Data analysis, 1980.
175. Phelps CD: Glaucoma: General concepts, in Duane TD (ed.): *Clinical Ophthalmology* vol. 3. Philadelphia, Lippincott, 1988, ch. 42, pp 1–8.
176. Bengtsson B: The prevalence of glaucoma. *Br J Ophthalmol* 1981;65:46–49.
177. Phelps CD: Examination and functional evaluation of crystalline lens, in Duane TD (ed.): *Clinical Ophthalmology*, vol. 1. Philadelphia, Lippincott, 1988, ch. 72, pp 1–23.
178. Luntz MH: Clinical types of cataract, in Duane TD (ed.): *Clinical Ophthalmology*, vol. 1. Philadelphia, Lippincott, 1988, ch. 73, pp 1–20.
179. Olson L: Anatomy and embryology of the lens, in Duane TD (ed.): *Clinical Ophthalmology*, vol. 1. Philadelphia, Lippincott, 1988, ch. 71, pp 1–52.
180. Katz M: The human eye as an optical system, in Duane TD (ed.): *Clinical Ophthalmology*, vol. 1. Philadelphia, Lippincott, 1988, ch. 33, pp 1–52.
181. Gates GA, Caspary DM, Clark W, Pillsbury HC, Brown SC, Dobie RA: Presbycusis. *Otolaryngol Head Neck Surg* 1989;100:266–271.
182. Dawson DA, Adams PF: National Center for Health Statistics. Current estimates from

the Health Interview Surgery, United States, 1986. Vital and Health Statistics Series 10, no. 164, DHHS publication no. (PHS) 87-1592. Washington, D.C., U.S. Department of Health and Human Services, 1987.
183. Peterson FT: Accuracy of a 40 dB HL audioscope and audiometer screening for adults. *Ear Hear* 1987;8:180–183.
184. Snyder JM: Office audiometry. *J Fam Pract* 1984;19:535–548.
185. Uhlmann RF, Rees TS, Psaty BM, Duckert LG: Validity and reliability of auditory screening tests in demented and nondemented older adults. *J Gen Intern Med* 1989;4:90–96.
186. ASHA Committee on Audiometric Evaluation: Guidelines for determining the threshold level for speech. *ASHA* 1979;21:353–356.
187. American Academy of Otolaryngology—Head and Neck Surgery: *Five Minute Hearing Test*. Washington, D.C., 1989.
188. Hatton ER, Cogan CM, Hatton MN: Common oral conditions in the elderly. *AFP* 1989;40:149–162.
189. Mashberg A, Barsa P: Screening for oral and oropharyngeal squamous carcinomas. *Cancer* 1984;34:262–268.
190. Blazer D: Depression in the elderly. *N Engl J Med* 1989;320:164–166.
191. American Psychiatric Association: *Diagnostic and Statistical Manual of Mental Disorder*, ed. 3. Washington, D.C., American Psychiatric Association, 1980.
192. Mortimer JA: Alzheimer's disease and senile dementia: Prevalence and incidence, in Reisberg B (ed.): *Alzheimer's Disease: The Standard Reference*. New York, Free Press, 1983.
193. Blessed G, Tomlinson BE, Roth M: The association between quantitative measures of dementia and of senile change in the cerebral grey matter of elderly subjects. *Br J Psychiatry* 1968;114:796–811.
194. Lishman WA: Cerebral disorder in alcoholism: Syndromes of impairment. *Brain* 1981;104:1–20.
195. Perry EK, Curtis M, Dick DJ, et al: Cholinergic correlates of cognitive impairments in Parkinson's disease: Comparisons with Alzheimer's disease. *J Neurol Neurosurg Psychiatry* 1985;48:413–421.
196. Larson EB, Reifler BV, Featherstone HJ, English DR: Dementia in elderly outpatients: A prospective study. *Ann Intern Med* 1984;100:417–423.
197. Clarfeld AM: The reversible dementias: Do they reverse? *Ann Intern Med* 1988;109:476–486.
198. Strachan RW, Henderson JG: Psychiatric syndromes due to avitaminosis B12 with normal blood and bone marrow. *QJ Med* 1965;34:303–309.
199. Folstein MF, Folstein SE, McHugh PR: Mini-mental state: A practical method for grading the cognitive state of patients for the clinician. *J Psychiatr Res* 1975;12:189–198.
200. U.S. Department of Health and Human Services: The health consequences of smoking: Cardiovascular disease. Rockville, Maryland, 1983.
201. U.S. Department of Health and Human Services: The health consequences of smoking: Cancer. Rockville, Maryland, 1982.
202. U.S. Department of Health and Human Services: The health consequences of smoking: COPD. Rockville, Maryland, 1984.
203. State-specific estimates of smoking attributable mortality and years of potential life lost—United States 1985. *MMWR* 1988;37:689–692.
204. Paulozzi L: The costs of smoking for Washington. *Wash Morb Rep* 1984;1:4.
205. Friedman GD, Petitti DB, Bawol RD, Siegelaub AB: Mortality in cigarette smokers and quitters. *N Engl J Med* 1981;304:1407–1410.
206. Smoking and cardiovascular disease. *MMWR* 1984;32:677–679.
207. Willet WC, Green A, Stampfer MJ, et al: Relative and absolute excess risks of coronary heart disease among women who smoke cigarettes. *N Engl J Med* 1987;317:1303–1309.

208. Rosenberg L, Palmer JR, Shapiro S: Decline in the risk of myocardial infarction among women who stop smoking. *N Engl J Med* 1990;322:213–217.
209. Rogers RL: Abstention from cigarette smoking improves cerebral perfusion among elderly chronic smokers. *J Am Med Assoc* 1985;253:2970–2974.
210. Neighbor WE: The physician's role in smoking cessation. *UW Medicine* 1989;15:22–24.
211. Pederson LL: Compliance with physician advice to quit smoking: A review of the literature. *Prev Med* 1982;11:71–84.
212. Ockene JK: Smoking intervention: The expanding role of the physician. *Am J Pub Health* 1987;77:782–783.
213. Greene HL, Goldberg RJ, Ockene JK: Cigarette smoking: The physician's role in cessation and maintenance. *J Gen Intern Med* 1988;3:75–87.
214. Risser NL, Belcher DW: Adding spirometry, carbon monoxide and pulmonary symptom results to smoking cessation counselling: A randomized trial. *J Gen Intern Med* 1989;5:16–22.
215. U.S. Preventive Services Task Force: Recommendations for physical exercise in primary prevention. *JAMA* 1989;261:3588–3589.
216. Harris SS, Caspersen CJ, DeFriese GH, Estes EH: Physical activity counseling for healthy adults as a primary preventive intervention in the clinical setting. *JAMA* 1989;261:3590–3598.
217. Sorock GS, Bush TL, Golden AL, Fried LP, Breuer B, Hale WE: Physical activity and fracture risk in a free-living elderly cohort. *J Gerontol* 1988;43:M134–139.
218. Koplon JP, Caspersen CJ, Powell KE: Physical activity, physical fitness and health: Time to act. *JAMA* 1989;262:2347.
219. Surgeon General's Workshop on Health Promotion and Aging: Summary recommendations of the physical fitness and exercise working group. *MMWR* 1989;38:700–707.
220. The President's Council on Physical Fitness and Sports: Progress toward achieving the 1990 national objectives for physical fitness and exercise. *MMWR* 1989;38:449–453.
221. Gotto AM, Scott LW, Foreyt JP: Diet and health. *West J Med* 1984;141:872–877.
222. Worthington-Roberts B: Diet and health. *UW Medicine* 1989;15:13–17.
223. U.S. Department of Health and Human Services, Public Health Service: *The Surgeon General's Report on Nutrition and Health*. Superintendent of Documents, Washington D.C., U.S. Government Printing Office, 1988.
224. Committee on Diet and Health: *Diet and Health: Executive Summary*. Washington D.C., National Academy Press, 1989.
225. Food and Nutrition Board, National Research Council: *Recommended Dietary Allowances*, ed. 10. Washington D.C., National Academy Press, 1989.
226. Calcium Supplements. *Med Lett* 1989;31:101–103.
227. Pennington JAT, Church HN: *Bowes and Church's Food Values of Portions Commonly Used*, ed. 13. New York, Harper & Row, 1980.
228. Gebhardt SF, Mathews RH: *Nutritive Value of Foods*. Washington, D.C., U.S. Department of Agriculture, U.S. Government Printing Office, 1981.
229. Brody JE: Changing nutritional needs put the elderly at risk because of inadequate diets. *New York Times*, February 8, 1990, p B7.
230. Andres R: Mortality and obesity: The rationale for age-specific height-weight tables, in Andres R, Bierman EL, Hazzard WR (eds.): *Priniciples of Geriatric Medicine*. New York, McGraw-Hill, 1985.
231. Bloom BS: Risk and cost of gastrointestinal side effects associated with nonsteroidal anti-inflammatory drugs. *Arch Intern Med* 1989;149:1019–1022.
232. Sandler DP, Smith JC, Weinberg CR, et al: Analgesic use and chronic renal disease. *N Engl J Med* 1989;320:1238–1243.
233. Friedman GD, Goldberg M, Ahuja JN, Siegelaub AB, Bassis ML, Collen MI: Biochem-

ical screening tests: Effect of panel size on medical care. *Arch Intern Med* 1972;129:91–97.
234. Cebul RD, Beck JR: Biochemical profiles. *Ann Intern Med* 1987;106:403–413.
235. Canadian Task Force on the Periodic Health Examination: The periodic health examination. *Can Med Assoc J* 1979;121:1193–1254.
236. Medical Practice Committee, American College of Physicians: Periodic health examination: A guide for designing individualized preventive health care in the asymptomatic patient. *Ann Intern Med* 1981;95:729–732.
237. Harris MI, Hadden WC, Knowler WC, Bennett PH: Prevalence of diabetes and impaired glucose tolerance and plasma glucose levels in US population aged 20–24 years. *Diabetes* 1987;36:523–534.
238. Kaplan SE, Lippe BM, Brinkman CR, Davidson MB, Geffner ME: Diabetes mellitus. *Ann Intern Med* 1982;96:635–649.
239. Rotter SI, Vadheim CM: Diabetes mellitus, in King RA, Rotter JI, Motulsky AG (eds.): *The Genetic Basis of Common Disease*. New York, Oxford University Press, 1990. In press.
240. Singer DE, Samet JH, Coley CM, Nathan DM: Screening for diabetes mellitus. *Ann Intern Med* 1988;109:639–649.
241. Bennett PH, Knowler WC: Early detection and intervention in diabetes mellitus: Is it effective? *J Chronic Dis* 1984;37:653–666.
242. National Diabetes Data Group: Classification and diagnosis of diabetes mellitus and other categories of glucose tolerance. *Diabetes* 1979;28:1039–1057.
243. Morris LR, McGee JA, Kitabachi AE: Correlation between plasma and urine glucose in diabetes. *Ann Intern Med* 1981;94:469–471.
244. Davidson MB: The effect of aging on carbohydrate metabolism: A review of the English literature and a practical approach to the diagnosis of diabetes mellitus in the elderly. *Progress in Endocrinology and Metabolism* 1979;28:688–705.
245. Expert Committee on Diabetes Mellitus, World Health Organization: *WHO Technical Report Series 646*. Geneva, World Health Organization, 1980, pp 1–80.
246. Nathan DM, Singer DE, Hurxthal K, Goodson JD: The clinical information value of the glycosylated hemoglobin assay. *N Engl J Med* 1984;310:341–346.
247. Forrest RD, Jackson CA, Yudkin JS: The glycohaemoglobin assay as a screening test for diabetes mellitus: The Islington Diabetes Survey. *Diabetic Med* 1987;4:254–259.
248. Singer DE, Coley CM, Samet JH, Nathan DM: Tests of glycemia in diabetes mellitus: Their use in establishing a diagnosis and treatment. *Ann Intern Med* 1989;110:125–137.
249. O'Sullivan JB, Mahan CM: Prospective study of 352 young patients with chemical diabetes. *N Engl J Med* 278:1038–1011.
250. Keen H, Jarrett RJ, McCartney P: The ten year follow-up of the Bedford Survey (1962–1972): Glucose tolerance and diabetes. *Diabetologia* 1982;22:73–78.
251. Atkinson RL: Occult thyroid disease in an elderly hospitalized population. *J Gerontol* 1978;33:372–376.
252. Robuschi G, Safran M, Braverman LE, Gnudi A, Roti E: Hypothyroidism in the elderly. *Endocr Rev* 1987;8:142–153.
253. Klein I, Levey GS: Unusual manifestations of hypothyroidism. *Arch Intern Med* 1984;144:123–128.
254. Schectman JM, Pawlson G: The cost-effectiveness of three thyroid function testing strategies for suspicion of hypothyroidism in a primary care setting. *J Gen Intern Med* 1990;5:9–15.
255. Morrow LB: How thyroid disease presents in the elderly. *Geriatrics Apr* 1978;33:42–45.
256. Davis PJ, Davis B: Hyperthyroidism in patients over the age of 60 years. *Medicine* 1974;53:161–181.
257. Thomas FB, Mazzafern EL, Skillman TG: Apathetic thyrotoxicosis: A distinctive clinical and laboratory entity. *Ann Intern Med* 1970;72:679–687.

258. Boonstra CE, Jackson CE: Serum calcium—Survey for hyperparathyroidism: Results in 50,000 clinic patients. *Am J Clin Pathol* 1971;55:523–526.
259. Heath H III, Hodgson SF, Kennedy MA: Primary hyperparathyroidism: Incidence, morbidity, and potential economic impact in a community. *N Engl J Med* 1980;302:189–193.
260. Ferero MS, Klein RF, Nissenson RA, Nelson K, Heath H III, Arnaud CD, Riggs BL: Effect of age on circulating immunoreactive and bioactive parathyroid hormone levels in women. *J Bone Min Res* 1987;2:363–366.
261. Von Hoff W, Ballardie FW, Bicknell EJ: Primary hyperparathyroidism: The case for medical management. *Br Med J (Clin Res)* 1983;287:1605–1608.
262. Wilson RJ, Rao DS, Ellis B, Kleerekoper M, Parfitt AM: Mild asymptomatic primary hyperparathyroidism is not a risk factor for vertebral fracture. *Ann Intern Med* 1988;109:959–962.
263. Bilezikian JP: The medical management of primary hyperparathyroidism. *Ann Intern Med* 1982;96:198–202.
264. Wesson LG: *Physiology of the Human Kidney*. New York, Grune & Stratton, 1969.
265. Rowe JW, Andres R, Tobin JD, Norris AH, Shock NW: The effect of age on creatinine clearance in man: A cross-sectional and longitudinal study. *J Gerontol* 1976;31:155–163.
266. Rowe JW, Andres R, Tobin JD, Norris AH, Shock NW: Age-adjusted normal standards for creatinine clearance in man. *Ann Intern Med* 1976;84:567–569.
267. Epstein M, Hollenberg NK: Age as a determinant of renal sodium conservation in normal men. *J Lab Clin Med* 1976;87:411–417.
268. Elwood PC, Waters WE, Green WJ, Wood MM: Evaluation of a screening survey for anemia in adult non-pregnant women. *Br Med J* 1967;4:714–717.
269. Shapiro MF, Greenfield S: The complete blood count and leukocyte differential count: An approach to their rational application. *Ann Intern Med* 1987;106:65–74.
270. Kaplan EB, Sheiner LB, Boeckmann AJ, et al: The usefulness of preoperative laboratory screening. *JAMA* 1985;253:3576–3581.
271. Kiel DP, Moskowitz MA: The urinalysis: A critical appraisal. *Med Clin North Am* 1987;71:607–624.
272. Is routine urinalysis worthwhile? *Lancet* 1988;1:747.
273. Akin BV, Hubbell FA, Frye EB, Rucker L, Friis R: Efficacy of routine admission urinalysis. *Am J Med* 1987;82:719–722.
274. Carel RS, Silverberg DS, Kaminsky R, Aviram A: Routine urinalysis (dipstick) findings in mass screening of healthy adults. *Clin Chem* 1987;33:2106–2108.
275. Bard RH: The significance of asymptomatic microhematuria in women: Its economic implications—A ten-year study. *Arch Intern Med* 1988;148:2629–2632.
276. Shorliffe L: Asymptomatic bacteriuria: Should it be treated? *Urology* 1986;27S:19–25.
277. Benbassat J, Froom P, Feldman M, Margoliot S: The importance of leukocyturia in young adults. *Arch Intern Med* 1985;145:79–80.
278. Abuelo JG: Proteinuria: Diagnostic principles and procedures. *Ann Intern Med* 1983;98:186–191.
279. Ginsberg JM, Chang BS, Matarese RA, Garella S: Use of single voided urine samples to estimate quantitative proteinuria. *N Engl J Med* 1983;309:1543–1546.
280. Medical Practice Committee, American College of Physicians: Periodic health examination: A guide for designing individualized preventive health care in the asymptomatic patient. *Ann Intern Med* 1981;95:729–732.
281. Sox HC, Garber AM, Littenberg B: The resting electrocardiogram as a screening test. *Ann Intern Med* 1989;111:489–502.
282. Tape TG, Mushlin AI: The utility of routine chest radiographs. *Ann Intern Med* 1986;104:663–670.
283. Strand J: The living will: The right to death with dignity? *Case Western Reserve Law Rev* 1976;26:485–526.

284. Finucane TE, Shumway JM, Powers RL, D'Alessandri RM: Planning with elderly outpatients for contingencies of severe illness. *J Gen Intern Med* 1988;3:322–325.
285. Lo B, McLeod GA, Saika G: Patient attitudes to discussing life sustaining treatment. *Arch Intern Med* 1986;32:930–934.
286. Goldberg RJ: Training family members of high-risk cardiac patients in cardiopulmonary resuscitation. *Arch Intern Med* 1989;149:25–26.
287. Dracup K, Heaney DM, Taylor SE, Guzy PM, Breu C: Can family members of high-risk cardiac patients learn cardiopulmonary resuscitation? *Arch Intern Med* 1989;149:61–64.
288. Brody EM: Women in the middle and family help to older people. *Gerontologist* 1981;25:19–29.

Chapter 7

Hypertension

G. Aagaard, MD

Hypertension is a major risk factor for stroke, coronary heart disease, congestive heart failure, and kidney failure. For several years an intensive educational campaign has been waged to make physicians and the public more aware of hypertension and its possible consequences. One positive result of these efforts has been that many people have become aware of their elevated blood pressure. A questionable outcome is that many patients with mild hypertension may have received drug therapy when other methods of treatment may have been more appropriate. This is an important problem, since 70% of newly discovered hypertension is in the "mild" range (diastolic 90 to 104 mm). This discussion of hypertension will suggest ways in which physicians can help older women with high blood pressure.

The determination of blood pressure is an important part of the examination of an older woman. It is important to give the patient an opportunity to relax for 5 minutes in the sitting or supine position. My usual practice is to take a series of readings first in the supine position, continuing until the pressure is stabile. Next, the pressure is checked in the standing position. Going from supine to standing in that order gives the best opportunity to detect a postural drop in pressure, which is not uncommon in older patients. Finally, blood pressure is taken in the sitting position with a series of readings until it is stabile.

Blood pressure may vary considerably between visits, and will usually be higher on the first visit. Therefore, if blood pressure is elevated on the initial visit, it should be rechecked at two subsequent visits.

In dealing with populations, blood pressure differs slightly with age and between males and females. The National Health and Nutrition Survey of 1971 to 1974 showed that the average systolic pressure increased from age 7 years to age 74 years, while diastolic pressure tended to peak at 50 years. Hamilton reported mean blood pressures of 159.1/92.4 mm in females, aged 60 to 64 years, and 175.3/93.1 mm for ages 70 to 74 years.[1]

Systolic pressure probably reflects aging changes in the large arteries. The mean systolic pressure of women is slightly lower than that of men until 50 years of age. Diastolic pressure of women averages slightly lower than men until the seventh decade.

In evaluating older women, it is important to recognize that a falsely high diastolic pressure is not uncommon. Spence et al have pointed out that pseudohypertension should be considered if diastolic pressure is 110 mm or greater, and there are no clinical signs of secondary hypertensive change (fundiscopic changes, abnormal electrocardiogram, cardiomegaly by chest x-ray, or impaired kidney function).[2] Spence studied 24 subjects who were over 60 years of age. In 12, diastolic pressure (measured by the indirect method with a regular size adult cuff), was 30 mm or more greater than the direct arterial reading.

Messerli has suggested a clinical test for pseudohypertension, which he has called the Osler Maneuver.[3] The examiner identifies the pulsating radial or brachial artery. The pressure in the cuff is then pumped up until it exceeds the systolic pressure, obliterating the pulse. If the artery (no longer pulsating) is definitely palpated, the test is positive. The assumption is that the thickened and stiff arterial wall resists the external pressure of the cuff, resulting in a falsely high reading.

Prevalence of Hypertension

The prevalence of hypertension in the 1976 to 1980 National Health Survey was 44% in whites ages 65 to 74 years, and 60% in blacks. Hypertension was diagnosed when three readings taken on a single visit averaged 160/95 mm or greater. The World Health Organization has also recognized 160/95 as the beginning level of hypertension. The high prevalence of hypertension may be due, in part, to pseudohypertension.

Risks to Health of Hypertension

It is important to consider the risks associated with hypertension because physicians must evaluate the hazards of an illness in making a decision regarding therapy. Life insurance data show that mortality increases with both systolic and diastolic pressure independently. The increased mortality begins at 128 to 137 mm systolic and 78 to 82 mm diastolic, well within the normal range. In such studies the mortality of a group with blood pressure in a given range is compared to the mortality of the general population of the same age.

It is difficult to separate the effect on mortality of age and elevated blood pressure. Mortality increases sharply with each decade after middle age. Hypertension has an unfavorable effect on mortality in the aged but its effect appears to be less marked than it is in middle-aged women.

The Framingham (Figure 7.1) study reported increased annual mortality and increased incidence of cardiovascular disease (coronary heart disease, congestive heart failure, cerebrovascular disease, and intermittent claudication) with increased blood pressure in women.[4] The unfavorable influence of an elevated diastolic pressure appeared to be less marked in women age 65 to 74 years than in those age 55 to 64 years.

Other studies also suggest that hypertension has relatively less impact on older than middle-aged women. Fry observed 704 hypertensives in a London suburban practice over a 20-year period.[5] He found that in hypertensives the ratio of observed to expected deaths was 6.21 in women age 30 to 39 years and 0.80 in women 70 years and older. This suggests that the older hypertensives had a more favorable outlook than the normotensive women of their own age.

Matilla et al followed 561 elderly people for 5 years—all were 85 years of age or older.[6] The greatest mortality was observed in those with the lowest systolic and diastolic pressures. Mortality was lowest in subjects with systolic

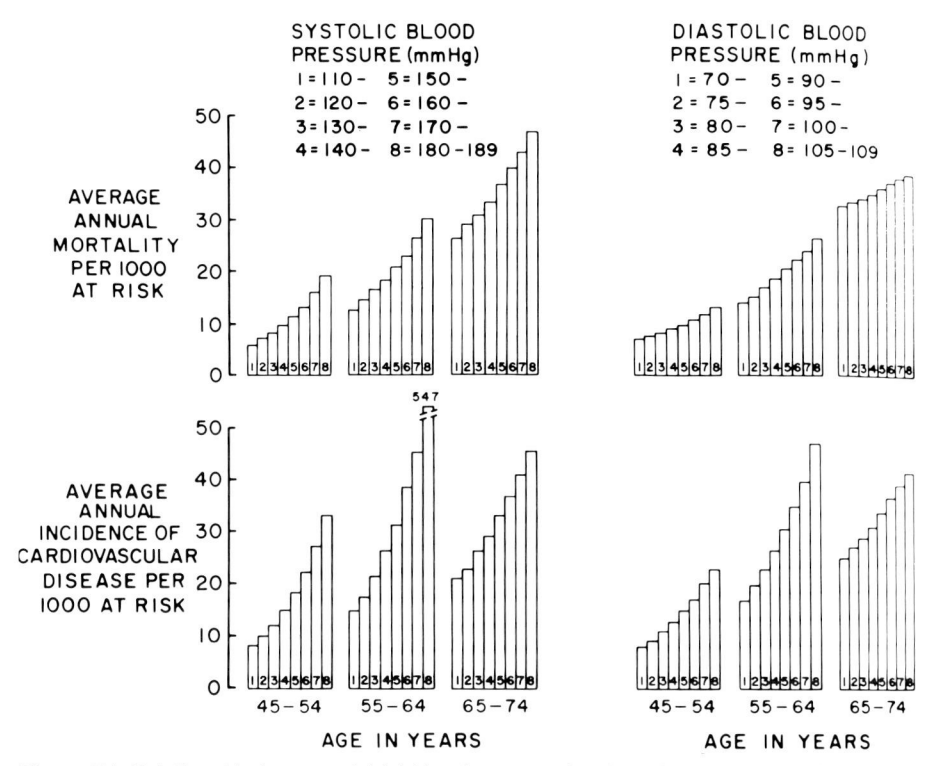

Figure 7.1 Relationship between initial blood-pressure levels and average annual mortality and incidence of cardiovascular disease in Framingham males followed for an 18-year period. Cardiovascular disease represents the occurrence of coronary heart disease, congestive heart failure, cerebrovascular disease, or intermittent claudication. [From Whelton PK: Principles of geriatric medicine, in Andres R, Bierman CL, Hazzard WR (eds.): *Hypertension in the elderly*. New York, McGraw-Hill, 1985, p 544.]

pressure of 160 mm or greater and with diastolic pressure of 90 mm or greater. Those with lower blood pressure were leaner, and had lower levels of blood glucose, serum cholesterol, and hematocrit. This suggests that the subjects with the lowest blood pressure were in a poorer state of health and that this may have contributed to their poor survival rate. However, it is important to note that the elderly subjects with blood pressure greater than 160 systolic and 90 diastolic had the best 5-year survival record.

Anderson and Cowan examined 432 men and women aged 70 to 89 years.[7] Mean systolic and diastolic blood pressures were 167.1 and 87.3, respectively. They found no relationship between systolic or diastolic pressure and survival.

It is difficult to interpret these studies which suggest that hypertension has less impact on older women. In cross-sectional studies it is possible that the most vulnerable subjects have been eliminated, leaving a more resistant population. This could make the incidence of complications or the death rate appear to be falsely low. However, this criticism does not apply to the prospective-survival-type study.

Another factor that may confound the studies on the influence of hypertension on health in the elderly is the possibility of pseudohypertension. It is possible that many of the subjects who apparently had higher readings were really normotensive. As far as we can determine from the reports referred to above, no effort was made to rule out the possibility of falsely high diastolic pressure.

Efficacy of Drug Treatment

Great controversy exists over the blood-pressure level at which drug therapy of hypertension is indicated. There is no doubt that hypertension is a risk factor for stroke, coronary heart disease, and congestive heart failure. The difficult questions are: Does drug treatment of hypertension reduce morbidity and mortality? And, at what level of blood pressure does this favorable effect occur? The answers to these questions are a matter of considerable controversy at present.

In general, it is true that the higher the pretreatment diastolic pressure, the greater the favorable effect of drug treatment. The VA Study of moderate-to-severe hypertension (diastolic pressure 115 mm and greater) showed a profound effect of drug treatment on deaths and complications in treated subjects as compared to controls.[8] However, in the mild-to-moderate hypertensives, drug therapy did not have a significant effect on subjects with entering diastolic pressure of 90 to 104 mm but did cause a decrease in morbidity and mortality in subjects in the 105 to 114 mm stratum.[9]

Many clinical trials have been reported since the VA Study. They vary considerably in design and in results. The U.S. Public Health Service study of mild-to-moderate hypertension showed no significant effect of drug treatment in a group of subjects, 80% of whom had baseline diastolic pressure 90 to 104 mm and 20% 105 to 114 mm.[10] The Australian Study of mild hypertension had subjects with entry pressures of 95 to 109 mm.[11] A small but significant benefit was found in complication rate. It is interesting to note that, in 50% of the placebo-treated subjects, diastolic pressure fell below 95 mm and remained there for the 3-year study period.

The British Medical Research Council study had subjects with entry diastolic pressures of 90 to 109 mm.[12] They found a small but significant reduction in strokes in the subjects who received the active drugs. However, the report states that one would have to treat 850 patients for 1 year to prevent one stroke.

The data summarized above suggest that drug treatment of hypertension should be reserved for patients with diastolic pressure consistently above 100 mm, despite the use of the hygienic measures of treatment.

Does Drug Treatment of Hypertension Increase Risk of Myocardial Infarction

A disappointing finding of most clinical trials of hypertension treatment has been the failure to show that drug treatment will reduce the frequency of manifestations of coronary heart disease. In fact, there is growing evidence that drug treatment may have an adverse effect.

Stewart followed 169 patients with severe hypertension.[13] He found that those whose diastolic pressure was below 90 mm under treatment had a greater risk of having a myocardial infarction than those with 100 to 109 mm pressure.

The Multiple Risk Factor Intervention Trial also showed that the intensively treated subjects had an increased death rate from coronary heart disease.[14] The report suggests that this may have been due to cardiac arrhythmias secondary to diuretic therapy. However, the data in the report also suggest that low treatment blood pressure may have been a factor.

Cruickshank found that mortality from myocardial infarction followed a J-shaped curve in hypertensives receiving drug therapy.[15] Below a diastolic pressure of 85 mm mortality increased. This was true for subjects who had some evidence of ischemic heart disease on entry into the study. Samuelsson et al in a 12-year study of hypertensive men found that cardiovascular morbidity was lowest at a treatment diastolic of 86 to 89 mm, and increased when diastolic pressure was below 86 mm.[16] This was true across all subjects in the study, and not limited to those who had evidence of ischemic heart disease on entry.

It appears that patients with coronary heart disease may be more likely to suffer a myocardial infarction if blood pressure is lowered excessively with drug therapy. Since older women are more likely to have coronary artery narrowing than younger women, it seems wise to be cautious in our use of drug therapy. This is especially true in those with mild hypertension, since in such patients drug therapy may more readily reduce diastolic pressure to levels at which risk of myocardial infarction may be increased.

Hygienic Methods of Treatment

Hygienic methods of treatment of hypertension include weight reduction in patients who are over ideal body weight, restriction of dietary salt, recreational exercise, and psychological and behavioral methods. In general, these measures promote health and make patients feel and function better. Properly applied, they do not have troublesome adverse effects. Some, such as restricting diet, may require a measure of self-discipline. Recreational exercise, on the other hand, may give pleasure and entertainment and add to the enjoyment of life.

Hygienic methods will bring the blood pressure of most women with mild hypertension to a satisfactory level without the need for drugs. In patients with moderate or severe hypertension they may make it possible to control blood pressure with fewer drugs and with smaller doses of drugs. Hygienic methods should, therefore, be the foundation stones of every treatment program for hypertension.

Reduction of Body Weight

In populations, there is a correlation between body weight and blood pressure. It is also true that, in populations, an upward change in body weight correlates with an increase in blood pressure. Conversely, reduction of body weight is a powerful method of lowering blood pressure. Stamler followed a group of overweight men for 5 years.[17] Their average weight loss was 12 pounds. The average blood pressure decrease was 13/10 mm. Reisin reported a significant decrease in blood pressure in hypertensives who had an average weight loss of 10 kg over a 6-month period.[18] In general, it can be said that a reduction of 10 to 15 pounds in weight will reduce blood pressure to the same degree as the administration of full doses of an antihypertensive drug.

It is possible that weight loss causes a decrease in sympathetic nervous system activity or catecholamine metabolism. Young and Landsberg measured norepinephrine turnover rate in cardiac muscle.[19] They found an increase with forced feeding and a decrease with fasting. Jung et al followed obese women on a low-carbohydrate diet.[20] They found a decrease of urine 4-hydroxy-3-methoxy-mandelate and in plasma norepinephrine concentration.

Many physicians take a pessimistic view of the prospects of helping patients to reduce body weight. Perhaps, they are influenced by results reported in the management of morbid obesity. Fortunately, in hypertension, we are dealing with patients who are, on the average, only 25% over ideal body weight. They have a powerful motivation for weight reduction in their elevated blood pressure. An additional inducement is the fact that a reduction in weight is likely to have a favorable effect on blood lipids.

It is important for physicians to take an active and continuing role in helping the hypertensive patient to reduce weight and to monitor weight carefully, so that the benefits of a lowered blood pressure may continue. I recommend that patients check their weight each morning under standard conditions. If weight goes more than two pounds above the maximum which the patient has set, diet should be restricted until weight is back within the desired range.

Restriction of Dietary Salt

Population studies show a correlation of salt intake and blood pressure. Page has published an excellent review of this subject.[21] Oliver et al observed people of the Yanomamo Tribe who live in the area of the Venezuelan and Brazilian border.[22] Salt had never been introduced into their culture. Blood pressure did not rise on the average after the second decade of life. Averages for females over 50 years of age were 106 mm systolic and 64 mm diastolic.

An increase in salt intake in individuals may cause an increase in blood pressure. Mark et al gave young men with borderline hypertension an oral salt load.[23] Blood pressure and vascular resistance was increased and blood flow was decreased. These responses were not observed in normotensive controls.

Dietary salt restriction was reported by Allen to be effective in lowering blood pressure in hypertensives.[24] Some of his subjects had extremely high diastolic pressures. Kempner described dramatic reduction in blood pressure following the use of the rice-fruit diet.[25] Both the Allen diet and the Kempner diet were very low in sodium. The rice-fruit diet was also extremely monotonous. This approach to the treatment of hypertension has been judged impractical by some because of the extremely low-sodium content of the above-mentioned diets.

However, Morgan et al obtained an average decrease of 7.3 mm diastolic in subjects who followed a diet with 70 to 100 mEq of sodium.[26] Hunt and Margie had good results in subjects who reduced salt intake so that sodium excretion was consistently 75 mEq or less per day.[27] Eight-five percent of subjects with entry diastolic pressure at 90 to 104 mm became normotensive over the 4-year study. A satisfactory result was obtained in 50% of those subjects who had entry pressures of 115 mm or more. It should be noted that these subjects also lost weight during the study (an average of 12 pounds during the first 3 months).

My practice has been to suggest a diet with approximately 45 mE (1000 mg) of sodium. This is attainable if the patient can avoid processed foods with a

Table 7.1 Sodium Content of Basic Foods

Milk—2 glasses	260 mg
Bread—2 slices	250 mg
Butter—2 pats	100 mg
Meat—6 oz.	150 mg
Egg—1	60 mg

high sodium content, such as cold meats, ham, and most canned vegetables. Foods must be prepared without using salt. It is possible to prepare tasty meals without salt if creative use is made of spices, wine, tomato, onions, and other sources of flavoring. Table 7.1 shows the sodium content of some foods which are basic to the American diet and illustrates that an attractive diet can be possible. Today, chefs in many restaurants and in the airlines will make low-sodium foods available to their patrons.

Differences exist between hypertensive patients in their sensitivity to salt. In general, older patients tend to show a greater response than younger. This may be related to the increased blood volume and decreased renin level which are common in older hypertensives.

Exercise

In general, an exercise program of 30 minutes followed 3 to 7 days per week will be associated with a decrease in blood pressure. Boyer and Kasch observed middle-aged men over a span of 6 months in an exercise program.[28] Blood pressure was reduced by 13.5/11.8 mm.

Hagberg et al worked with hypertensive adolescents who followed an endurance exercise training program for 8 months.[29] Diastolic pressure decreased an average of 7 mm. Subjects with increased cardiac output or peripheral resistance on entry also showed a decrease in these measures.

Korner et al used a bicycle ergometer in an exercise program for mild hypertensives.[30] Subjects did 30 minutes of exercise at a workload of 60% to 70% of their calculated capacity. The exercise was preceded and followed by a 5-minute warm-up and cool-down period. Patients participated 3 or 7 days per week and showed an average diastolic decrease of 11/9 mm or 16/11 mm, respectively. They also observed a decrease in peripheral resistance and plasma norepinephrine, and an increase in cardiac output.

Exercise has other benefits which may be significant to the older hypertensive woman. It may help to reduce body weight. This is important since many older women can maintain weight on very modest energy intake. Exercise will help them burn additional calories. It has been estimated that adding a 1-mile walk to the daily activity, while keeping the food intake constant, will cause a weight reduction of 1 pound per month, or 12 pounds per year.

Exercise may also have beneficial psychological effects. Patients may feel more relaxed. A walking program may offer a chance to expand the horizons of daily life. Many older women are sedentary because no one has ever suggested a program of exercise. An 80-year-old woman did not like to walk in the rainy winter weather. A program of dancing in her living room to the music of a record player was suggested and followed. She found that she loved to dance the hula and was soon dancing for 45 minutes daily.

An exercise program should be started with minimal intensity and duration and slowly increased as tolerated. Walking is the best exercise because most patients have the necessary skill, and no special equipment or facility is required. Ten minutes of walking is a good beginning for a sedentary woman. The duration can be increased by 1 minute each day, if tolerated, until the patient is walking 20 or 30 minutes daily. The pace should always be comfortable; never at a level which causes shortness of breath or discomfort. A good guide is to walk at a pace at which one can carry on a conversation with a companion.

Patients who cannot walk because of disabilities may be able to use a stationary bicycle. One can exercise in front of the television set and be informed or entertained while fulfilling an exercise program. Swimming is an excellent exercise for some of those who cannot walk, but pools are not always readily available. Many women who cannot walk may exercise their shoulders and arms by sitting on a small chair or stool and swinging small weights. The number of repetitions and the amount of the weight load can be gradually increased as tolerated. If possible, an exercise program should be comfortable, convenient, enjoyable, and readily available.

Games, such as tennis or golf, are excellent supplements to an exercise program because of the companionship and the competition they provide. However, they do not serve well for a basic exercise program.

Psychological and Behavioral Methods

Blood pressure is markedly influenced by emotions; going up with anger and fear and going down in relaxed states and during sleep. Any form of stress may raise blood pressure. In hypertensives, even mild and moderate, the blood-pressure increase caused by stress is likely to be greater and to last longer.

Older hypertensive women may be under considerable stress. Theirs may not be the placid rocking-chair existence. Older women may be lonely because of loss of spouse, family, and friends. There may be insecurity and isolation because of fear to go outside the home. Intergenerational relationships may deteriorate because of differences in tastes or in standards of behavior. The need for understanding and support may be great, and the physician should provide this and also help his patient to find additional assistance if needed.

Suggestions can be made which will help the patient to avoid stressful situations. It may be possible to help the patient to more effectively cope with the situation, or to perceive it in a less-disturbing light. It is important to try to help the patient to avoid anger, anxiety, and a sense of hurry or time pressure—and to recognize these feelings even when they occur to a mild degree.

Meditation, relaxation, and biofeedback techniques have been studied in hypertension. Studies differ widely in design and in the adequacy of baseline readings, duration of treatment and follow-up, and in well-matched control subjects. Shapiro reviews these techniques in detail.[31]

In my experience these techniques have not had a significant blood-pressure-lowering effect. However, I believe that they may be useful in some patients who achieve a sense of quietness when practicing relaxation or meditation. These patients may become more sensitive to their own feelings of anger, anxiety, or time pressure, and as a result may be more successful in avoiding the situations which cause these feelings.

The support of an interested physician is an important element in the treatment of the hypertensive older woman. Two noteworthy studies suggest that psychosocial support may have a significant beneficial effect in preventing the development of coronary heart disease manifestations. Medalie and Goldcourt followed a large group of men at high risk for coronary heart disease.[32] Men who had a loving and supportive wife had a lower incidence of angina. Frasure-Smith and Prince followed a large group of patients who had been hospitalized for acute myocardial infarction.[33] Patients in the experimental group were called by telephone once a month to administer a short questionnaire designed to detect stress. Those subjects who showed an increase in stress since the previous monthly score were visited at home by a nurse who explored the cause of stress and continued monthly visits for the remainder of the 1-year follow-up period. The experimental group had a decrease in cardiac deaths of 47% as compared to the control group.

Drug Treatment of Hypertension

The decision to initiate drug therapy in a woman with hypertension should be based on the total health picture of the patient and on the published results of efficacy and safety of drug therapy. In summary of the discussion given above, drugs should not be prescribed unless diastolic pressure is consistently above 100 mm in a patient who has made a sincere effort to follow the hygienic measures.

Start slowly with drug therapy. Use small initial doses and increase slowly with small increments and at long intervals. Ambulatory hypertension is not an emergency. The chance of obtaining the patient's compliance with the drug-treatment program is increased if disturbing adverse effects can be avoided in the beginning. Fatigue, lassitude, disturbed sleeping patterns, impaired sexual desire and/or function, and postural hypotension are common, unless skill is used in beginning drug therapy. In general, older patients are more vulnerable to the adverse effects of antihypertensive drugs. They are also more likely to have silent coronary heart disease. One should avoid lowering blood pressure too quickly or too much.

The pattern of drug treatment has changed in recent years because the majority of hypertensives have mild-to-moderate blood-pressure levels when first diagnosed. These patients are more likely to respond satisfactorily to a single drug. One can, therefore, prescribe a single drug with the expectation that it will be effective in reducing blood pressure to a satisfactory level. If the response is not adequate or if adverse effects are significant, the first drug may be discontinued and another drug prescribed in its place. A few years ago, common practice was to go through a series of steps, adding drugs until a satisfactory response was obtained. The first step in the stepped care plan was usually a mild diuretic. The second step was an adrenergic-inhibiting drug such as reserpine, methyl-dopa, or a β blocker. The third step was the vasodilator, hydralazine. Drugs were added in sequence until blood pressure was at a satisfactory level.

Drugs which are useful in the management of hypertension will be discussed below. Table 7.2 summarizes key information regarding the different groups of drugs. An effort will be made to suggest the situations in which drugs may be of special value. No mention will be made of drugs which, although of historical importance, are infrequently used today.

Diuretics

The *mild diuretics* have diuretic, natriuretic, and chloruretic effects; however, they may vary in promptness of onset and in duration of action. These drugs reduce extracellular volume and plasma volume. They may also act by reducing the sodium content of vascular smooth muscle. With chronic use, peripheral resistance may be reduced. Diuretics, in addition to their own blood-pressure-lowering effect, may increase the blood-pressure reduction of other drugs, such as some of the adrenergic inhibitors and the vasodilators. They will usually prevent salt and water retention which may occur if other types of antihypertensive drugs are given alone. The effects of these drugs are quite limited in patients with impaired renal function. Increased dosage will usually not increase the response.

In general, these drugs are well-tolerated, especially if used in small doses. Hypokalemia is a significant risk, particularly in older women. The cause for their vulnerability is not known. It may be because of an inadequate diet. It is important to check serum potassium before prescribing. This is especially important in women who are receiving digitalis.

Other adverse effects are hyperuricemia, hyperglycemia, skin rashes, GI distress, and vasculitis. These drugs may also cause an increase in total cholesterol and triglycerides.

Loop diuretics usually cause a prompt and copious diureses. This may be a disadvantage in some women, especially those who have questionable urinary sphincter control. They may be immobilized until this surge of diuresis is spent. These drugs can cause fluid and electrolyte depletion. With increased dosage, they are usually effective even in patients with impaired renal function. In women with normal renal function they have no advantages over the mild diuretics, and may cause significant problems.

Potassium-sparing diuretics include Triamterene and Amiloride. They are weak diuretics and natriuretics, and are usually given with a diuretic such as hydrochlorothiazide because of their potassium-sparing properties.

Adverse effects include nausea and leg cramps. Renal failure has been attributed to these drugs. This hazard may be increased by concomitant use of nonsteroidal antiinflammatory drugs.

Spironolactone is an aldosterone antagonist. It causes sodium excretion and potassium retention. It is often used with a mild diuretic such as hydrochlorothiazide. It should not be used in patients with impaired renal function, nor together with potassium supplementation because of the possibility of hyperkalemia. Breast tenderness may be a problem.

Adrenergic-Inhibiting Drugs

The sympathetic nervous system is obviously important in the regulation of blood pressure. Drugs may reduce sympathetic nervous system activity in various ways, many of them involving some aspect of the synthesis or release of

Table 7.2 List of Drugs, Dosages, and Side Effects

Drug	Adult daily dose (mg)	Remarks*
Diuretics		
Hydrochlorothiazide	12.5–50	AE: Hypokalemia in older women; lethargy, depression; hyperurecemia
Chlorthalidone	12.5–50	AE: As above; other mild diuretics are also available; effectiveness limited with impaired renal function
Loop diuretics		
Bumetanide (Bumex)	0.5–2.0	Powerful agents; dehydration a hazard; best reserved for impaired renal function when larger doses are required; may limit mobility by rapid copius response
Furosemide	20–40	
Potassium-sparing diuretics		
Amiloride (Midamor)	5–10	Hyperkalemia; do not use with potassium supplements; GI distress, rash, headache
Spironolactone (Aldactone)	25–100	As above plus menstrual irregularities
Triamterene (Dyrenium)	50–100	As with Amiloride; renal stones have been reported
Adrenergic-inhibiting drugs		
β-adrenergic blockers		
Propranolol (Inderal)	20–320	Fatigue, depression, may increase symptoms of peripheral vascular disease; bradycardia; contraindicated with a history of asthma
Acebutolol (Sectral)	200–1200	See propranolol; some degree of cardioselectivity and intrinsic sympathomimetic (ISA) effect
Atenolol (Tenormin)	50–100	See propranolol; cardioselective
Carteolol (Cartrol)	2.5–10	See propranolol; has ISA; caution in renal impaired
Metoprolol (Lopressor)	25–100	See propranolol; cardioselective
Nadolol (Corgard)	20–160	See propranolol
Penbutolol (Levatol)	10–40	See propranolol
Pindolol (Visken)	5–30	See propranolol; has ISA
Timolol (Blocadren)	5–40	See propranolol
Labetol (Normodyne)	100–800	See propranolol; risk of postural hypotension is increased by α-1 blocking action
Clonidine (Catapres)	0.1–0.6	Sedation, dry mouth, sudden withdrawal may give rebound hypertension
Methyldopa (Aldomet)	250–750	Sedation, orthostatic hypotension; hemolytic anemia and hepatitis were reported early, not recently
Guanabenz (Wytensin)	4–16	See clonidine
Guanfacine (Tenex)	1–3	See clonidine
Guanethidine (Ismelin)	10–50	Orthostatic and exertional hypotension, diarrhea, and exacerbation of asthma may occur
Guanadrel (Hylorel)	10–35	Like guanethidine but less severe
Prazosin (Minipress)	1–15	Take first dose in bed in PM; postural dizziness may occur
Terazosin	1–5	Like prazosin

Table 7.2 (*continued*)

Drug	Adult daily dose (mg)	Remarks*
Vasodilators		
Hydralazine (Apresoline)	30–300	Headache, tachycardia, aggravation of angina
Minoxidil (Loniten)	2.5–40	Diuretic and a β blocker or other adrenergic inhibitor should be given with drug
Calcium channel blockers		
Diltiazem (Cardizem and SR)	30–120	Use with caution in patients with conduction defects and left-ventricular weakness
Nicardipine (Cardene)	60–120	Like nifedipine
Nifedipine (Procardia XL)	30–120	AE: Dizziness, flushing, headache, edema, may relate to vasodilator action
Verapamil (Calan and Calan SR)	120–440	Like diltiazem; constipation, dizziness, nausea
Angiotensin-converting enzyme inhibitors		
Captopril (Capoten)	25–150	Observe response to first dose carefully; excess BP drop may occur in patients who are volume-depleted or who have bilateral renal artery stenosis as a cause of their hypertension; cough is a dose-related AE
Enalapril (Vasotec)	5–40	Like captopril; with moderate to severe renal function impairment reduce first dose to 2.5 mg
Lisinopril	5–40	Like captopril and enalapril

* AE, adverse effects.

norepinephrine. Drugs may block adrenergic receptors or in other ways prevent sympathetic stimulation of end-organs.

Beta-Adrenergic Blockers

See Table 7.2 for list of drugs. These drugs reduce the rate and force of cardiac contraction. This may be the mechanism through which they lower blood pressure. They also reduce renin release. Some β blockers are cardioselective, blocking β-1 receptors but not β-2 receptors. These drugs should cause less bronchoconstriction. However, freedom from bronchoconstriction is only relative. Even cardioselective β blockers may cause bronchoconstriction in asthmatic patients. Intrinsic sympathomimetic activity is present in some β blockers. This may permit blood-pressure reduction without significant reduction of heart rate. Beta blockers have been shown to reduce recurrance rates of myocardial infarction, and are commonly used in the treatment of angina and cardiac arrhythmias. However, they have not been shown to reduce the frequency of coronary heart disease complications in hypertension.

These drugs should not be used in patients with a history of asthma or of chronic obstructive pulmonary disease, nor in patients with a slow initial heart rate or with heart block. Patients who experience an upper-respiratory infection with bronchitis while taking a β blocker may have persistent cough, which may not stop until the drug is discontinued.

Other adverse effects include disturbances of sleep, cognitive function, and memory, as well as lassitude. Gastrointestinal complaints, especially flatulence, are common. Many patients will tolerate the lassitude and other complaints if the drug is started in low doses. These drugs may cause an increase in triglyceride concentration, a decrease in high-density lipoproteins, and a reduction in the ratio of total cholesterol to high-density lipoproteins. In diabetics, β blockers may accentuate the degree of hypoglycemia with insulin overdosage and mask the symptoms and signs (tachycardia and anxiety). Cardioselective β blockers have a theoretical advantage in diabetics.

Labetolol (Normodyne)

This drug acts both as a noncardioselective β blocker and as an α-1 blocker. Flamenbaum et al reported that labetolol was equally effective as monotherapy in blacks and whites.[34] A multicentered study showed that it was effective when used with small doses (25 mg bid) of hydrochlorothiazide. Standing blood pressure is reduced more than supine, which means that postural hypotension may be a problem. Lund-Johanson in a long-term study reported that peripheral resistance was reduced, and that cardiac output, which had been reduced early in the study, was increased at the end of the study.[35]

Adverse effects include dizziness, which is probably related to its α-1 blocking effect. The adverse effects ascribed to the β blockers may also be a problem. These include fatigue, sleep disturbances, and gastrointestinal distress. McGonigle et al have reported a reduction in total cholesterol without any change in high-density lipoproteins,[36] while Frishman et al have reported no change.[37]

Clonidine

This drug acts centrally on α-2 receptors and causes a reduction in sympathetic outflow, in norepinephrine release, and in plasma level, a decrease in peripheral resistance, a small decrease in cardiac output, and a decrease in renin release. This drug does not have a great blood-pressure-lowering effect as monotherapy but may be quite effective when used with a mild diuretic.

Adverse effects of clonidine include dry mouth and drowsiness, which may be a difficult problem for those who work at desks or who must drive. Taking 75% of the daily dose before bedtime may be useful in reducing the daytime drowsiness. However, sleep disturbance may also be a problem with this drug.

Withdrawal hypertension may be a problem with clonidine. If the drug is abruptly discontinued after a significant blood-pressure reduction has been achieved with clonidine, the result may be a sharp increase in blood pressure and heart rate. Because of the possibility of a withdrawal reaction, clonidine is not recommended for older women who might forget to take daily drug doses.

Transdermal clonidine is now available. Patches may be applied once weekly. More consistent plasma levels of the drug may be an advantage. However, a significant number of patients may have local skin reactions. This method of administration may be useful in forgetful patients.

Methydopa

The exact mechanism of action is still uncertain but this drug probably acts through central depression of sympathetic activity. For many years it was widely used as a step-two drug, following a diuretic. Sedation, fatigue, and loss of libido must be avoided by careful dosing. Postural hypotension may be a problem in some patients.

Guanabenz and Guanfacine

These centrally acting drugs are similar to clonidine in actions and in adverse effects.

Guanethidine

This drug probably acts at the sympathetic neuroeffector junction by inhibiting norepinephrine release. It was once widely used as a step-four drug when the first three drugs did not lower blood pressure satisfactorily. Postural and exertional hypotension are significant problems. Diarrhea may be severe. It may aggravate bronchial asthma. Guanadrel is similar to guanethidine in action and may cause postural hypotension.

Prazosin (Minipress)

This drug acts as a selective antagonist to peripheral postsynaptic α-1 receptors. This selective action leaves the presynaptic α-2 receptors able to inhibit release of norepinephrine, thus decreasing the tachycardia which often occurs with α-1 blockade. Another explanation may be that prazosin acts on both resistance and capacitance vessels, and thus reduces venous return to the heart. Prazosin has been reported to cause a reduction in total cholesterol and triglycerides and an increase in high-density lipoproteins.[38]

Adverse effects of prazosin include a marked hypotensive response after taking the first dose (probably 5% of patients). To minimize the danger of this response, the first dose can be given in the evening, when the patient is ready to get into bed. Profound hypertension can also occur if a β blocker is added to prazosin or if prazosin is added to a treatment program with a β blocker. Other adverse effects which have been reported are headache, drowsiness, nervousness, and lassitude.

Vasodilators

Hydralazine

This direct vascular smooth muscle vasodilator effects mainly the arterial side of the circulation, and has little effect on the capacitance vessels. Hence, return venous flow is increased with increased heart rate and cardiac output. Therefore, angina may occur in patients with coronary heart disease. This drug has been widely used as a third-step drug, and still may be useful when blood pressure is difficult to control. It should usually be given along with a diuretic and an adrenergic inhibitor.

Adverse effects are tachycardia, angina, headache, and sodium and water retention. Headaches can usually be avoided if the drug is started in small doses. Some patients acetylate hydralazine at a slow rate, and show a therapeutic response and/or adverse effect at low doses.

Minoxidil

This very potent vasodilator is useful in severe hypertension. It is usually given with a β blocker and a diuretic as noted above with hydralazine. Abnormal hair growth may be a distressing adverse effect, especially in women.

Calcium Channel Blockers

Calcium ions play an important role in the function of cardiac and vascular tissues and the specialized cardiac conduction system. Reduction of calcium concentration within the cell will reduce activity. Thus vasodilation, reduced force of cardiac contraction, or slowed sinus node firing or AV conduction may be caused by this group of drugs. They differ in the extent to which they effect various functions.

Verapamil, nifedipine, and diltiazem have been available the longest. All have vasodilator effects, with nifedipine being the most potent. Verapamil and diltiazem both cause negative chronotropism and inotropism. Thus, they are less likely to cause a reflex increase in heart rate. In hypertensive patients with impaired left-ventricular function, they could theoretically cause further impairment. However, the reduced left-ventricular afterload and the improved coronary circulation might compensate for such effects. Verapamil and diltiazem should be used with caution in such patients.[39]

These drugs will probably have an important place in the treatment of hypertensives with cardiovascular complications or associated diseases. Hypertensives with angina may benefit from the coronary vasodilation, which is a part of the main action of these drugs.[40] Calcium antagonists have great advantages over the β blockers in hypertensives with asthma or diabetes. Thus far, they do not appear to have any adverse effects on plasma lipids, which may give them an advantage over diuretics and β blockers. These drugs appear to have a special place in the treatment of older hypertensives.

Adverse effects of the calcium antagonists vary considerably. In general, they are well-tolerated. Constipation has been a common complaint for verapamil. Tachycardia, headaches, and palpitation are more common for nifedipine. Flushing, dizziness, and skin rashes are not uncommon. Swelling of the feet may require stopping the drug. It is probably related to vasodilation and not to sodium retention. In fact, in some patients these drugs cause a natriuresis.

Some patients complain of fatigue and reduced tolerance for exercise, especially with verapamil. Verapamil and diltiazem should be used only with great caution if at all with β blockers. Increased atrioventricular block may occur. These drugs may reduce the renal clearance of digoxin and cause an increase in plasma digoxin levels. Therefore, the dose of digoxin should be reduced or the plasma level carefully monitored.

Angiotension-Converting Enzyme Inhibitors (ACEI)

These drugs reduce the production of angiotensin II, a potent vasoconstrictor which also causes the increased release of aldosterone and stimulation of the sympathetic nervous system. Angiotensin II also causes the degradation of bradykinin, an endogenous vasodilator. Thus, inhibitors of ACE may lower blood pressure through at least two mechanisms: reducing angiotensin II, and increasing bradykinin. These drugs are effective in reducing peripheral resistance. They may also dilate the large arteries.

One would expect that ACEIs would be most effective in high renin hypertension; and, therefore, less effective in the elderly and in blacks in whom low renin is common. Nonetheless, these drugs are often effective in, and well-tolerated by, elderly patients.

Initially, captopril, the first of these drugs to become available, was used almost exclusively in severe hypertension, and almost always with a diuretic and an adrenergic inhibitor. It is clear now that these drugs can be effective as monotherapy in older patients.

ACEIs cause a blood-pressure decrease similar to the β blocker.[41] The VA study of captopril showed a good response at a daily dose of 37.5 mg. The addition of hydrochlorothiazide increased the blood-pressure response by 4 to 6 mm diastolic.[42]

Adverse effects of the ACEIs appear to be about half as frequent as with the β blockers. Early reports of skin rash and loss of taste sensation with captopril have declined with the use of smaller doses. Neutropenia and proteinuria are uncommon but are more likely to occur in patients with decreased renal function and/or collagen diseases (ie, lupus or scleroderma). These adverse effects may be related to the SH group in captopril. They are less common with enalapril, which has no SH group. Neutropenia, when it has occurred, has usually resolved quickly when the drug was stopped.

The most common adverse effects of the ACEIs appear to be dizziness, headache, fatigue, diarrhea, and upper-respiratory symptoms. Cough is fairly common and is dose-related. The drug has been discontinued in approximately 6% of patients because of adverse effects.

Conclusions

Hypertension is a common finding in older women. It deserves careful and thoughtful consideration. Initial efforts at treatment should focus on hygienic measures because they are frequently effective in lowering blood pressure, and have a beneficial effect on quality of life, mental status, and plasma lipids.

If drug therapy is needed, it should be started at a small initial dose. The patient should be followed carefully for the blood-pressure response and for any adverse effects. Increments in dose should be small, and should be made at long intervals.

References

1. Hamilton M, et al: Etiology of essential hypertension: Arterial pressure in the general population. *Clin Sci* 1954;13:11.
2. Spence JD, Sibbald WJ, Cape RD: Pseudohypertension in the elderly. *Clin Sci Molecular Med* 1978;55:399S.
3. Messerili FH, et al: Osler's maneuver and pseudohypertension. *N Engl J Med* 1985; 1548.
4. Kannel WB, Gordon T (eds.): *Framingham Study: An Epidemiological Investigation of Cardiovascular Disease.* Sec. 30 NIH 74-599, 1974.

5. Fry J: Natural history of hypertension: A case for selective non-treatment. *Lancet* 1974;431.
6. Matilla K, et al: Blood pressure and five year survival in the very old. *Brit Med J* 1988;296:887.
7. Anderson F, Cowan NR: Survival of healthy older people. *Brit J Prev Soc Med* 1976;30:231.
8. VA Cooperative Study Group on Antihypertensive Agents: Effects of treatment on morbidity in hypertension: Results in patients with diastolic blood pressures averaging 115 through 129 mm Hg. *JAMA* 1967;202:1028.
9. VA Cooperative Study Group on Antihypertensive Agents: Effects of treatment on morbidity in hypertension: II. Results in patients with diastolic blood pressure averaging 90 through 114 mm Hg. *JAMA* 1970;213:1143.
10. U.S. Public Health Service Hospitals Cooperative Study Group: Treatment of mild hypertension: Results of a ten-year intervention trial. *Circ Res* 1977(Suppl I)40:1–98.
11. Australian Therapeutic Trial in Mild Hypertension. *Lancet* 1980;1261.
12. Medical Research Council Working Party: MRC trial of treatment of mild hypertension: Principal results. *Brit Med J* 1985;291:97.
13. Stewart I, McD. G: Relation of reduction in pressure to first myocardial infarction in patients receiving treatment for severe hypertension. *Lancet* 1979;861.
14. Multiple Risk Factor Intervention Trial Research Group, 1982: Multiple risk factor intervention trial: Risk factor changes and mortality results. *JAMA* 1982;248:1465.
15. Cruickshank JM, et al: Benefits and potential harm of lowering high blood pressure. *Lancet* 1987;581.
16. Samuelsson O, et al: Cardiovascular morbidity in relation to change in blood pressure and serum cholesterol levels in treated hypertension. *JAMA* 1987;258:1768.
17. Stamler J, et al: Prevention and control of hypertension by nutritional-hygienic means. *JAMA* 1980;243:1819.
18. Reisin E, et al: Effect of weight loss without salt restriction on the reduction of blood pressure in overweight hypertensive patients. *N Engl J Med* 1978;298:1.
19. Young JB, Landsberg L: Suppression of sympathetic nervous system during fasting. *Science* 1977;196:1473.
20. Jung RT, et al: Role of catecholamines in hypotensive response to dieting. *Brit Med J* 1979;12.
21. Page LB, et al: Antecedents of cardiovascular disease in six Solomon Islands societies. *Circulation* 1974;49:1132.
22. Oliver W, et al: Blood pressure, sodium intake and sodium related hormones in the Yanomamo Indians, a "no-salt" culture. *Circulation* 1975;52:146.
23. Mark AL, et al: Effects of high and low sodium intake on arterial pressure and forearm vascular resistance in borderline hypertension. *Circ Res* 1975(Suppl I)36&37:194.
24. Allen FM: Arterial hypertension. *JAMA* 1920;74:652.
25. Kempner W: Treatment of hypertensive vascular disease with rice diet. *Am J Med* 1948;545.
26. Morgan T, et al: Hypertension treated by salt restriction. *Lancet* 1978;227.
27. Hunt JC, Margie JD: Influence of diet on hypertension management, in Hunt JC (ed.): *Hypertension Update: Dialogues in Hypertension*, 1980, p. 197.
28. Boyer JL, Kasch FW: Exercise therapy in hypertensive men. *JAMA* 1970;211:1668.
29. Hagberg JM, et al: Effect of weight training on blood pressure and hemodynamics in hypertensive adolescents. *J Pediatrics* 1984;147.
30. Korner PI, et al: Long-term antihypertensive action of regular exercise: Its role in a new treatment strategy, in Yamori, Lenfant (eds.): *Prevention of Cardiovascular Diseases: An Approach to Active Long Life*. New York, Elsevier, 1987, p. 213.
31. Shapiro AP, et al: Behavioral methods in the treatment of hypertension: A review of their clinical status. *Ann Int Med* 1977;86:626.
32. Medalie JH, Goldbourt U: Angina pectoris among 10,000 men: II. Psychosocial and

other risk factors as evidenced by a multivariate analysis of a five year incidence study. *Am J Med* 1976;60:910.
33. Frasure-Smith N, Prince R: The ischemic heart disease life stress monitoring program: Impact on mortality. *Psychosomatic Med* 1985;47:431.
34. Flamenbaum W, et al: Monotherapy with labetalol compared with propranolol. *J Clin Hyper* 1985;1:56.
35. Lund-Johansen P: Short- and long-term (six-year) hemodynamic effects of labetalol in essential hypertension. *Am J Med* 1983;24.
36. McGonigle RJS, et al: Labetalol and lipids. *Lancet* 1981;1:163.
37. Frishman WH, et al: Multiclinic comparison of labetalol to metroprolol in treatment of mild to moderate systemic hypertension. *Am J Med* 1983;54.
38. Weinberger MH: Antihypertensive therapy and lipids: Evidence, mechanisms and implications. *Arch Int Med* 1985;145:1102.
39. Van Zweiten PA, et al: Pharmacology of calcium entry blockers: Interaction with vascular alpha adrenoreceptors. *Hypertension* 1983(Suppl 5):8.
40. Kaplan NM: Calcium entry blockers in the treatment of hypertension: Current status and future prospects. *JAMA* 1989;262:817.
41. VA Cooperative Study Group on Antihypertensive Agents: Low-dose captopril for the treatment of mild to moderate hypertension: I. Results of a 14-week trial. *Arch Intern Med* 1984;144:1947.
42. VA Cooperative Study Group on Antihypertensive Agents: Captopril: Evaluation of low doses, twice-daily doses and the addition of diuretic for the treatment of mild to moderate hypertension. *Clin Sci* 1982;63:443S.

Chapter 8

Genitourinary Changes and Incontinence

Morton Stenchever, MD

Profound changes take place in the genitourinary tract during the aging process. These changes are influenced by a number of circumstances, including physical stress, hormonal withdrawal, and the effects of a variety of medications that the patient may need for other health problems at this stage of life. The result of the interplay of many of these factors may be urinary incontinence. Incontinence occurs, conservatively, in at least 10% of all women during their lifetime, becoming more common as the woman ages. The maintenance of continence depends on a number of factors, including the neurologic control of micturition, specific anatomical relationships, and the effects on these of various acute and chronic pathologic conditions. This chapter will review the physiology of micturition, the anatomical relationships of the female genitourinary tract, and the diagnosis and therapy of conditions which effect continence.

Anatomy and Physiology of Micturition

Continence is a function of the urethra's ability to prevent the flow of urine and the bladder's ability to store urine. Micturition is dependent on the ability of the urethra to relax and the detrusor muscle of the bladder to contract. Both the urethra and the bladder are under neurologic control via the autonomic nervous system. Simply stated, the sympathetic portion of the autonomic nervous system maintains continence because the stimulation of α-adrenergic receptors, which occur primarily in the urethra, and, rarely, in the bladder, causes contraction of the urethral musculature and stimulation of the β-adrenergic receptors, which occur primarily in the bladder and, rarely, in the urethra, causes relaxation when stimulated. The neurotransmitter for the sympathetic system is norepinephrine. On the other hand, the parasympathetic nervous system stimulates contraction of the detrusor muscle and relaxation of the urethral musculature. The neurotransmitter involved here is acetyl choline (Figure 8.1).

The factors that affect urethral closure involve urethral tone, which is affected by the elasticity of the urethral wall, the presence of smooth and striated muscle in the urethra and the vascular component supplying the urethra and bladder neck. In addition, urethral pressure is supported by the vaginal levator muscle attachments, which DeLancey has shown are primarily supportive of the

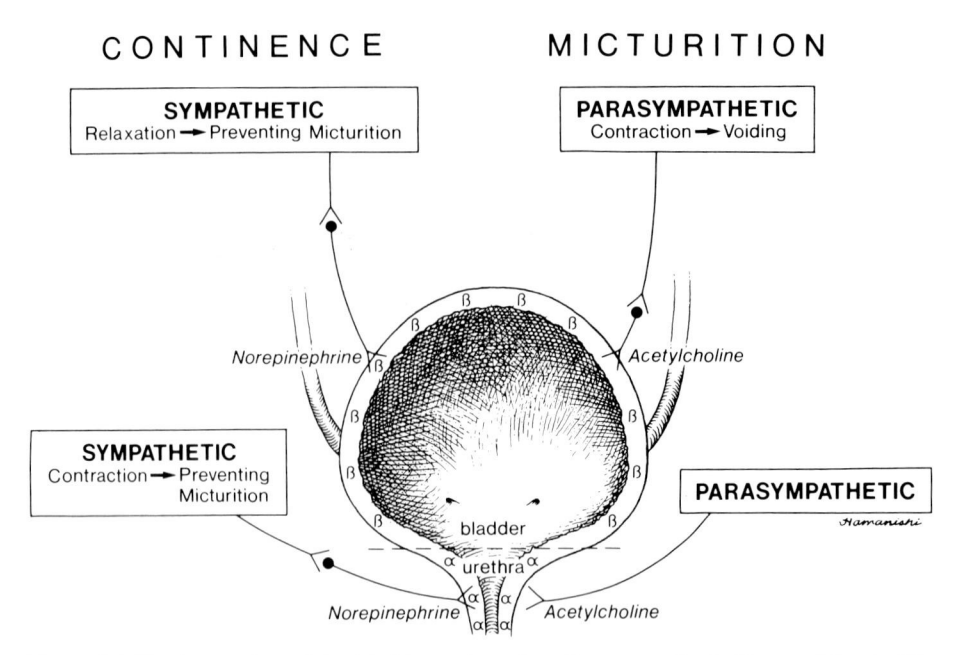

Figure 8.1 The innervation of the bladder and urethra. Parasympathetic fibers arising in S2 through S4 have long preganglionic fibers and pelvic ganglia close to the bladder and urethra. These parasympathetic fibers excrete acetyl choline. Sympathetic fibers that have long postganglionic fibers discharge norepinephrine to β receptors, primarily in the bladder, and α receptors, primarily in the urethra. (Redrawn and modified from Raz S: *Urol Clin North Am* 1978;5:323.)

mid-60% of the urethral length.[1] The fascial and connective tissue supports which suspend the urethra to the posterior region of the pubic symphysis are important because they maintain the proximal urethra and the bladderneck in an intraabdominal position.

The act of voiding involves four basic autonomic and somatic nervous system feedback loops.[2] The first (loop I) connects the cerebral cortex to the brain stem, and inhibits micturition by modifying sensory stimuli which emanate from the second loop. The second loop (loop II) originates in the sacral micturition center (S-2 through S-4) and the detrusor muscle wall itself. Sensory fibers of this loop run to the brain stem, where a modulation by loop I takes place. If cerebral inhibition is not imposed via loop I, the stimuli return to the sacral micturition center and allow activation of loop III. This loop involves the sensory nerve flow from the bladder-wall pressure receptors to the sacral micturition center with return motor fibers to the urethral sphincter striated muscle. This allows the voluntary relaxation of the urethral sphincter as the detrusor contracts. Loop IV is initiated in the frontal lobe of the cerebral cortex and extends to the sacral micturition center and on to the urethral striated muscle, allowing urethral voluntary muscles to relax, thus initiating the voiding mechanism (Figure 8.2). A variety of conditions, such as demyelinating diseases, Parkinson's disease, cerebral vascular conditions, disease of the lower urinary tract, and CNS tumors, may interfere with any or all of these loops and cause malfunction of the system. Table 8.1 summarizes the importance of each loop and the way in which pathological conditions may affect them. Furthermore, medications

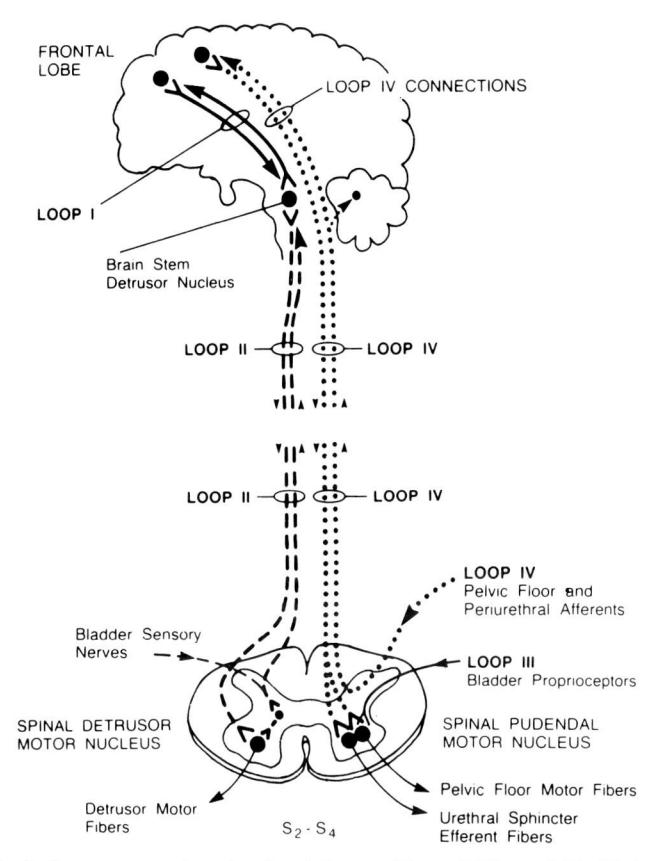

Figure 8.2 Central nervous system feedback loops. (From Williams ME, Fitzhugh CP: *Ann Intern Med* 1982;97:895.)

which affect the autonomic nervous system by stimulating or blocking either the action of acetyl choline or norepinephrine, thereby affecting CNS transmission, may affect micturition and continence. Table 8.2 lists a number of common medications often used by aging patients, and the specific effects they may have on the micturition process.

Sympathetic receptors are influenced by estrogen and progesterone with estrogen-stimulating α receptors and progesterone-influencing β receptors. Hormone withdrawal during the aging process will effect these, and hormone replacement may reverse the effects that are observed.

Asmussen and Ulmsten consider the bladder and urethra a functional unit with the bladder's subfunction to store urine and the urethra's to allow it to pass.[3] For urine to exit the urethra, the maximum urethral pressure must be lower than the intravesicular pressure. Intravesicular pressure depends upon the volume of urine in the bladder, the part of the intraabdominal pressure that is transmitted to the bladder, and the tension in the bladder wall that is related to muscular and nervous system activity. Normal resting pressure within the bladder is 20 cm to 30 cm of water.

The intraurethral pressure depends upon striated and smooth muscle fibers within the urethral wall, the vasculature of the urethral submucosal cavernous

Table 8.1 Neurologic Control of Micturition: Clinical Considerations on Central Nervous System Reflex Loops

Loop	Origin	Termination	Function	Associated conditions
I	Frontal lobe	Brainstem	Coordinates volitional control of micturition	Parkinson's disease, brain tumors, trauma, cerebrovascular disease, MS, lower urinary tract disease
II	a. Brainstem	Sacral micturition center	Detrusor muscle contraction to empty bladder	Spinal cord trauma, MS, spinal cord tumors
	b. Bladder wall	Brainstem		
III	Sensory afferents of detrusor muscle	Striated muscle of urethral sphincter via pudendal motor nervous and micturition center	Allows relaxation of urethral sphincter in synchrony with detrusor contraction	MS, spinal cord trauma or tumors, diabetic neuropathy, local urinary tract disease
IV	Frontal lobe	Pudendal nucleus	Volitional control of striated external urethral sphincter	Cerebral or spinal trauma or tumor, MS, cerebrovascular disease, lower urinary tract disease

From Ostergard DR: The neurologic control of micturition and integral voiding reflexes. *Obstet Gynecol Surv* 1979; 34:417.

Table 8.2 Drugs with Possible Effects on the Lower Urinary Tract

Class	Possible side effects	Drug and usual indication	Action
Antihypertensives	Incontinence	Reserpine—hypertension Methyldopa—hypertension	Pharmacologic sympathectomy by depleting catecholamines
Dopaminergic agents	Bladderneck obstruction	Bromocriptine—galactorrhea Levodopa—Parkinson's disease	Increased urethral resistance and decreased detrusor contractions
Cholinergic agonists	Decreased bladder capacity and increased intravesical pressure	Digitalis—cardiotropic	Increased bladder wall tension
Neuroleptics	Incontinence	Major tranquilizers: prochlorperazine, promethazine, trifluoperazine, chlorpromazine, haloperidol	Dopamine receptor blockade, with internal sphincter relaxation
β-adrenergic agents	Urinary retention	Isoxsuprine—vasodilator Terbutaline—bronchodilator Ritodrine—tocolytic agent	Inhibited bladder muscle contractility
Xanthines	Incontinence	Caffeine	Decreased urethral closure pressure

From Corlett RC: Gynecologic urology: I. Urinary incontinence. *Female Patient* 1985; 10:20.

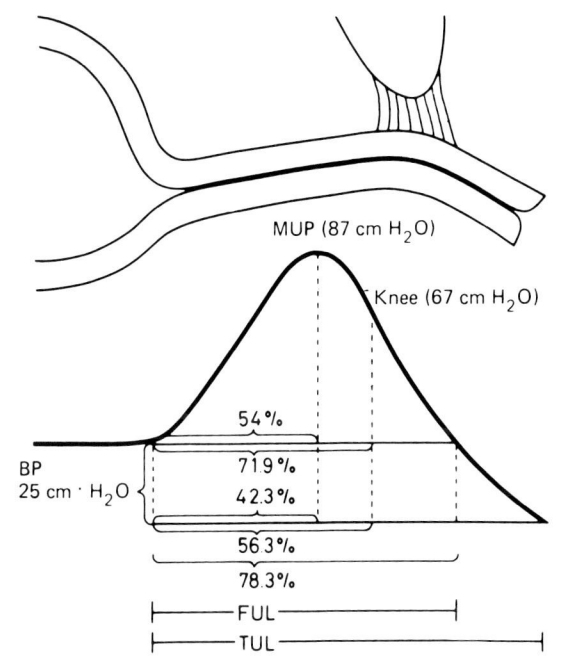

Figure 8.3 The location of maximum urethral pressure in relation to the urogenital diaphragm (average value of 25 normal women). KNEE indicates the location of the urogenital diaphragm seen on x-ray film and transformed to the pressure curve. (From Asmussen M, Ulmsten U: On the physiology of continence and pathophysiology of stress incontinence in the female. *Contrib Gynecol Obstet* 1983;10:32–35.)

plexus, the elasticity of the urethral wall, and the part of the intraabdominal pressure which is transmitted to the urethra. The urethral closure pressure is defined as the maximum urethral pressure minus the bladder pressure. For continence to be present, the urethral closure pressure (UCP) must be greater than the intracystic pressure. Asmussen and Ulmsten have demonstrated that the highest pressure zone in the urethra is just proximal to the mid-point of the total length of the urethra, and just above the urogenital diaphragm (Figure 8.3). Enhorning et al[4] and Asmussen and Ulmsted[3] have noted that the submucosal cavernous plexus of vessels, the bulk of smooth and striate musculature, and the majority of autonomic nervous system fibers are the most prominent in this area. In addition, pressure recording within this area oscillates in synchrony with the heartbeat, making it likely that the submucosal cavernous plexus is important in helping to maintain continence. The structure is also under the influence of estrogen. The oscillations which correlate with heartbeat in young women can be as great as 25 cm of water. In postmenopausal women not on estrogen replacement, it may be as little as 5 cm of water. In addition, this cavernous plexus is more thick-walled and less elastic in older women. Therefore, estrogen is important to the urethral closure mechanism because of its effect upon the α-adrenergic receptors, the elasticity and maintenance of the subcavernous plexus, and, also, because of its positive effect on the epithelium of the urethra, itself. When the urethra is properly supported and the majority of the functional urethra is in its normal position above the urogenital diaphragm, it will receive an increase in intraabdominal pressure simultaneously with the effect of the increase on the bladder. Thus, a sudden increase in intraabdominal pressure should not, under normal circumstances, cause incontinence. If the functional urethra is displaced from its usual anatomical relationships, it is now below the urogenital diaphragm. Then an increase in intraabdominal pressure to the bladder will not equally affect the urethra but, rather, will be additive to the intravesicular pressure. In such instances, stress incontinence is a common finding. These issues will be discussed later in the chapter when incontinence is considered.

Diagnostic Tests and Procedures

A great number of tests and procedures are available to the physician for the evaluation of urinary tract symptoms and incontinence. These range from very simple tests which can be performed in the doctor's office to more sophisticated tests which require specialized equipment and expertise. Several of these will be discussed.

Urinalysis and Culture

Urine may be collected for analysis and culture either by catheterizing the patient or by collecting a clean voided sample. Such a sample can be collected by first preparing the periurethral area of the vulva with an antiseptic solution. The presence of red blood cells, white blood cells, or bacteria may suggest a urethritis, trigonitis, cystitis, or an infected diverticulum of the urethra as well as the possibility of upper urinary tract infection, such as pyelonephritis. Lower urinary tract infection will often be accompanied by the symptoms of urgency, frequency, dysuria, and, at times, incontinence. Treating the infection with specific antibiotic therapy may alleviate the symptoms completely. Elderly women may be more prone to urinary tract infections because of a loss of resistance created by urethral epithelial changes, decrease in blood supply to the region, change in vaginal pH to a more neutral pH, and a change in vaginal bacteria flora as a result. Debilitation with decreased activity may also contribute. Estrogen-replacement therapy may alleviate some of these conditions.

Test for Residual Urine

This test can be very helpful in evaluating a patient with a cystocele or one who may have overflow incontinence. The patient voids and the amount of urine is measured. She is then catheterized and the residual urine left in the bladder is measured and may be sent for culture and analysis. If the patient has voided at least 100 mL to 150 mL, the residual urine should be less than 50 mL. Larger residuals are suggestive of inadequate bladder emptying, and large amounts may indicate overflow incontinence. This may be seen in patients with a neurogenic bladder. Inadequate bladder emptying may be seen with anatomical abnormalities, such as large cystocele or vaginal prolapse, or may occur as a result of medications affecting micturition. In the case of neurogenic bladder, the patient may have a demyelinating disease, diabetic neuropathy, Parkinson's disease, or a tumor or vascular accident involving the brain or spinal cord.

Office Cystometrics

A good deal of information can be gained about bladder capacity and bladder function quite simply in an office setting. After the patient is catheterized to obtain a residual urine, the catheter is left in place and attached to a graduated asepto syringe without bulb. Warm sterile saline is then infused through the syringe, carefully measuring the amount introduced. When the patient first has the urge to void, the amount can be noted. In a normal patient, this urge generally occurs with 150 mL to 200 mL of saline in the bladder. Following this, saline infusion continues until the patient has a strong urge to void. This usually occurs when 400 mL to 500 mL has been infused. Women with irritated bladders or bladder dyssynergia frequently have their first urge to void at levels far below 150 mL and have bladder capacities considerably less than 400 mL to 500 mL. Patients with neurogenic bladder will often be able to tolerate much larger volumes. Normal women can maintain bladder capacities of greater than 500 mL but generally with great conscious effort.

Stress (Bonney) Test

To perform this test, 250 mL of saline is left in the bladder and the catheter is removed. The patient is asked to cough while in the recumbent position. If urine spurts from the urethral meatus, stress incontinence may be present. Gentle elevation of the bladderneck using the index finger and the middle finger on either side of the urethra may then be performed. Care should be taken not to obstruct the urethra, only to replace it behind the pubic symphysis. The patient is then asked to cough and is observed for loss of urine. If the urine is not lost, the Bonney test is said to be positive. This test can be repeated with the patient in the standing position, as it frequently requires this to demonstrate stress incontinence. Urine loss in the case of stress incontinence is always instantaneous and usually in small amounts. If an instable detrusor muscle is present, there may be a spurt of urine after a slight delay following the cough. The amounts of urine lost are usually much larger. Although the differences may be quite subtle between the performance of the Bonney test in the stress incontinent woman as compared to the woman with a dyssynergic bladder, careful observation may give the operator a clue as to which problem is prominent.

There is a good deal of controversy as to whether or not the Bonney test is of value. This is because it is difficult to compare the results of a Bonney test with more sophisticated cystometric studies. Nevertheless, in the hands of an experienced gynecologist, the information gained may be helpful in determining which steps to follow next in the workup of the patient.

Urethroscopy

This technique allows the operator to visualize the urethra, and therefore offers information about the possibility of an inflammatory reaction, a diverticulum, or other pathology, as well as allowing the operator to note urethral tone, presence of estrogen effect, and other anatomical defects that may be present. A gas medium is usually used, with carbon dioxide being the most common. Currently available equipment allows for the performing of pressure readings within the urethra and the bladder but caution must be exercised to avoid rapid installation of carbon dioxide into the lower urinary tract. This may in itself stimulate detrusor contraction and lead to a reflex opening of the vesicle neck, thus giving the operator a false impression of function and pathology. Equipment is relatively simple to operate and quite inexpensive, and can easily be applied to office evaluation.[5]

Cystoscopy and Cystometry

Cystoscopy can be performed using either a water system or carbon-dioxide gas system. The former is probably better in diagnosing detrusor hyperactivity because it is less irritating to the detrusor muscle. With either system the bladder may be visualized and pathology noted.

Cystometry involves the simultaneous recording of pressure within the urethra, the bladder, and the abdominal cavity, and the evaluation of how changes within one area affect others. This can be accomplished with a variety of equipment, ranging from the very simple to the very sophisticated. It is possible to combine these pressure readings with a video cinematography instrument which makes it possible to record the pressure changes during micturition. Since some women are incontinent because of both a stress urinary incontinence component and a bladder dyssynergia component, it is important to define the causes of incontinence for the individual patient before undertaking therapy. This will be discussed more thoroughly when the specific types of incontinence are considered.

Lower Urinary Tract Infections

At least 25% of all women develop urinary tract infections at some time during their life, and by age 70 as many as 10% will have developed chronic urinary tract infections. The inflammation generally involves the urethra, the trigone area of the bladder, and the bladder itself. Symptoms of frequency, urgency, dysuria, pyuria, hematuria, and even pelvic pain and back ache, as well as fever, may occur. Occasionally, incontinence is associated with acute or chronic infection. A variety of organisms including *Klebsiella, Pseudomonas, Proteus, Streptococcus fecalis, Staphylococcus,* and *Chlamydia* are found, but *Escherichia coli* is probably the most commonly encountered organism. Bacteria may be present in the urine (bacteriuria), but a clinical infection usually involves a concentration of organisms of at least 1×10^5 per mL of urine. However, in cases of urethritis and trigonitis, as few as 1×10^2 organisms per mL may be found in infection because of a dilution factor from bladder urine. White blood cells (pyuria) are found with urinary tract infections, and red blood cells may be present as well in either microscopic or macroscopic numbers, especially when the infection is acute.[6]

It is not clear why women are susceptible to urinary tract infections and why older women may actually be more vulnerable. The reasons advanced include: a shortened urethra in the female often made apparently shorter by hormone withdrawal; the close proximity of the vulva, vagina, and rectum to the urethra (areas where multiple bacterial flora is present); poor hygiene brought about because of physical or mental incapacitation; the habit some women have of wiping their anus toward the urethra; chronic mild trauma from sexual intercourse; and the loss of estrogen effect on the reproductive and urinary tract in postmenopausal women. Urinary tract obstruction that may occur because of pelvic relaxation problems may also play a role in some women.[6]

The treatment of infections of the lower urinary tract involve culture and identification of the appropriate organism, followed by appropriate antibiotic therapy. In the acute situation, a culture may be obtained and the patient begun on a general antibiotic regimen known to be effective against most urinary pathogens, such as a sulfa preparation or a nitrofurantoin. A variety of other antibiotics could be used as substitutes, including tetracycline, ampicillin, a cefalosporin, or NegGram. After the culture report is available and the sensitivities of the organism are known, the appropriate antibiotic may be substituted, if necessary. While most authorities accept the fact that appropriate treatment for 10 days is generally adequate for most acute infections, it may be possible to sterilize the urine and clear the infection in less time under some circumstances. Chronic recurrent infections may be the result of undertreatment. Since many individuals will stop using their therapy after 48 hours if the symptoms have disappeared, if the same organism is found in a recurrent infection, it is likely that this is the case. However, if different organisms are found, a recurrent infection may have been what has occurred. For such individuals, long-term use of lower-dose antibiotics may be appropriate.[6]

Frequent catheterization and manipulation of the lower urinary tract may lead to urinary tract infections. In general, indwelling catheters left in place for 24 hours will lead to bacteriuria in as many as 50% of the patients. When left in place for 96 hours, they will cause bacteriuria in almost everyone. There is no good evidence that prophylactic antibiotic use for chronically catheterized patients prevents infection. The patients with catheters should be monitored for the presence of infection. Postoperative and debilitated patients seem to be at the greatest risk.[7]

Elderly patients with chronic urinary tract infections almost always benefit from estrogen replacement. This should be considered as part of the therapy. Sexually active elderly women who note flare-ups of urinary tract infections after coitus can be encouraged to void immediately after intercourse. This tends to wash bacteria from the urethra and may cut down on the incidence of urinary tract infections.

Urethral Diverticulum

Urethral diverticula have been reported in women of all ages, with the majority occurring between the ages of 30 and 50. Nonetheless, elderly women often develop diverticula and, as many as 3% to 4% of women will actually develop this problem sometime during their life. The disease occurs more frequently in Blacks than Caucasians, with a ratio as high as 6:1.[8]

Proposed etiologies for urethral diverticula include congenital, acute and chronic inflammatory conditions, and trauma. While a variety of etiologic conditions may be responsible, an infectious etiology is probably the most common, perhaps stemming from infection and obstruction of the peri-urethral glands. Resultant retention cyst formation and rupture into the lumen of the urethra could give rise to the diverticulum. Although *N. gonococcus* has been implicated as the cause of this condition by some authors, *E. coli* and other organisms have often been found in diverticula.

Inflamed diverticula generally cause urgency, frequency, dysuria, and sometimes dyspareunia. Recurrent urinary tract infections, dribbling, and even incontinence have been noted. Occasionally, hematuria is present. The majority of patients complain of a tender suburethral mass and, occasionally, the diverticulum may protrude from the vagina.

The diagnosis may be suspected on physical examination and can be confirmed by cystourethroscopy or by voiding cystourethrogram. The technique of double-catheter balloon insufflation to demonstrate the diverticulum at the time of cystogram is frequently helpful in making the diagnosis. Therapy for diverticulum of the urethra requires identification of the diverticulum using urethroscopy and operative excision and repair. It is important to investigate for the possibility of multiple diverticula. Lee noted 18 such instances in 85 patients investigated by the Mayo Clinic.[9]

Major complications following the repair of a urethral diverticulum include urethrovaginal fistula, which has been reported in about 5% of repairs, and stricture of the urethra which occasionally occurs. Recurrence rates have been estimated to be 5% to 10%. If a diverticulum recurs immediately following the operation, it probably represents a second diverticulum that was overlooked or an inappropriate repair. If there is a recurrence after 1 year, it is probably a new lesion. Occasionally, stress incontinence secondary to the dissection of the bladderneck may occur.

Genuine Stress Incontinence

Genuine stress incontinence is defined as a condition of immediate involuntary loss of urine when intravesicular pressure exceeds the maximum urethral closure pressure in the absence of detrusor activity. In the continent woman in the resting state, the urethra closure pressure is greater than the intravesicular pressure, and the sudden increase in the intraabdominal pressure generated by either a cough or the strain of lifting something is generally transmitted equally to both the bladder and the bladderneck and urethra. This is true because the bladderneck and proximal urethra are above the urogenital diaphragm and essentially above intraabdominal organs. This phenomenon was demonstrated by Enhorning et al[4] using simultaneous intraurethral and intravesicle pressure measurements. In the woman with genuine stress incontinence, the proximal urethra and bladderneck are frequently displaced below the urogenital diaphragm and are no longer intraabdominal organs. With an increase in intraabdominal pressure, the force generated is additive to the intravesicle pressure, and is usually enough to overcome urethral closure pressure. These anatomical changes may come about because of relaxation of pelvic-support structures, including the urogenital diaphragm musculature, or because of damage to the supports of the urethra and upper vagina to the pubic symphysis. Childbearing, trauma, loss of hormonal support to these tissues, and general stress and strain over the years may cause or accentuate this process.

In the past, a number of other reasons have been given for the cause of stress incontinence. One of these was felt to be the shortening of the urethra which occurred with time. Lapides et al measured urethral length before and after operations for correction of stress incontinence using calibrated intraurethral catheters and found that, in incontinent cases, the urethra did appear to be shorter. However, during the procedure, downward traction was exerted in order to give the most accurate measurement.[10] Since the bladderneck of many women will funnel, the accuracy of their measurements has been suspect. In studies using bead-chain cystourethrocystography by multiple investigators, no difference in length of the urethra has been noted before or after surgical repair. Thus, urethral length does not seem to be a major factor in the cause of stress incontinence.[11]

Jeffcoate and Roberts[12] introduced the concept of the importance of the posterior urethral vesicle angle for the maintenance of stress incontinence. They believed that a normal posterior urethrovesicle angle (PUV) of less than 120° was an important aspect for the maintenance of continence, since this angle was usually greater than 120° in patients suffering from stress incontinence. They had noted that the relationship of the bladderneck and the urethra to the pubic symphysis was not the major anatomic feature in the etiology of stress incontinence, since many patients with bladder descent but with normal PUV angles were continent, whereas some incontinent women had bladders and urethras reasonably well positioned to the pubic symphysis but had lost their PUV angle. Normal continent women will demonstrate a bladder base nearly parallel to the horizontal in the standing position, and will have a PUV angle of 90° to 100°. Such bladders, when visualized on cystourethrocystography will be noted to have this angle maintained with cough, and funneling of the bladderneck does not occur. With stress incontinence, there is almost a complete loss of the PUV angle, and funneling and posterior descent of the vesicle neck does occur. Attempts to measure the PUV angle using chain cystourethrocystography and the Q-tip test, in which a Q-tip is placed in the urethra and the angle measured both in the standing relaxed position and with cough, have demonstrated that the change in the PUV angle is not a predictive finding in patients with genuine stress incontinence. Recently, Montz and Stanton[13] reevaluated the Q-tip test and discovered that 32% of patients with a positive Q-tip test had either pure detrusor instability or pure sensory urgency after complete urologic workup. Twenty-nine percent of the patients who had a negative Q-tip test were diagnosed as pure genuine stress incontinence. Fantel et al[11] demonstrated that 83 cystourethrograms, done by the chain cystourethrogram technique and interpreted by three radiologists utilizing five specific radiologic landmarks, failed to identify any agreement in interpretation with a variation in interpretation being from 19.3% to 54.2%. Fantel's group could find no statistically significant difference in the distribution of radiographic characteristics between patients with stress incontinence and detrusor instability using this test. Therefore, it must be concluded that tests that measure PUV angle are not sensitive enough to determine whether or not the patient has stress incontinence, and a complete urologic urodynamic workup is indicated in most instances. It is fairly well accepted that PUV angle is not as critical as the position of the bladderneck within the abdominal cavity.

Many women with pelvic relaxation have large cystoceles. A cystocele is a herniation of the bladder into the vagina and can be seen with the patient in the lithotomy position or standing as a bulge in the anterior vaginal wall. If these patients have well-supported bladdernecks, they will usually be continent. On the other hand, if the urethra and bladder are involved in the anatomical defect forming a cystourethrocele, the patient will often be incontinent. Incontinence in a patient with a cystocele is rare, whereas in patients with cystourethroceles it is quite common.

Therapy for stress incontinence can be divided into nonoperative and operative approaches. In the older woman, this would include estrogen replacement therapy, which increases the vasculature and tone of the bladderneck and the pelvic supports and thereby increases urethral closure pressure. Estrogen also stimulates an increase in β receptors, which tend to quiet the bladder and increase the contractility of the urethra. In addition, isometric exercises first described by Kegel may increase the muscular tone of the urogenital diaphram. Kegel[14] in 1956 suggested that patients contract their pubococcygeal muscles five times upon awaking, five times upon arising, and five times every half hour throughout the day. These muscles can be demonstrated to the patient by asking her to contract the muscles that it takes to stop the urinary stream during urination. Once she knows which muscles to contract, Kegel exercises may be performed. Since most patients will not follow a rigorous schedule as laid down by Kegel, it will probably suffice to ask them to exercise these muscles by contracting them 10 times to the count of 10 several times a day. A combination of Kegel exercises and estrogen replacement may be enough to overcome milder forms of genuine stress incontinence.

Other drugs and combinations of drugs have been studied to determine whether or not they are of aid in preventing stress incontinence. Kiesswetter et al[15] studied 30 stress incontinent women with clinical and urodynamic assessment. These authors compared a continence profile before and after treatment with an α-adrenergic stimulant, midodrine; a cholinesterase inhibitor, distigmine bromide; a tricyclic antidepressant, imipramine; or an estriol, triodurin. In each case, the patients were treated for 4 weeks and reevaluated. Finally, a suspensory sling operation was performed. The continence profile as described by the authors improved 45% with the sling procedure as compared with an improvement of 9% for midodrine; 8.9% for imipramine, and 7.9% for a combination of estriol and distigmine bromide. Urethral pressures increased by a mean value of 8.1% after operation, 8.3% after midodrine, 7.9% after imipramine, and 3.5% after the estrogen and distigmine bromide combination. The combination of estriol plus midodrine and estriol plus imipramine were favored by patients over single-drug therapy, but little difference was noted in urodynamic assessment. Imipramine is a tricyclic antidepressant but does have α-adrenergic enhancement characteristics.

Before 1950, the operative procedure of choice for treating stress incontinence was primarily a vaginal procedure which included plication of the bladderneck (Kelly procedure) with an anterior colporrhaphy to reduce a cystocele, if it existed. However, with Green's[16] attempt to grade degrees of PUV angle loss, Bailey[17] and others stated that success rates for curing stress incontinence using the vaginal approach varied according to the etiology of the stress incontinence. Patients showing a complete loss of PUV angle had a 90% success rate when followed for 5 to 10 years after bladderneck plication and anterior colporrhapy, but only 50% of patients with lesser PUV angle loss remained continent over that time period. With the introduction of the suprapubic urethrovesicle suspension operations, the 5-year cure rate for these latter patients has passed 90% in most series. It did seem important to workers at that time to determine the type of anatomical defect the patient had and to design appropriate operative management. Today, the general consensus is that women with definite anterior vaginal-wall relaxation and bladderneck displacement into the lower pelvis do best with anterior colporrhaphy and plication of the bladderneck.

Since many of these patients have uterine prolapse, these operations are frequently performed in conjunction with a vaginal hysterectomy and posterior colporrhaphy. However, vaginal hysterectomy should be performed only if indicated.

Newer polyglycol suture has made it possible to improve the success rate with anterior colporrhaphy and bladderneck plication, and many operators will suspend the upper vagina and bladderneck to the pubic symphysis during a vaginal procedure. One such procedure is that designed by Pereyra,[18] in which a special needle is used to guide sutures from the paracervical tissue through the space of Retzius and through the rectus fascia on both sides. The sutures are then tied above the anterior rectus fascia via a small suprapubic incision. Stamey's[19] modification of the Pereyra procedure utilizes a small tube of dacron material to buttress the suture, thereby keeping it from pulling through. Stamey reports about 3% of patients in his series require removal of this suprapubic suture because of pain or infection.

For patients without significant anterior vaginal-wall relaxation but with genuine stress incontinence, a suprapubic urethropexy is the best procedure. Basically, two procedures are in common use. The first is the Marshall–Marchetti–Krantz suprapubic urethrovesicle suspension operation, which was first reported in 1949,[20] and may be performed either by itself or in conjunction with other abdominal procedures, such as hysterectomy. In this respect, paravaginal tissue adjacent to the bladderneck is sutured bilaterally to the pubic symphysis utilizing two or three interrupted sutures on either side. Today, polyglycol suture is the most ideal for this procedure, but permanent sutures such as silk or nylon may also be used.

The second procedure in common use was first described by Burch[21] in 1961. In this case, the upper vaginal wall is sutured to Cooper's ligaments on either side, also using a polyglycol suture. These operations have a success rate in excess of 90% when performed properly.

In situations where these procedures fail to alleviate the stress incontinence, the operations may be reperformed or a urethral sling procedure using a variety of materials may be fashioned. Currently, the most popular of these is the use of a strip of anterior rectus fascia. Although the sling procedure has been reported to have uniformly good results, it is more of an operative procedure than the Marshall–Marchetti–Krantz or Burch procedures because of the necessity of dissecting the bladderneck free by both a vaginal and abdominal approach and a greater instance of morbidity and infection. In most instances, it is reserved as a back-up procedure.

In a study of 29 women investigated urodynamically before and after a Marshall–Marchetti–Krantz by Beisland et al[22] no major changes in urethral pressure profile could be demonstrated. These authors did demonstrate a good correlation between the clinical results and the changes in transmission of increased abdominal pressure to the urethra. The procedure did not increase urethral pressure. Those patients with low maximal urethral pressure preoperatively continued to have insufficient urethral sphincter function after the operation. These authors concluded that patients with a low urethral closure pressure, but with good transmission to the urethra of pressure, are not suitable candidates for urethropexy. Insufficiency of the urethral sphincter in postmenopausal women is most often associated with atrophy of the urethra and vaginal epithelium as well as decreased blood supply to the periurethral tissue. Beisland et al, therefore, suggested that such patients should be treated with a combination of α-receptor-stimulating drugs and estrogen and not by operation. Further studies have demonstrated that Marshall–Marchetti–Krantz and Burch procedures most likely work by partially mechanically obstructing the bladderneck in addition to replacing the bladderneck behind the pubic symphysis.

Detrusor Dyssynergia

Detrusor dyssynergia is defined as involuntary contraction of the bladder during distension with urine or other fluids. It is usually associated with urge incontinence, which is the involuntary loss of urine associated with a strong desire to void. This may be divided into motor urge incontinence, which is associated with uninhibited detrusor contractions, and sensory urge incontinence which is not caused by uninhibited detrusor contractions. Fifty to eighty percent of detrusor dyssynergic patients have an underlying functional or psychosomatic component, but patients may suffer from generalized diseases which effect the bladder or its innervation. Often, the loss of urine is painless and consists of a large volume. Leakage may occur in any position and often with a change of position. In stress situations, such as running, walking, coughing, sneezing, or laughing, the incontinence may be triggered, but is usually followed by a general delay of seconds after the stress has occurred. On the other hand, urine loss with stress incontinence occurs immediately following the stress. Stress incontinence disappears at night but urge incontinence or detrusor dyssynergia continues with nocturia. Detrusor dyssynergia patients are rarely able to stop their stream during the act of voiding, whereas women with stress incontinence can often accomplish this. The loss of urine in detrusor dyssynergia is usually triggered by a sudden inhibited stimulation of receptors in the bladder wall. These receptors may be hyperactive due to emotional reasons or due to chronic irritation, such as urinary tract infection. The condition may also be secondary to a breakdown of normal neurologic and inhibitory reflexes.[22]

The diagnosis is made using electronic urethrocystometry or fluid cystometrography, which detects spontaneous involuntary pressure changes within the bladder as the bladder is filled. These techniques will also allow for the detection of a detrusor dyssynergia component in patients with genuine stress incontinence, so that both issues may be addressed.

Treatment of detrusor dyssynergia is not surgical. Although patients with both stress incontinence and detrusor dyssynergia may require an operation after medical therapy has been tried, it is not infrequent, however, to find that when the detrusor dyssynergic component is treated that the operative procedure is not necessary. In like manner, individuals with both components who are subjected to surgery first may find they are still incontinent after the procedure because of the detrusor dyssynergia component. In some instances, when the anatomical defect is repaired, the dyssynergia component gradually disappears.

Detrusor dyssynergia may be due to an irritated bladder. An inspection for urinary tract infection and for intrinsic bladder disease should be carried out. Obviously, such infections should be treated, if found, and other bladder pathology noted on cystoscopy can be treated as well.

Since the majority of patients with detrusor dyssynergia have psychosomatic problems, retraining or bladder drills may be of use. These take the form of a program of progressively lengthening the period between voiding with or without the addition of medications or biofeedback techniques. Millard and Oldenburg[24] demonstrated improvement in 74% of women with detrusor dyssynergia using such techniques. Cystometic studies before and after therapy revealed a reversion to stable bladder function.

Estrogen is a major part of the therapy of detrusor dyssynergia in the elderly, since not only will it improve the vasculature of the bladderneck and urethra and improve the condition of the epithelium of the urethra and trigone, it will also stimulate the development of α-adrenergic receptors.

Anticholinergic drugs or β-adrenergic-stimulating agents will help relax detrusor muscle and may be useful in the therapy of detrusor dyssynergia. Propantheline (Pro-Banthine) at doses of 15 mg to 30 mg 4 times per day, oxybutynin chloride (Ditropan) 5 mg every 8 to 12 hours, flavoxate (Uripas) 200 mg every 6 hours, imipramine (Tofranil) 50 mg every 8 hours, or ephedrine sulfate 25 mg every 6 hours may be tried with or without bladder training. Most elderly women with detrusor dyssynergia will respond very well to a combination of estrogen replacement and an anticholinergic drug. On the other hand, since anticholinergic drugs are contraindicated in women with glaucoma, this possibility should be addressed in prescribing for an older woman.[6]

True Incontinence

True incontinence is the loss of urine without abnormal bladder function. It is usually seen in the case of fistulas or other damage to the urinary tract. Such damage may be congenital or secondary to trauma, such as that occurring secondary to injury, operative procedures, or irradiation.

The diagnosis of a fistula should be aimed at determining the site of the fistula (ie, vesicovaginal, urethrovaginal, or ureterovaginal). Each will need to be corrected surgically in a different fashion. Urethrovaginal fistulas are generally seen following the repair of a urethral diverticulum or postoperatively following surgery to correct incontinence. These injuries are rare and must be repaired operatively.

Vesicovaginal fistulas are diagnosed by instilling toluidine blue dye into the bladder and noting that it passes directly into the vagina. Cystoscopy and intravenous pyelogram should be carried out to determine that the ureters are not involved and to identify the site of the fistula. If the fistula is free of the ureteal orifices, it may lend itself to vaginal repair. If the fistula is near the ureteral openings, it is probably best to repair via a transvesicle approach. This approach is often most suited to repeat attempts at repair. Ureterovaginal fistuli most often require a mobilization of the ureter and reimplantation into the bladder.

In all cases of fistula, the operator must ensure that the blood supply to the area is adequate. For fistuli that follow trauma or operative injury, generally this is not a serious problem. However, for fistuli secondary to irradiation injury, the blood supply is generally compromised. Procedures to cover a vesicovaginal fistula with a myelo-cutaneous flap are probably the best solution to correcting the problem. For ureterovaginal fistuli following irradiation therapy, reimplantation of the ureter into the bladder is appropriate.

Overflow Incontinence

This condition occurs when a bladder is overdistended because of its inability to empty. The problem is most often neurologic and is seen in conditions which interfere with normal bladder reflexes or to partial obstruction of the urethra. The patient generally complains of voiding small amounts of urine and still having the feeling that there is urine in the bladder. The patient may lose small amounts of urine frequently. The condition is commonly seen in patients with multiple sclerosis, diabetic neuropathy, trauma, or tumors of the central nervous system. A complete general medical and neurologic evaluation is necessary to identify the cause of the problem. Therapy is generally directed at the primary cause. The patient may need to be trained in techniques of intermittent self-catheterization.

References

1. DeLancey JO: Correlative studies of periurethral anatomy. *Obstet Gynecol* 1986;68:91.
2. Williams ME, Fitzhugh CP: Urinary incontinence in the elderly. *Ann Intern Med* 1982; 97:895.
3. Asmussen M, Ulmsten U: On the physiology of continence and pathophysiology of stress incontinence in the female. *Controversies Gynecol Obstet* 1983; vol. 10.
4. Enhorning G, et al: Simultaneous recording of intravesicle and intraurethral pressure. *Acta Chir Cand* 1971;276(Suppl):1.
5. Hodgkinson CP, Cobert N: Direct urethrocystommetry. *Am J Obstet Gynecol* 1960; 79:648.
6. Droegemueller W, Herbst AL, Mishell DR, Stenchver MA: *Comprehensive Gynecology*. St. Louis, CV Mosby, 1987.
7. Buchsbaum HJ, Schmidt JD (eds.): *Gynecologic and Obstetric Urology*. Philadelphia, WB Saunders, 1982.
8. Andersen MTF: The incidence of diverticula in the female urethra. *J Urology* 1967; 98:96.
9. Lee RA: Diverticulum of the female urethra: Postoperative complications and results. *Obstet Gynecol* 1983;61:52.
10. Lapides J, Ajemian EP, Stewart EH, et al: Physiopathology of stress incontinence. *Surg Gynecol Obstet* 1960;11:224.
11. Fantl JA, Beachley MC, Bosch HA, et al: B-chain cystourethrogram: An evaluation. *Obstet Gynecol* 1981;58:237.
12. Jeffcoate TNA, Roberts H: Observations of stress incontinence of urine. *Am J Obstet Gynecol* 1952;64:721.
13. Montz FJ, Stanton SL: Q-tip test in female urinary incontinence. *Obstet Gynecol* 1986; 67:258.
14. Kegel AH: Stress incontinence of urine in women: Physiologic treatment. *J Int Coll Surg* 1956;25:487.
15. Kiesswetter H, Hennrichs F, Englisch M: Clinical and urodynamic assessment of pharmacologic therapy of stress incontinence. *Urol Int* 1983;38:58.
16. Green TH Jr: Development of a plan for diagnosis and treatment of urinary stress incontinence. *Am J Obstet Gynecol* 1962;83:632.
17. Bailey KV: The clinical investigation into uterine prolapse with stress incontinence: Treatment of modified Manchester colporrhaphy. *Br J Obstet Gynaecol* (Part I) 1954; 61:291; (Part II) 1956;63:663; (Part III) 1963;70:947.
18. Pereyra AJ: A simplified surgical procedure for the correction of stress incontinence in women. *Western J Surg* 1959;67:223.

19. Stamey TA: Endoscopic suspension of the vesicle neck for urinary incontinence in females: A report of 203 consecutive cases. *Ann Surg* 1980;192:465.
20. Marchetti AA, Marshall VF, Shultis LD: Simple vesicle urethral suspension for stress incontinence of urine. *Am J Obstet Gynecol* 1957;74:57.
21. Burch JC: Cooper's ligament urethrovesicle suspension for stress incontinence. *Am J Obstet Gynecol* 1968;100:764.
22. Beisland HO, Fossberg E, Sander S: Urodynamic studies before and after retropubic urethropexy for stress incontinence in female. *Surg Gynecol Obstet* 1982;155:333.
23. Frewen WK: Urgency incontinence. *Br J Obstet Gynaecol* 1972;79:77.
24. Millard RJ, Oldenburg BF: The symptomatic urodynamic and cyclodynamic results of bladder re-education programs. *J Urol* 1983;130:715.

Chapter **9**

Problems of Loss of Pelvic Support

Morton Stenchever, MD

Pelvic-support structures frequently weaken as women age. Such stresses as congenital anatomical weakness, childbirth, physical injury, and damage sustained by chronic straining or by surgical intervention, all contribute to this phenomenon. In addition, the withdrawal of estrogen stimulation to pelvic-support tissue and its blood supply further aids this weakening. This chapter will address the specific conditions which are a result of the weakening of the pelvic-support structures, and discuss their diagnosis and treatment.

Anatomical Considerations

Pelvic Diaphragm

The pelvic diaphragm is the major muscle group that with its fascia supports the pelvic organs. It consists of two muscles: the coccygeus and levator ani muscles. These muscles have evolved from the tail-wagging musculature of quadrupeds. They are strong muscles with interwoven bundles and they completely close off the pelvis except for openings for the urethra, vagina, and rectum, which they encircle. The levator ani muscle is the largest and has three components named for their origin and insertion: pubococcygeus, puborectalis, and iliococcygeus. The total muscle mass extends from the pubic symphysis to the coccyx, and from lateral sidewall to lateral sidewall. The coccygeus is a triangularly shaped muscle that extends between both ischial spines and to the coccyx as the apex of the triangle. The levator ani muscles functioning jointly play a major role in the control of urination, in the birth process, in maintaining fecal continence, and in supporting abdominal and pelvic viscera (Figure 9.1).

Urogenital Diaphragm

A second musculofascial diaphragm important in pelvic support is the more superficial diaphragm extending from the pubic symphysis to a line between the two ischial tuberosities. It supports the anterior segment of the pelvic outlet and consists of three muscle bundles: the ischiocavernosus, which extends between the pubic symphysis and the ischial tuberoscity along the pubic ramus;

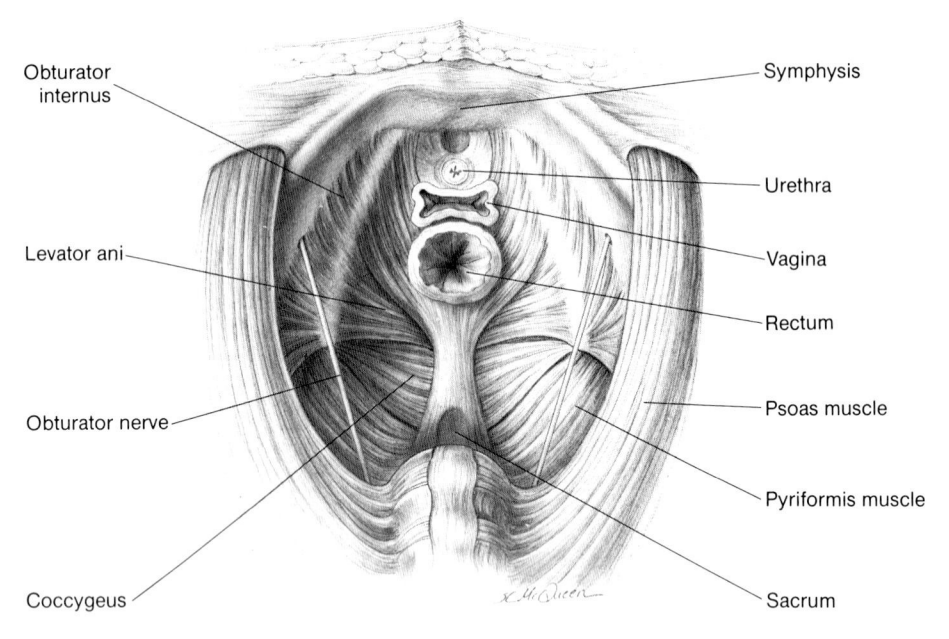

Figure 9.1 A superior view of the pelvic diaphragm, demonstrating the levator ani and coccygeus muscles. (From Droegemueller W, Herbst AL, Mishell DR, Stenchever, MA: Disorders of abdominal wall and pelvic support, in *Comprehensive Gynecology*, Ch. 19. St. Louis, CV Mosby, 1987.)

the bulbocavernosus, which extends between the pubic symphysis and the perineal body surrounding the vaginal outlet; and the deep transverse perineal muscle, which extends from the ischial tuberosities to the perineal body. These join with the external anal sphincter muscles that surround the rectum but blend into the perineal body. The urogenital diaphragm supports the external urethra and the introitus to the vagina. The urogenital diaphragm contains the pudendal blood vessels and nerves, the external sphincter of the urethra, and the dorsal nerve to the clitoris. The urogenital diaphragm is extremely important in maintaining the position of the bladderneck (Figure 9.2).

Supporting Ligaments

Although pelvic ligaments are called ligaments, they are really thickenings of the retroperitoneal fascia. Nonetheless, these structures tend to surround the vagina and cervix as an endopelvic fascia. The layer that separates the vagina and the cervix from the bladder is commonly called the pubocervical fascia, and tends to support the bladder from herniating into the vagina. This blends laterally with the cardinal ligaments (Mackenrot's ligaments) which extend from the lateral aspect of the upper vagina and cervix to the lateral pelvic wall bilaterally. The cardinal ligaments, as such, form the base of the broad ligament which is a tent of peritoneum draped across the round ligament in which are found the uterine artery and vein and the ureter. The ureter transverses the cardinal ligament adjacent to the cervix. Posteriorly, the endopelvic investment fascia thickens into the uterosacral ligaments which join the cervix to the sacrum. Within these ligaments run nerve bundles that supply the uterus and cervix.

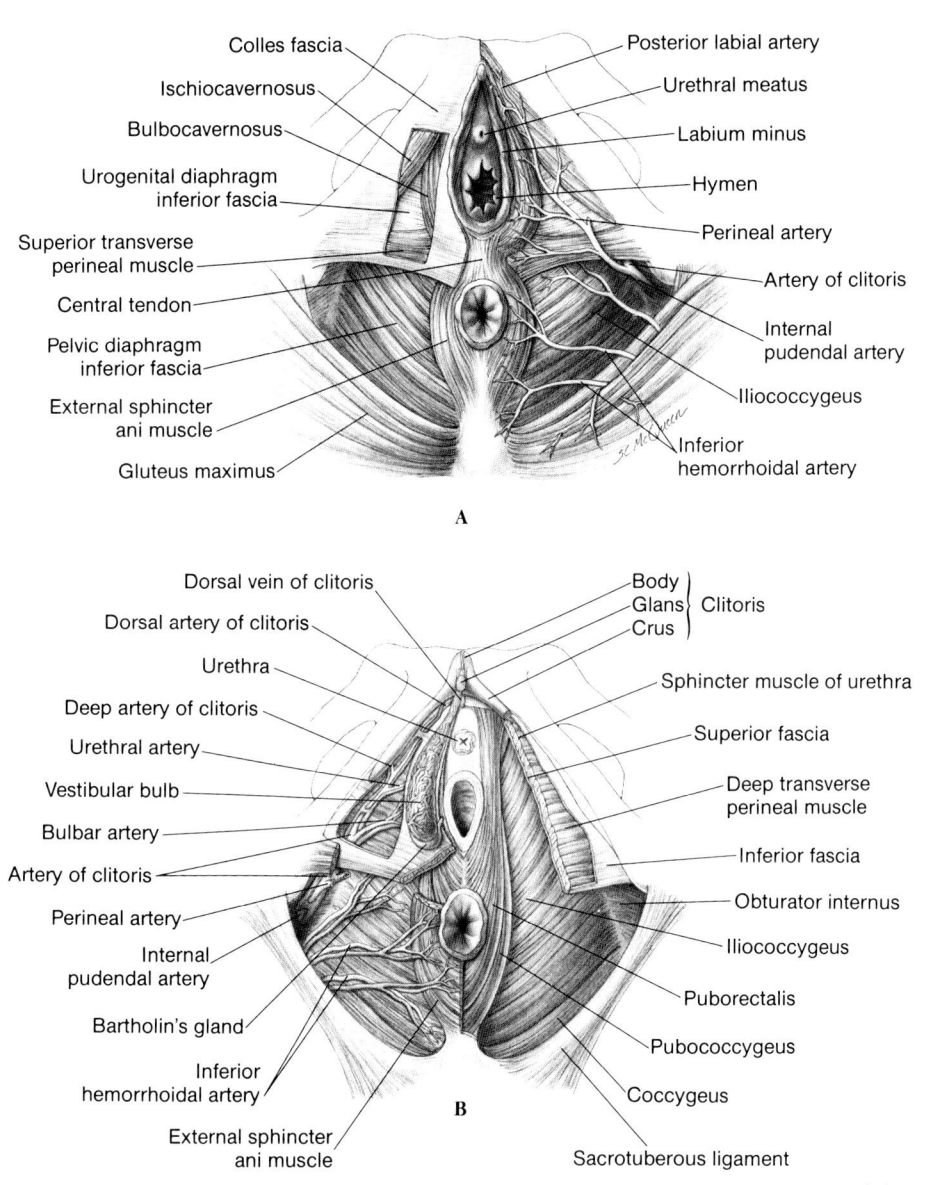

Figure 9.2 (A) Schematic view of the perineum, demonstrating superficial structures of the urogenital diaphragm. **(B)** Schematic view of the perineum, demonstrating superficial structures and deeper structures showing the relationship of the levator, ani, and coccygeus muscles. (From Droegemueller W, Herbst AL, Mishell DR, Stenchever, MA: Disorders of abdominal wall and pelvic support, in *Comprehensive Gynecology*, Ch. 19. St. Louis, OV Mosby, 1987.)

The endopelvic fascia jointly offers support to the pelvic structures that it invests and contributes via the uterosacral ligament to the support of the cul de sac. The round ligament extends from the fundus of the uterus into the inguinal canal, and has little support function other than to help to hold the uterus forward in an anteflexed position. It does, however, make up the apex of the tent of the broad ligament.

Changes with Estrogen Withdrawal

Estrogen withdrawal may have a profound effect on pelvic-support structures. Not only does the loss of estrogen lead to atrophy of the epithelium of the vagina, bladderneck, and urethra, it also relates to the loss of elastic tissue and collagen in the endopelvic support fascia. Such changes can often be reversed, at least in part, by utilizing estrogen-replacement therapy. In general, estrogen-replacement therapy should be prescribed whenever patients are undergoing treatment for pelvic relaxation, unless, of course, there is a contraindication to this therapy.

Pelvic-Support Disorders

If weakening of pelvic-support structures occurs, the resultant problem may be urethrocele, cystocele, rectocele, enterocele, or descensus of the uterus and cervix. Often a variety of these conditions occur in the same patient.

Urethrocele and Cystocele

Weakening of the pubocervical fascia may allow for a herniation of the urethra (urethrocele), bladderneck, or bladder (cystocele) into the vagina. When the urethra and bladderneck remain supported but a cystocele develops, the patient often does not suffer from urinary incontinence. On the other hand, when the support structures beneath the urethra and bladderneck are weakened, urinary stress incontinence may be present. Women with gynecoid-type pelvises, whose subpubic arches are wide, may be at greatest risk for damage to the pubocervical fascia since the pressure of the fetal head at the time of vaginal delivery may be brought to full bear against this region. However, women with narrower pelvic arches may be afforded a degree of protection to this structure.

The symptoms associated with urethrocele and cystocele may include stress incontinence, often a feeling of urgency or a sensation of incomplete emptying after voiding, and a sensation that a structure is falling out of the vagina. The patient may be aware of a soft, bulging mass from the anterior vaginal wall and occasionally will need to replace this mass before being able to void. With strain and cough, the mass is accentuated and may remain present outside the introitus. When the physician examines such a patient, either in a standing position or in lithotomy with straining, the bulge will be apparent (Figure 9.3).

Although urethroceles and cystoceles are almost always found in parous women, they have been noted in nulliparous women who have poor structural supports. This may be associated with congenital malformations or weakness of the musculature and connective tissue of the pelvic floor secondary to chronic strain, trauma, or other forces. Cystoceles are quite common and, in patients without symptoms, therapy may not be required.

For specific diagnosis, the patient is placed in lithotomy position, a posterior blade of a vaginal speculum is inserted to depress the posterior wall, and the patient is asked to strain. The degree of cystocele and/or urethrocele may then be noted. The physician should palpate the bladderneck and estimate the degree of its support. Generally, if the bladderneck is well-supported, the urethra will be as well. In order to best assess the degree of cystocele and urethrocele, the exam is best performed with the bladder at least partially filled (100 to 250 mL).

Urethroceles must be differentiated from inflammation and enlargement of

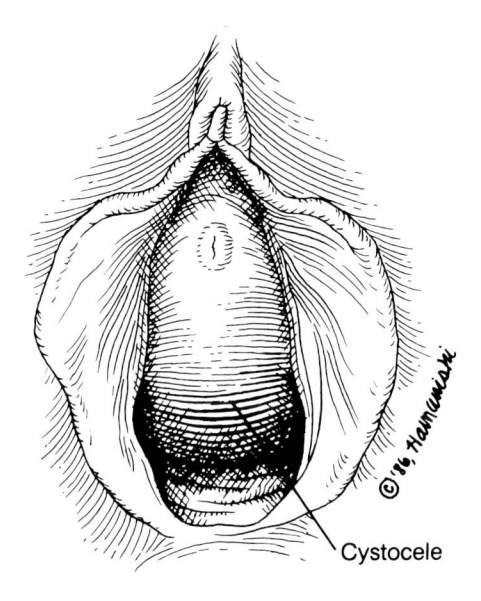

Figure 9.3 Cystocele. (From Droegemueller W, Herbst AL, Mishell DR, Stenchever, MA: Disorders of abdominal wall and pelvic support, in *Comprehensive Gynecology*, Ch. 19. St. Louis, CV Mosby, 1987.)

the Skene's glands and from urethral diverticulum. Bladder tumors and bladder diverticula, which are both rare, may masquerade as cystoceles. Although diverticula of the urethra or the bladder may be reduced, there is generally the sensation of a mass on palpation. Inflamed Skene's glands are tender, and it may be possible to express pus from the urethra when they are palpated. Pus may be expressed from urethral diverticula as well. When such is found, cultures, specifically for chlamydia and gonococcus, are appropriate. Although these organisms are less likely to be found in older than younger women, the possibility still exists.

Therapy for urethrocele and cystocele may be nonoperative or operative. The former consists of supporting the herniation of the bladder using a pessary of the Smith Hodge or inflatable type. Occasionally, in less symptomatic women, even a large tampon may suffice. Kegal exercises (see Chapter 8) will help to strengthen pelvic floor muscles and, therefore, may relieve some of the symptoms of pressure, but will not address the problem of endopelvic fascial damage. In postmenopausal women, estrogen should be prescribed either as a vaginal cream or systemically. This should help to strengthen pelvic-support structures and to improve their vascular supply. Even if a surgical procedure is contemplated, a prethcrapy treatment with estrogen should improve the outcome and aid the healing process.

Cystocele and urethrocele repair may be performed separately or in conjunction with repair of other pelvic-relaxation problems. It is most common, at least, to perform a rectocele repair as well. Often, when a large cystocele with small rectocele is present, if only the cystocele is repaired, the subsequent weakening of the posterior wall will lead to a need for further repair of the posterior wall at a later date. If uterine descensus is noted, this may be addressed operatively as well. Frequently, an enterocele accompanies a cystocele and rectocele and should always be sought during the procedure. When it is present, the enterocele sac should be excised and repair effected.

Anterior wall repair (colporrhaphy) is performed by incising the vaginal

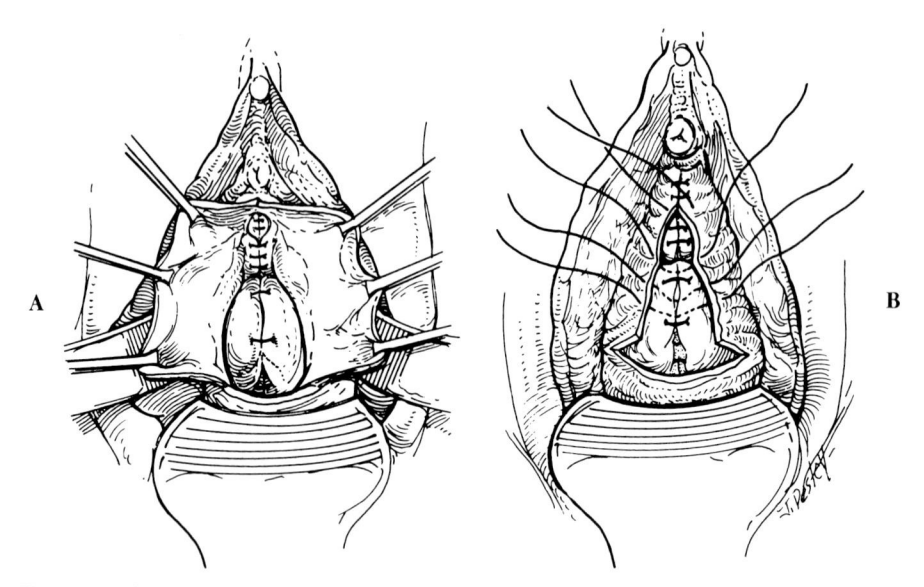

Figure 9.4 Cystourethrocele repair. **(A)** Appearance of a cystourethrocele after plication of bladderneck and repair of cystocele; cut edges of vagina are held apart above repair. **(B)** Repair of vagina over cystocele is noted. (From Symmonds RE: Relaxation of pelvic supports, in Benson RC (ed.): *Current Obstetrics and Gynecologic Diagnosis and Treatment*, ed. 5. Los Altos, California, Lange Medical Publications, 1984.)

epithelium transversely just above the anterior lip of the cervix in the region of the bladder reflection. If a previous hysterectomy has been performed, the incision may be made 1 cm to 1.5 cm anterior to the vaginal scar. The vagina is then incised longitudinally from the transverse incision to the level of the bladderneck. If no urethrocele is present, this is a sufficient extent for the incision. If a urethrocele is present, the incision must be continued under the urethra as well. When a longitudinal incision is complete, the cut edges of the vagina are separated by blunt and sharp dissection from the pubocervical fascia, which is attached to the bladder. This procedure is repeated on both sides and, at this point, the bladder and pubocervical fascia are free of the vaginal wall. The operator then places a suture at the level of the bladderneck (Kelly stitch), bringing together the pubocervical fascia from either side (Figure 9.4). This stitch is placed in such a fashion that pubocervical fascia is sutured as far away from the cut edge as possible in a parallel fashion to the mid-line incision. Zero polyglycol suture is most appropriate for this closure. With the bladderneck identified and supported, the pubocervical fascia is then closed with progressive similar stitches in a fashion that completely imbricates the fascia over the bladder. If a urethrocele is present, it, too, may be repaired in a similar fashion. If a major stress incontinence problem is present, the bladderneck may be further supported to the pubic symphysis using sutures that connect the perivaginal tissue on either side of the urethra to the pubic symphysis. A Pereyra or Stamey modification of the Pereyra procedure is a reasonable alternative. After completing the imbrication of the pubocervical fascia, vaginal edges are trimmed and the vagina is closed with a row of interrupted 2-0 polyglycol or catgut sutures.

The bladder should be drained for about 5 days postoperatively, and this may accomplished in a number of different manners. The first would be to leave a no. 16 Foley catheter in place for 5 days, remove it on day 5, and allow the patient to try to void. If voiding occurs, to the amount of 100 mL to 200 mL, the patient would be catheterized for the presence of residual urine. If residual urine is found in a quantity of greater than 150 mL on two successive voidings, or if the amount of voiding is less than 100 mL, the physician should consider replacing the catheter for an additional 24 to 48 hours. If residual urines are less than 150 mL on two consecutive voidings, no further steps are necessary. Occasionally, patients have difficulty voiding even after an additional 2 days, and may be followed with Foley catheter to continuous drainage into a leg bag or may have the catheter clamped and may empty it when the need to void is noted. After 5 to 7 days, a further attempt to remove the catheter may be carried out. Prophylactic antibiotics are rarely necessary, but lower urinary tract infections are common in elderly women and should be treated if they occur. At the time of the removal of the catheter, the urine should be sent for culture and sensitivity. In the occasional patient with a chronic urinary tract infection, prophylactic antibiotics, such as a sulfa preparation or furadantin, may be administered.

Alternatives to the previously mentioned regimen of catheter control include: suprapubic catheter drainage or the placement of an infant feeding tube (no. 5) through the urethra attached to the labia with a suture. In both methods, the drainage tube can be clamped, allowing the patient to void when she can and for residual urines to be measured. Suprapubic technique is simple to use and seems to have a lower incidence of infection. However, patients may complain of extravasation of urine around the site and occasionally hematoma formation. The selection of a means of draining the bladder after repair is generally determined by the experience of the surgeon and the custom of the hospital.

Since it is imperative that healing be allowed to be completed before increasing stress and strain on the operative area, the patient must be cautioned to do no heavy lifting, straining, or prolonged standing for at least 3 months. Estrogen therapy should be maintained and, as a rule, coitus is not resumed until that 3-month period is past, in the older woman.[1]

Rectocele

A patient with a rectocele will often complain of heaviness in the pelvis or a sensation that her rectum is falling out of her vagina. She may have constipation, and occasionally state that she needs to splint her vagina with her fingers in order to effect a bowel movement. She, too, may have a feeling of incomplete emptying of the rectum after a bowel movement.

A rectocele may be identified by retracting the anterior vaginal wall upward and having the patient strain (Figure 9.5). The rectum may bulge into the vagina and, if the rectocele is large enough, the bulge may protrude through the introitus. The physician may place one finger in the rectum and one in the vagina and palpate the hernia. The rectovaginal septum may appear to be paper thin and the entire limits of the rectocele may be palpated. If an enterocele is present, with straining it may be possible to differentiate this sac from the rectocele. Small enteroceles will escape detection by this method and may only be found at the time of operation.

The rectocele may be treated with pessary, Kegal exercises, and estrogen

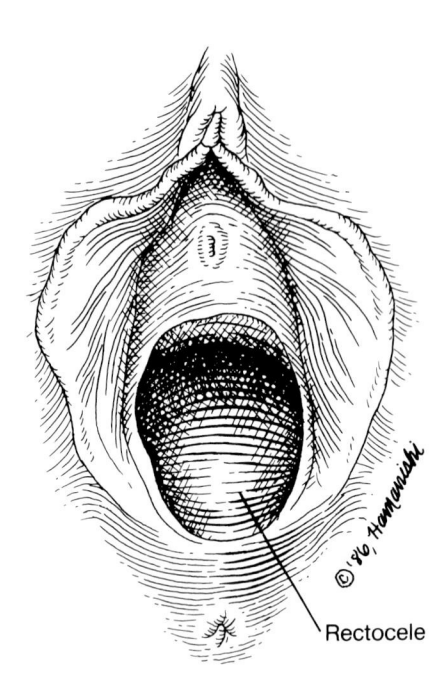

Figure 9.5 Rectocele. (From Droegemueller W, Herbst AL, Mishell DR, Stenchever, MA: Disorders of abdominal wall and pelvic support, in *Comprehensive Gynecology*, Ch. 19. St. Louis, CV Mosby, 1987.)

in appropriate situations. As with cystocele, estrogen replacement may help tissue strength and vascularity.

Operative management (posterior colporrhaphy) is often performed at the time of an anterior colporrhaphy with or without enterocele repair or operation for descensus of the uterus. Most women with rectoceles will also have weakened perineal bodies leading to gaping vaginas and, therefore, will require a perineorrhaphy at the time of the procedure. Therefore, when operatively repairing a rectocele, the surgeon should estimate at the beginning of the posterior wall repair what degree of perineorrhaphy is desirable. The margins of the perineum to be narrowed are marked with Allis clamps at their extremes, and the skin of the introitus between these clamps is then incised. The vaginal wall is then separated from the underlying tissue with a progressive longitudinal incision in the mid-line beginning at the introital incision and being carried to the apex of the vagina above the limit of the rectocele. This is best performed with Metzenbaum scissors in a similar fashion to the cystocele repair. The vaginal wall is completely incised, and the vagina is separated from the rectum by blunt and, if necessary, sharp dissection. This is continued until the operator can palpate the perirectal space on each side, exposing the region of the levator muscles. There is little endopelvic fascia in this region. If an enterocele is present, it will generally be observable at this point. The enterocele sac, if present, must then be dissected free as will be described later.

The operator then places a finger of the nondominant hand into the rectum using a double-glove technique, while an assistant picks up perirectal tissue on either side. The operator then places an 0 suture of either nonabsorbable type (silk or dermalon) or a polyglycol slow-absorbing suture into the perirectal tissue on either side, attempting to get portions of the levator muscle. Approximately three or four of these sutures are required but, in the case of a large defect, more may be necessary. The operator should use the finger in the rectum to ensure that no suture is placed into the rectum. The sutures are then tied interposing perirectal tissue and levator muscle fibers between the rectum and the vagina, thus reducing the rectocele. These sutures will also serve to tack the vagina to the levator ani area thereby avoiding future vaginal prolapse if a hysterectomy has also been performed. The vaginal edges are then trimmed and the vagina closed with either a row of continuous or interrupted polyglycol or catgut sutures.

The perineorrhaphy is then closed by placing 0 polyglycol suture into the lateral margins of the transverse incision, essentially bringing bulbocavernousal muscles from either side together in the mid-line. The operator should be sure that the bulbocavernousal muscle insertions are included in the sutures by pulling on the suture as they are placed, and noting whether there is tension in the muscle bundles. The remainder of the perineal incision is then closed using a row of 2-0 polyglycol or catgut suture in the deep tissue. The skin of the perineum may be closed with an interrupted or continuous subcutaneous suture of 3-0 catgut out to the margin.[1]

Enterocele

An enterocele is a true hernia of the peritoneal cavity from the pouch of Douglas (cul de sac) between the uterosacral ligaments and into the rectovaginal septum (Figure 9.6). The contents of an enterocele are always small bowel and may include omentum. Patients with enteroceles also note a heaviness in their pelvis and may detect a bulge coming from their introitus, frequently quite large. The enterocele is not always easy to diagnose. It may be detected as a separate bulge from a rectocele at the time of a rectovaginal examination. If large enough, it may be possible to transilluminate the sac, seeing small bowel shadows within the sac. It may be possible to reduce the hernia; however, at times, the small bowel contents are fixed to the peritoneum of the sac by adhesions.

While an enterocele may be supported as part of a total prolapse using a pessary, it is most effectively treated operatively. The repair may be carried out separately or at the time of a posterior colporrhaphy. The sac is visualized as

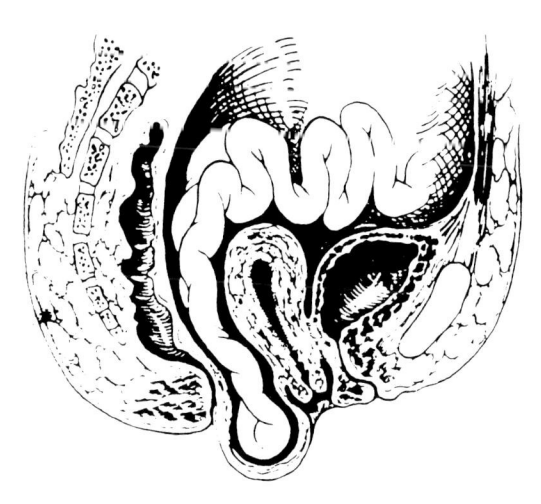

Figure 9.6 Enterocele and uterine prolapse. (From Symmonds RE: Relaxation of pelvic supports, in Benson RC (ed.): *Current Obstetrics and Gynecologic Diagnosis and Treatment*, ed. 5. Los Altos, California, Lange Medical Publications, 1984.)

the vagina is separated from the rectum. It must be dissected free of the underlying tissue and isolated at its neck. It should be opened to ensure that all contents are replaced into the peritoneal cavity. The neck of the hernia is then sutured with a purse string 0 chromic or polyglycol suture and the sac wall excised. In some cases where the sac neck is large, multiple progressive purse-string sutures may be necessary.

Enteroceles often occur after abdominal or vaginal hysterectomies, and generally are due to the fact that support of the pouch of Douglas is weakened. In order to prevent enteroceles at the time of hysterectomy, the uterosacral and cardinal ligaments are extremely important structures and should be incorporated into the vaginal vault repair. The ligaments from each side may be joined together.

Enteroceles may also be reduced transabdominally at the time of other abdominal procedures or as a primary procedure. The sac should be reduced upward and, if uterosacral ligaments can be identified, these should be brought together in the mid-line. If uterosacral ligaments cannot be identified as with large enteroceles following previous hysterectomy, the cul de sac may be obliterated by concentric purse-string sutures in the endopelvic fascia. Care must be taken to avoid damaging the ureters, rectum, and sigmoid colon. Permanent suture or polyglycol sutures are best used for this procedure. For large or multiple recurrent enteroceles, both a vaginal and abdominal approach may be necessary.

Pitfalls in enterocele repair, which may lead to a recurrence, often are related to the operator not isolating the neck of the sac adequately. This is an extremely important aspect of the procedure.[1]

Uterine Prolapse (Descensus, Procidentia)

Descensus of the uterus and cervix into or through the barrel of the vagina is often associated with injuries of the endopelvic fascia, including cardinal and uterosacral ligaments as well as injury or relaxation of the pelvic floor muscles, particularly the levator ani muscles. Prolapse may occur because of increased intraabdominal pressure, such as may be seen with ascites, or a large pelvic or intraabdominal tumor superimposed on poor pelvic supports. Occasionally, sacral nerve disorders, especially injuries to S1 through S4, or diabetic neuropathy may be responsible. Factors which increase tension of pelvic floor musculature, such as chronic respiratory disease (including asthma, bronchitis, and bronchiectasis) or morbid obesity, may be associated. Congenital damage or relaxed pelvic-floor supports may cause prolapse in young nulliparous women. Often, patients with descensus are multiparous, and the problem may be related to childbirth trauma. Descensus is almost always associated with other forms of pelvic relaxation, including cystocele and rectocele. Enterocele may be present as well.

Descensus is graded in the following manner. A prolapse into the upper barrel of the vagina is defined as first-degree. A prolapse through the barrel of the vagina to the region of the introitus is defined as second-degree. If the cervix and uterus prolapsed through the introitus, it is defined as a third-degree or total prolapse (Figure 9.7). Essentially, when a total prolapse occurs, the vagina is everted around the uterus and cervix and is completely exteriorized. Often, particularly in older women not on estrogen replacement, dryness rapidly de-

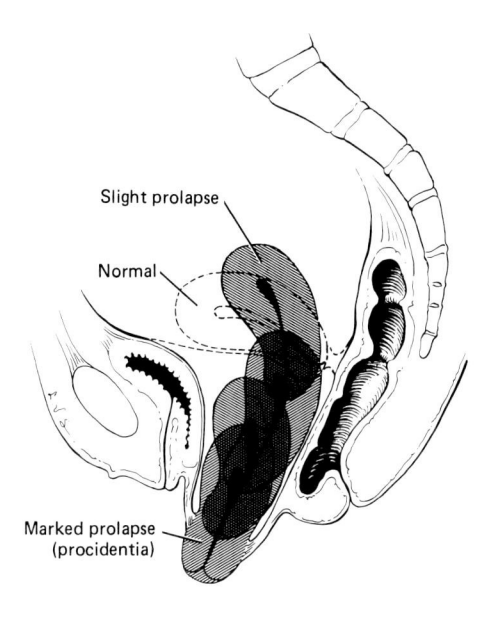

Figure 9.7 Various degrees of prolapse of the uterus. (From Symmonds RE: Relaxation of pelvic supports, in Benson RC (ed.): *Current Obstetrics and Gynecologic Diagnosis and Treatment*, ed. 5. Los Altos, California, Lange Medical Publications, 1984.)

velops with thickening and chronic inflammation of the vagina epithelium. Stasis ulcers may occur, and edema and interference with blood supply to the vaginal wall takes place. Rarely are these ulcers cancerous, but biopsies should be taken to ensure that they are not. Invariably, perineal supports are poor and the perineal body is damaged.

The major symptoms noted by patients with descensus are: a feeling of heaviness or fullness or feeling that something is falling out of the vagina. In second-degree prolapse, the cervix may be noted to be protruding from the introitus, giving the patient the impression that a tumor is bulging out of her vagina. Once total prolapse has occurred, the patient is aware that a mass is actually protruded from the introitus. Symptoms of cystocele and rectocele may also be present. With ulceration of the vaginal epithelium or of the cervix, pain and vaginal bleeding may occur. Discharge may also be present if infection has occurred.

First-degree prolapse may not need therapy unless the patient is very uncomfortable. As the degree of prolapse increases and the cervix is placed at or through the introitus, discomfort is generally more severe and therapy is indicated. Medical management of such conditions involves using a pessary. This requires the replacement of the uterus and cervix to their normal position in the pelvis and the institution of support using one of these devices. Pessary are available in various sizes and shapes. It is often necessary to consider the patient's anatomy and personal needs when selecting the appropriate pessary. This type of management is particularly of value in individuals of poor operative risk. Estrogen-replacement hormones are necessary in such patients as is the case for other pelvic-relaxation problems. Certainly, therapy with estrogen for at least 30 days should be undertaken before considering surgical repair. Repair should not be undertaken until all ulcers of the vagina and cervix are healed. Otherwise, there is risk of infection and breakdown of the repair.

Operative repair of a prolapse of the uterus and cervix generally involves a vaginal hysterectomy with anterior and posterior colporrhaphy. At the time of hysterectomy, cardinal and uterosacral ligaments are carefully isolated so that they may be used in support of the vaginal wall. Uterosacral ligaments and cardinal ligaments should be sutured carefully to the vagina and should be brought together in the mid-line to support the cul de sac. This will help to prevent enterocele in the future.

In some instances, a vaginal hysterectomy may not be advisable. These include previous intraabdominal surgery for an inflammatory process, such as pelvic inflammatory disease, endometriosis, etc. In such instances, an abdominal hysterectomy may be performed followed by a vaginal anterior and posterior colporrhaphy. Procedures that amputate the cervix and use the cardinal ligaments to support the bladder repair (Manchester procedure) may be instituted in certain situations. Most often, the best reason for performing a Manchester procedure is that the patient has an elongated cervix with a fairly well-supported uterus, and it is the cervix which is protruding from the introitus. This is seen not infrequently in elderly women.

In the very elderly, who are no longer sexually active, a simple procedure for reducing prolapse may be a partial colpocleisis. The classical procedure was described by Lefort and involves removal of a strip of anterior and posterior wall of the vagina with closure of the margins of anterior and posterior wall to each other. This procedure may be performed with or without the presence of a uterus and cervix. When it is completed, a small vaginal canal exists on either side of the septum, which is produced by the suturing of the lateral margins of the excision. The line of dissection of the vaginal wall should be carried out to the level of the bladderneck anteriorly, and to the reflection of bladder on to cervix in the depth of the vagina if the uterus is present.

Posteriorly, the dissection is carried from just inside the introitus to a position just posterior to the cervix, if the uterus is present. If the uterus is absent, the extent of the incision into the depth of the vagina should be to approximately 1 cm from the previous vaginal scar. Since the area of the bladderneck is avoided, urinary incontinence is generally not a consequence of this procedure. On the other hand, if stress urinary incontinence is a problem, bladderneck plication may be carried out as part of the procedure. After healing, a small introital area is noted which has cosmetic benefits in the older woman. Narrow canals are present on each lateral vaginal wall. If the cervix and uterus are still present and intrauterine pathology should occur, bleeding along these canals could take place, alerting the physician to the fact that a problem existed.

The Goodall–Power modification of a Lefort operation is essentially the removal of a triangular piece of vaginal wall beginning at the cervical reflection or 1 cm above the vaginal scar as the base of the triangle and the apex of the triangle just beneath the bladderneck anteriorly, and just at the introitus posteriorly. The cut edges of the vaginal wall making up the base of the triangle anteriorly are sutured to the similar wall posteriorly, and the vaginal incision is then closed with a row of interrupted sutures beginning beneath the bladderneck and being carried side to side to the area of the introitus. This procedure works well for relatively small prolapses, whereas the Lefort method is best for larger ones.[1]

At the time of colpocleisis, if an enterocele is found, it must be repaired. Failure to repair an enterocele at the time of colpocleisis will probably lead to a breakdown of the repair. In all cases, a perineorrhaphy is performed in order to reduce the size of the introitus.

Colpocleisis to reduce a prolapse and to prevent recurrence is generally quite effective. Ridley reports no prolapse recurrence in 58 patients unless an incomplete procedure was performed. Three patients in Ridley's series developed urinary stress incontinence where none had been present preoperatively.[2]

Prolapse of the vaginal stump at some time remote to the performance of either abdominal or vaginal hysterectomy has been reported as occurring in between 0.1% and 18.2% of patients. Such a prolapse may be total and may be accompanied by cystocele, rectocele, enterocele, or some combination thereof. In examining such patients, it is important to identify the upper scar of the vagina and then try to determine which contents are present within the stump (ie, cystocele, rectocele, or enterocele).[3] Richter, reporting on 97 vaginal stump prolapses, found 6.2% contained cystocele only, 5.1% rectocele only, 9.3% enterocele primarily, and 72% a mixture of contents.[4]

Vaginal stump prolapse probably occurs as a continuing pelvic-support weakness problem, and a failure of the cardinal and uterosacral ligaments to maintain their tone or attach to the vagina.

The symptoms and signs are the same as those delineated for descensus of the uterus, including pelvic heaviness, backache, and a mass protruding from the introitus. At times, stress incontinence, urgency, frequency, dribbling, vaginal bleeding, or discharge (if there is an ulcer) will occur. If the mass is large, there may be difficulty in sitting or walking.

Examination will help to differentiate the contents of the prolapse. Rectovaginal examination may help to delineate an enterocele from a rectocele.

In the planning of a repair of a vaginal prolapse, several principles should be kept in mind. The first is that the normal position of the vagina in a standing position is against the rectum and no more than 30° from the horizontal. Second, pelvic relaxation is a part of a problem which dictates an existing cystocele, rectocele, or enterocele must be repaired as part of the procedure. A third principle acknowledges that the perineal body is almost always weakened, and that in such individuals there should be reconstruction of this as well. The nonsurgical management of vaginal prolapse can include pessary, estrogen replacement, and the clearing up of ulcers when they are present. Pessaries are rarely retained in such individuals unless there is an adequate perineal body.

Surgical procedures to repair a vaginal prolapse are many. They include those which use an abdominal approach, vaginal approach, or some combination thereof. If the surgeon prefers an abdominal approach, a variety of procedures have been tried. These include fixation of the vaginal vault to the anterior abdominal wall, to the lumbar spine, to the sacral promontory, or to various tendonous lines in the musculature of the true pelvis or to the sacrospinous ligament. The anterior abdominal wall fixation increases the diameter of the pouch of Douglas and frequently helps create a subsequent enterocele. Fixation to the lumbar spine or sacral promontory is often difficult to achieve directly. Most often, it requires the interposition of a different material. In the past, ox fascia lata, fascial aponeurosis from the individual herself, or inert material (such as mersaline) have been utilized. If a stint is used, it should be covered with peritoneum—thereby rendering the stint retroperitoneal. Obliteration of the pouch of Douglas may be necessary as well in order to prevent a recurrent enterocele.

Fixation to the sacrospinous ligament has had some encouraging degrees of success.

Sacrospinous ligament fixation of the vaginal wall can be accomplished vaginally. Randall and Nichols reported excellent success with both abdominal and vaginal approaches. Of 18 patients treated with fixation of the vaginal wall to the sacrospinous ligament via the vaginal route, all had successful outcomes.[5]

Although a variety of vaginal procedures have been designed, the best success has been in those situations where adequate vaginal length is maintained and the vagina is positioned against the rectum in a nearly parallel to the horizontal manner.

Morley and DeLancey reported on 100 women who underwent repair of vaginal stumps using the vaginal sacrospinous ligament suspension with good and lasting success. Twenty-three had only the suspension performed, whereas 67 underwent a form of colporrhaphy as well. One-year follow-up revealed 67 of the 71 patients available had satisfactory results, four had developed sympathetic cystoceles, and three had had a recurrent prolapse.[6]

If a vaginal prolapse has occurred without a concordant cystocele and/or rectocele, a repair may be effected vaginally by making a transverse incision on the posterior wall of the vagina approximately 1 cm or 2 cm from the upper scar separating the rectum from the vagina by blunt dissection, splitting the perirectal tissue above the sacrospinous ligament on the right, and suturing the upper end of the vaginal vault to the sacrospinous ligament, using either 0 silk or a polyglycol suture of 0 strength. Generally two sutures are used. Following this the vagina is simply closed. In older women who are no longer sexually active, a colpocleisis procedure may be performed.

It is important that the operator determine the desires of the patient before deciding which procedure is best suited for her needs. This can be accomplished by careful preoperative counseling. Many elderly women, although no longer sexually active, do not wish to lose the potential use of their vaginas. Therefore, the physician caring for such women should not take for granted that their current circumstances of sexual inactivity dictate a colpocleisis as the appropriate therapy.

References

1. Droegemueller W, Herbst AL, Mishell DR, Stenchever MA: Disorders of abdominal wall and pelvic support, in *Comprehensive Gynecology*, Ch. 19. St. Louis, CV Mosby, 1987.
2. Ridley JH: Evaluation of the colpocleisis operation: A report of 58 cases. *Am J Obstet Gynecol* 1972;113:1114.
3. Randall CI, Nichols DH: Surgical treatment of vaginal inversion. *Obstet Gynecol* 1971; 38:327.
4. Richter K: Massive eversion of the vagina: Pathogenesis, diagnosis, and therapy of the true prolapse of the vaginal stump. *Clin Obstet Gynecol* 1982;25:897.
5. Nichols DH: Transvaginal sacrospinus fixation. *Pelvic Surgery* 1981;1:10.
6. Morley GW, DeLancey JOL: Sacrospinous ligament fixation for eversion of the vagina. *Am J Obstet Gynecol* 1988;158:872–881.

Chapter **10**

Vulva and Vaginal Conditions

Morton Stenchever, MD

A number of changes occur in the lower genital tract as part of the aging process. Many, but not all, are due to hormonal changes. This chapter will deal with the changes that take place in the vulva and vagina as a woman ages. It will discuss the management that is required to maintain comfort and normal function.

Vulva

Anatomically, the vulva includes the mons pubis, clitoris, labia majora and minora, external urethral opening, vestibule of the vagina, and the skin between the anus and the vagina. The mons pubis, which covers the pubic symphysis and the labial majora, are areas of skin covered with hair and contain a good deal of subcutaneous fat. The labia minora are devoid of hair follicles, and the two labia minora are joined at a point anterior which represents the position of the clitoris. The clitoris is normally covered with a partial skin hood and consists of two corpora cavernosa, which are vascular erectile structures composed of blood vessels and fibrous tissue. Beneath the clitoris and between the labia minora is the opening of the urethra. Just inside the urethral meatus are the openings of the Skene's glands. The glands themselves are present beneath the urethra on either side, approximately 1 cm from the meatus. The Bartholin glands are present in the labia majora but open into the vestibule of the vagina in the posterior third of the labia minora. The two labia join at the posterior junction of the vaginal vestibule known as the posterior fourchette (Figure 10.1). Blood supply to the vulva is from the pudendal artery, which is a branch of the hypogastric artery. The pudendal vein drains the area with rich anastamoses to the abdominal wall. Nerve supply to the vulva, which consists of both sensory and motor components, is from the second, third, and fourth sacral nerves. The tissue of the vulva is sensitive to estrogen, which is responsible for the integrity of the epithelium and the blood supply to the various layers. After estrogen withdrawal, the skin of the vulva often thins, subcutaneous fat of the labia majora and mons pubis frequently undergoes atrophy, and secretions from the vestibular glands decrease.

Vulvar Dystrophy

For many years, many elderly patients have complained of itching and burning of the vulva frequently associated with thinning of the skin of the vulva, at times intermingled with white vulvar skin patches. In 1875, Weir[1] described such le-

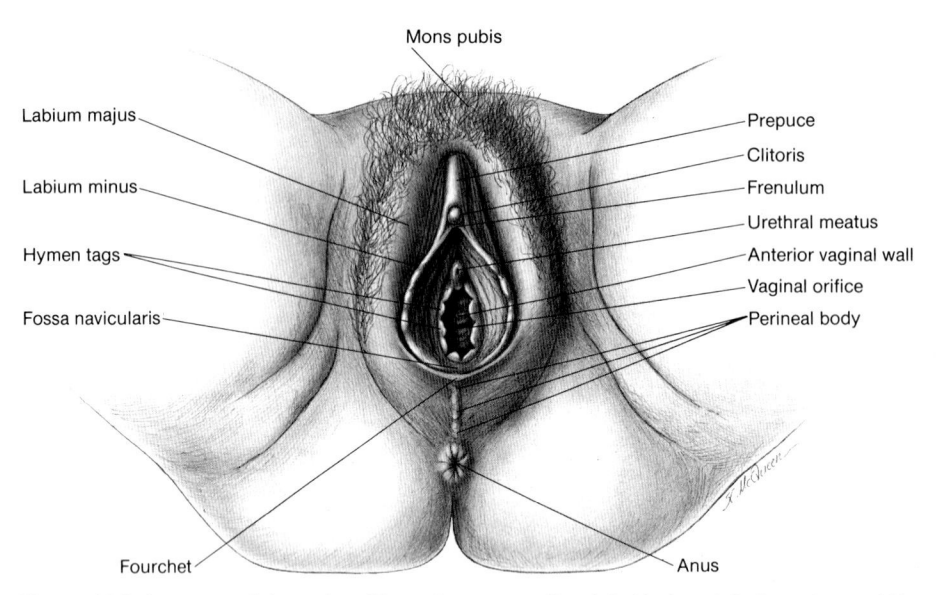

Figure 10.1 Anatomy of the vulva. (From Droegemueller, LO, Herbst, AC, Stenchever, MA, Mishell, DR: *Comprehensive Gynecology*. St. Louis, CV Mosby, 1987.)

sions and in 1929, Graves and Smith[2] discussed what they called kraurosis vulvae. They interpreted this as a shrinkage of the skin with precancerous aspects.

In 1961, Jeffcoate and Woodcock[3] suggested that the white lesions noted on the vulva of such women (leukoplakia) and shrinkage (kraurosis) were part of the same process which they called chronic epithelial dystrophy. They had followed a group of 98 women for over 25 years and had found no evidence of cancer at the time of their initial presentation nor during the observation period. Thus, they suggested that the treatment which was commonly followed for such conditions, namely, simple vulvectomy, was unjustified.

At the Tenth World Congress of FIGO (International Federation of Obstetricians and Gynecologists) in 1970, the International Society for the Study of Vulvar Disease was conceived and given the mission to define and promulgate a universal nomenclature for vulvar disease, which would be acceptable to gynecologists, dermatologists, and pathologists.[4] The society was represented by individuals from each of these specialties. The terms leukoplakia and kraurosis were abandoned as ambiguous and the term *dystrophy* was adopted. In 1975, the International Society for the Study of Vulvar Dystrophy developed a classification which was acceptable to all three groups (see Table 10.1). From a gynecologic standpoint, this is a good working classification and will be discussed further in this chapter. Dermatologists, however, felt that a broader classification was necessary in order to take into consideration the more commonly seen dermatologic abnormalities, and their extension of the classification is presented in Table 10.2. It is reasonable to state that a number of conditions and circumstances may lead to vulvar dystrophy and that correcting these may, at times, reverse the process. Elderly patients may have any of the infectious diseases of the vagina and vulva that anyone else may have. This would include: candidiasis, trichomonas vaginalis, tinnea cruris, psoriasis, intertrigo, seborrheic dermatitis, contact dermatitis, etc. When such conditions are found, ther-

Table 10.1 Vulvar Dystrophy

A. The 1975 Classification of the International Society for the Study of Vulvar Disease
  I. Hyperplastic dystrophy
    a. Without atypia
    b. With atypia
  II. Lichen sclerosis
  III. Mixed dystrophy (lichen sclerosis with foci of epithelial hyperplasia)
    a. Without atypia
    b. With atypia
B. 1985 (Current) Classification of Vulvar Atypias
  I. Intraepithelial atypias
    a. VIN I-Mild dysplasia
    b. VIN II-Moderate dysplasia
    c. VIN III-Severe dysplasia
  II. Lichen sclerosis
  III. Squamous hyperplasia-not otherwise specified
  IV. Specific diagnosis (i.e. Paget's disease)

apeutic approaches should be applied to eliminate them. Underlying conditions, such as diabetes, must also be treated in order to help alleviate chronic irritation to the vulva. Simple hygienic considerations—such as the use of hypoallergic underwear and the elimination of the use of detergents, medicated douches, feminine sprays, etc.—should also be encouraged.

What is left is vulvar dystrophy, which exists in two major forms. The first is hyperplastic dystrophy, which is recognized histologically as acanthotic and

Table 10.2 Vulvar Dystrophies and Intraepithelial Neoplasias

Nonneoplastic disorders of vulvar skin and mucosa (dystrophies)
  Hyperplastic dystrophies
    Psoriasis
    Lichen planus
    Tinea cruris
    Candidiasis
    Hailey and Hailey disease
    Intertrigo and seborrheic dermatitis
    Contact dermatitis
    Plasma cell vulvitis
    Nonspecific epithelial hyperplasia (lichen simplex chronicus, pruritus vulvae, localized neurodermatitis)
  Atrophic dystrophies
    Lichen sclerosis (and atrophicus)
  Mixed dystrophies
    Nonspecific epithelial hyperplasia superimposed on other dystrophies
Intraepithelial neoplasia of vulvar skin and mucosa
  Squamous intraepithelial neoplasia
    VIN I
    VIN II
    VIN III
  Nonsquamous intraepithelial neoplasia
    Paget's disease
    Melanoma in situ (level 1)

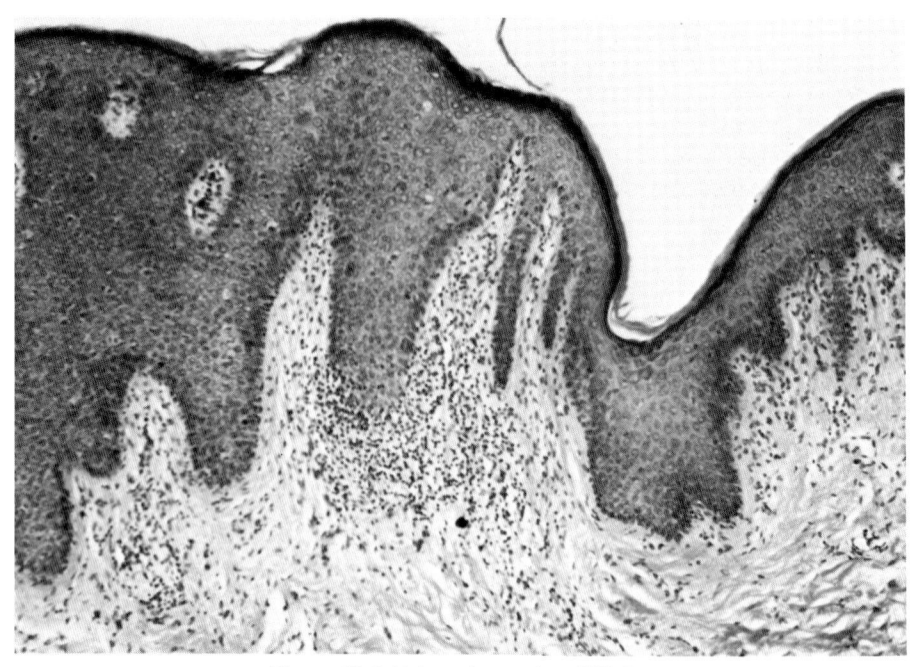

Figure 10.2 Vulvar dystrophy—VIN III.

hyperkeratotic changes in the vulvar epithelium with or without epithelial atypia, and lichen sclerosis, which is primarily thin epithelium beneath which there is a homogenous zone of dermis with deep lymphactic infiltration. Mixed varieties are frequently present. Friedrich[4] feels that these changes are generally related to a response to irritation which may be intrinsic or extrinsic. He points out that the vulva sweats more than any other skin area except the axilla, and that this may be accentuated by psychogenic factors. The continued moisture—coupled with a variety of chemical compounds introduced either via medications, soaps, or clothing, as well as irritating fibers from underwear—may contribute to an irritated vulva. It is then irritated more because of itching and excoriation from scratching. All such agents are potential causes of these changes, and it is difficult in clinical practice to identify a specific cause. Clinically, the hyperplastic vulva may appear pink or red with a gray–white keratin covering of variable thickness.

Microscopically, the epithelial layer is thickened by an increased number of cells with mitoses with an abundant keratin cover. Rete pegs are accentuated and dip deeply into the dermis (Figure 10.2). If atypia is present within the cell layer, it may be graded using current FIGO nomenclature into VIN I, VIN II, and VIN III. In VIN I, the active atypical area of epithelium is present at the basement membrane but is limited to the inner third of the epithelium. In VIN II, the condition continues through most but not all of the full thickness of the epithelium. VIN III involves atypical cellular activity through the full thickness of the epithelium, but there is no breakthrough of the basement membrane. VIN III is synonymous with intraepithelial carcinoma of the vulva.

Hyperplastic dystrophy without atypia often responds to corticosteroid therapy. It is wise to begin with a 1% hydrocortisone ointment or lotion which is applied to the affected area two to three times per day for 1 to 2 months. Often, if hygiene has been improved and irritating substances removed, the corticosteroid therapy is only necessary on an "as needed" basis. Fluorinated corticosteroids may be used but should be limited to short-term use. Fluorinated compounds frequently will accelerate atrophy of the skin of the vulva and some patients are sensitive to the fluorinated portion of the compound. It probably should be limited to use in patients who do not respond well to 1% hydrocortisone cream.

The treatment of hyperplastic vulvar dystrophy with atypia involves destruction of the lesion. VIN I and II can be managed after biopsy with local surgical excision, laser vaporization, or, in some cases, with the application of 5-fluorouridine (5-FU) cream. Careful follow-up is important to be sure that the entire lesion is irradicated. The treatment of VIN III also involves local excision or laser vaporization using the CO_2 laser. Extensive cases may be managed by simple vulvectomy but, in most situations, this is not necessary. Careful follow-up and reevaluation is necessary because of the recurring nature of the condition. Lesions which have become invasive require the usual management for invasive carcinoma of the vulva and specific therapy depends upon the size of the lesion and the staging involved.

Recently, the etiology of VIN III, at least in younger women, has been linked to infection with the human papilloma virus (HPV), particularly types 16, 18, and 32. Although these subtypes occur in only about 5% of genital warts, they are the most commonly associated with VIN lesions. While it is impossible to specifically identify a cause-and-effect relationship, the involvement may be part of a carcinogenic chain.[5] This relationship has not been seen in the elderly at this point. One could anticipate that, as women with HPV infections age, the relationship may be more commonly noted.

Lichen Sclerosis

Lichen sclerosis appears as white- to pink-colored flat macules, often symmeterically placed on the vulva. Frequently, these macules form into plaques. The skin appears thin, dry, occasionally scaly, and wrinkled—often resembling parchment. There may be edema of the underlying tissue and excorations noted as well. Fissures are often seen, particularly in the posterior fourchette and around the labia minor and clitoris (Figure 10.3). Lesions may be present on the vulva, the medial aspects of the thigh, and in the perianal region. Lichen sclerosis has been seen in other parts of the body, including the axilla. There is often little, if any, hair present on the affected areas. Telangiectasias and ecchymoses may be present if the area has been traumatized.

Lichen sclerosis has the appearance on histological section of atrophy. The cellular layer is thin. There are few mitoses. Rete pegs are generally missing and there is little keratin present. Studies would indicate that there is increased metabolic activity within the tissue, although there is no increased mitotic rate (Figure 10.4). Thus, from a histologic standpoint, the lesion is really not a lesion but rather a thin mature epithelium. The cause of lichen sclerosis is unknown. It does occur in prepubertal girls as well as postmenopausal women and rarely during the menstrual years. While hyperplastic dystrophy does occur in lichen sclerotic skin, it is impossible to know whether or not the etiology for both is the same or whether skin which is lichen sclerotic is simply sensitive to hy-

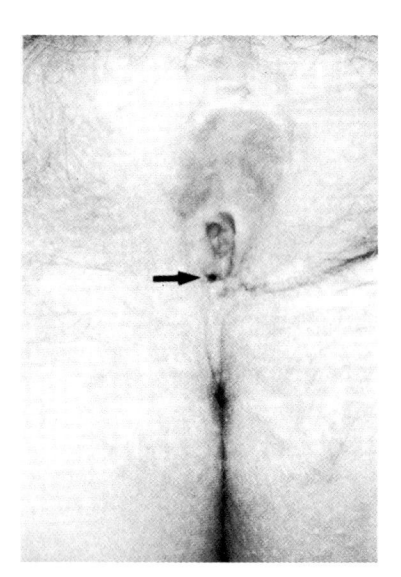

Figure 10.3 Lichen sclerosis. The introitus (arrow) of a parous elderly woman barely admitting one finger. (From Kaufman RH, Friedrich EJ Jr, Gardner HL: *Benign Diseases of the Vulva and Vagina*. Chicago, Yearbook Medical Publishers, 1989, p 308.)

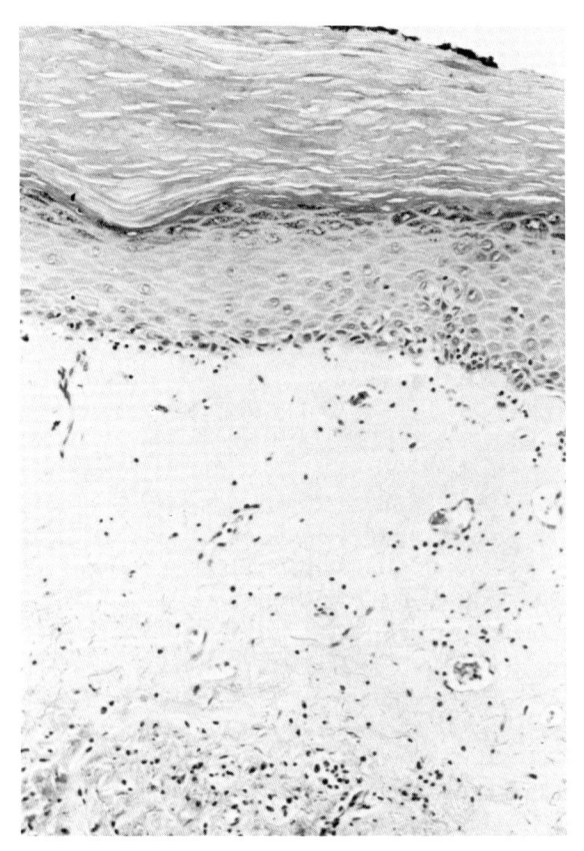

Figure 10.4 Lichen sclerosis of the vulva.

perplastic stimuli. One possible common denominator may be the fact that both lichen sclerosis and hyperplastic dystrophy seem associated with autoimmune disease, in general. Harrington and Dunsmore studied 50 women with lichen sclerosis and 50 age-matched controls. They noted a 34% incidence of clinical autoimmune disease in their patient group and only 4% in their controls. Seventy-four percent of their patients had autoantibodies in the circulation as compared with only 20% within the control group.[6]

A hormonal basis for lichen sclerosis was suggested by Friedrich and Kalra.[7] They discovered decreased levels of dihydrotestosterone, free testosterone, and androstenediol in patients with lichen sclerosis. Topical testosterone therapy caused an increase in all of these levels. They felt the abnormality might be a reduction of 5-α-reductase activity within the skin. Other theories of etiology have been put forward but, as yet, no specific cause is universally accepted.

The treatment of lichen sclerosis may be with testosterone cream, progesterone cream, or a combination of one of these plus a corticosteroid. Additionally, estrogen replacement systemically is probably wise if there are no contraindications. Testosterone 2% in petrolatum should be applied twice per day for approximately 2 months. If the lesion is relieved, the cream may be used once a day for 1 month then two or three times per week thereafter. Rarely are side effects noted with this therapy but some clinicians have reported increased hair growth, particularly on the upper lip and some decrease in voice tone. Jasionowski and Jasionowski have reported equally good results with progesterone cream.[8] In such cases, 200 mg of progesterone-in-oil is mixed with 2 ounces of hydrophilic ointment and applied twice daily to the lesions. Once satisfactory response is achieved, it is decreased to once per day. When the lesion is irradicated, it may be used every other day from then on.

One percent hydrocortisone cream should be used sparingly during the therapy if itching is the major continuing symptom. In most cases, it is unnecessary.

Mixed Dystrophy

The relative incidence of hyperplastic dystrophy, lichen sclerosis, and mixed dystrophy varies from clinic to clinic. The incidence of hyperplastic dystrophy has been reported to be between 24% and 54%; of lichen sclerosis, as high as 63%; and mixed dystrophies have been reported in various series from 15% to 30%.[4] The growth and histologic appearance of mixed dystrophy will depend upon the severity of the component. The treatment should be directed to the most severe of the components or, if atypia is not present, to the dominant component (ie, lichen sclerosis or hyperplasia).

Paget's Disease

Paget's disease of the vulva occurs exclusively in postmenopausal women. Grossly, the lesions are single or multiple, well-defined, erythematous plaques which may have a white velvety scaling and may demonstrate some degree of maceration (Figure 10.5). These occur on the labia majora and occasionally on the labia minora. They may also be present within the introitus and the entrance of the vagina or the genitocrural folds. Itching and burning may be present and excoriations may be noted. On histologic section, hyperkeratosis and paraker-

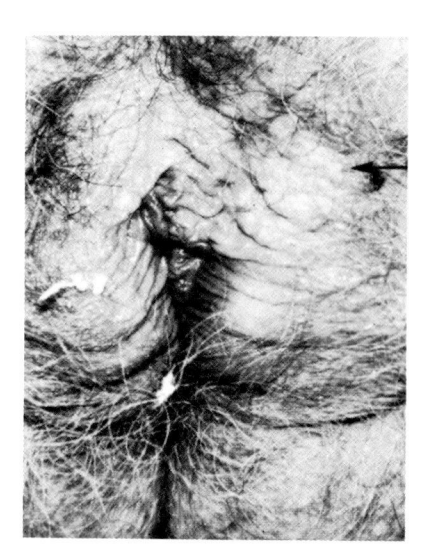

Figure 10.5 Paget's disease of the vulva. Grayish white poorly defined lesion (arrow) is visible. (From Kaufman RH, Friedrich EG Jr, Gardner HL: *Benign Diseases of the Vulva and Vagina.* Chicago, Year Book Medical Publishers, 1989, p 173.)

atosis with epidermal hyperplasia is noted. Paget cells are seen in disorganized array within the prickle layer of the skin. Erosion may be seen. Paget cells have foamy cytoplasm, are round or ovoid in shape, and have a rounded vesicular, hyperchromatic nucleus. They appear free-floating with little attachment to adjacent cells (Figure 10.6). On special stain with periodic acid-Schiff reagent, they are noted to contain acid mucopolysaccharide. Twenty-five percent of the lesions are associated with underlying carcinoma of the sweat glands. In addition, 25% of patients with extra mammary Paget's disease are at risk of having an underlying internal carcinoma, often of the breast, uterus, cervix, or bladder.[9]

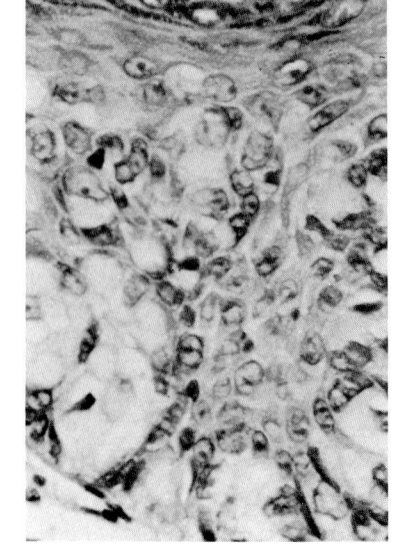

Figure 10.6 Paget's disease. Relatively normal squamous cells are seen between large vacuolated Paget's cells (Hard E stain). (From Kaufman RH, Friedrich EG Jr, Gardner HL: *Benign Diseases of the Vulva and Vagina.* Chicago, Year Book Medical Publishers, 1989, p 174.)

The actual etiology of Paget's disease is unknown. One theory states that it develops from a very specific clear cell of the epithelium that is readily found in nipple epithelium and in epithelium overlying the milk line of the trunk and groin. Most authorities believe that the tumor develops within the epithelium and extends into the underlying adnexal structures, but the reverse may be possible.

Treatment of Paget's disease involves excision and, of course, treatment of underlying or associated carcinomas.

Vaginal Conditions in the Elderly

Physiologic Changes in the Vagina of the Elderly

During the reproductive years, normal physiology of the vagina is maintained by the effects of endogenous estrogen. The first effect is that estrogen supports glycogen storage by vaginal epithelial cells. Lactobacillus and other vaginal bacteria metabolize this to lactic acid and other short-chain fatty acids and thereby create an acidic environment with a pH of between 3.8 and 4.2. This pH impedes the growth and proliferation of bacteria and protozoa, thereby protecting the vagina from infection. In the postmenopausal period, this protective mechanism is lost and the vaginal pH is therefore less acidic, allowing more easy invasion of bacteria that would have been suppressed by an acid environment.[10]

Estrogen also affects the vaginal epithelium by increasing stratification of squamous cells and producing a tendency toward cornification. In addition, estrogen supports the blood supply to the subepithelial portion of the vagina, ensuring adequate nourishment for vaginal epithelium. The thickening of the vaginal epithelium adds resistance to the invasion of bacteria; and several organisms, prevented from causing a vaginitis during the menstrual years, may actually be able to cause a vaginitis in the postmenopausal woman. The gonoccocus is an example of this. Thus, the postmenopausal vagina has a pH of 4.5 to 5.0, a decreased blood supply, a vaginal epithelium which is thinner, drier, and less cornified. Since vaginal secretions are reduced, the cleansing aspect of these is lost.

Atrophic (Senile) Vaginitis

Given the changes that occur in the postmenopausal woman without estrogen replacement, the stage is often set for infection with opportunistic organisms which normally would reside in the vagina without causing symptoms. These include facultative aerobic organisms, such as staphylococcus, streptococcus, *E. coli*, *Klebsiella*, etc., and anaerobic organisms, such as peptoccus, peptostreptococcus, bacteroids, etc. Symptoms and signs of atrophic vaginitis include a watery discharge, which may be foul-smelling, itching, and burning. Vulvitis may be present as well. The majority of patients with atrophic vaginitis will respond to estrogen therapy. It may be administered systemically or locally. Culturing for organisms may be helpful, but in most cases will not yield a single pathogen. If vaginal cream is used (ie, Premarin cream or Dienestrol cream), one applicator per night will usually bring relief in a short period of time. In most instances where there is no contraindication, systemic estrogen, either in the form of an oral preparation or as a transdermal patch, should be instituted. An example would be 0.625 mg per day of conjucated estrogen by mouth, 25 days out of each month. If the patient has a uterus, progestin therapy should also be given. An example of this would be 10 mg of medroxyprogesterone acetate orally for the last 10 to 13 days of estrogen therapy. The use of progesterone will prevent endometrial hyperplasia and possibly carcinoma of the endometrium. Many women will have periods, at least for a short time on this regimen. Eventually, these usually cease. The usual contraindications for estrogen therapy should be observed in deciding whether or not to begin the patient on such a regimen. Although vaginal estrogen therapy can be continued, in lieu of systemic therapy, there is probably little advantage since estrogen is absorbed through the vaginal epithelium and will have a systemic effect. Giving the estrogen systemically will probably ensure a maintenance of an appropriate drug level.

Generally, hormonal therapy is all that is necessary to correct the atrophic vaginitis. Occasionally, however, a specific organism, such as candida albacantes or trichomonas vaginilas, will be present and must be treated with appropriate medications.

Candida Vaginitis (Moniliasis)

Candida vaginitis infection can occur in women of any age group and may occur whether or not the patient is on estrogen maintenace therapy. It is frequently associated with obesity or undiagnosed or poorly controlled diabetes mellitus. The vulva and vagina appear reddened and irritated. There may be a thick white discharge resembling cottage cheese or there may be no discharge observed until the speculum examination is performed. Vaginial epithelium is often bright red and inflamed. The diagnosis is made by placing a drop of the discharge in a small amount of 10% to 20% potassium hydroxide solution and viewing under the microscope using low power. If candida is present, there will be stringy pseudomycelia noted. Frequently, these are accompanied by small budding organisms along the pseudomycelia. The organisms may be cultured in Nickerson and Sabouraud media. Culture requires 24 to 72 hours to grow in a flask kept at room temperature.

A variety of treatments are available for candida vaginitis. At the present time, the most popular is the use of one of the synthetic imidazoles, such as clotrimazole (Lotrimin or Mycelex), butoconazole (Femstat), miconazole (Monistat), or terconazole (Terazol). These are marketed in a variety of preparations requiring anything from a single treatment (Mycelex-G 500 mg) with a single suppository to a 7-night regimen using either cream or suppositories. Relief is generally rapid, but the recurrence rate in women is as high as 20%. In addition, as many as 25% of asymptomatic women will have organisms present in their vagina.[10] Follow-up after treatment is indicated. Antifungal preparations (nystatin) can be utilized for 2 weeks in a daily suppository or cream form or douches with povidone-iodine or the use of this agent in a jelly form may be utilized as can gentigen violet jelly (Gentigel).

Pockets of candida infection may remain in various parts of the body (ie, rectum, vagina, nasopharynx, etc.), requiring systematic therapy with nystatin.

Trichomonas Vaginitis

Infection with trichomonas vaginitis, a single-cell flagellated protozoa, can affect women of any age group. It is quite contagious and is passed by sexual contact or by contact with infected towels or water in a commode. In the case of the infected commode water, the women may become infected by a splash into the vagina at the time of urination or bowel movement. If sexual contact is not the means of transmission, there is generally an infected individual in the household or immediate environment.

Findings consist of a watery yellowish discharge which often contains small gas bubbles. There is a reddened vaginal epithelium and the vulva is often reddened and inflamed as well. A wet mount made of vaginal secretion using a drop of saline will frequently identify the organisms as single-cell flagellated mobile organisms.

Management consists of the use of metronidazole. A dosage schedule of 1 g followed by 1 g in 12 hours will cure about 90% of cases. Alternatively, metronidazole may be used as 250 mg three times a day for 7 days. In each case, active sexual partners should be treated as well to prevent reinfection.

In individuals who cannot take metronidazole, povidine-iodine douche or jelly, douching with hypertonic saline solutions (20%), or the use of topical clotrimazole for at least 1 week may bring relief.

Bacterial Vaginosis (Nonspecific Vaginitis)

Although bacterial vaginosis accounts for about 50% of the cases of vaginitis seen in the reproductive years, it can also occur in postmenopausal women. It is a sexually transmitted disease and is most likely related to a symbiotic infection of a variety of anaerobic and other organisms with *Gardnerella vaginalis*. The latter is a small gram-negative bacillus and, when present in bacterial vaginosis, produces a watery vaginal discharge with a "fishy" odor. The odor is due to a release of aromatic amines and is most severe in an alkaline environment. The discharge, which is thin, watery, and often grayish white in color, is frequently bubbly or frothy and is associated with a vulvar irritation as well.[11]

Diagnosis of bacterial vaginosis is made by observing a saline wet mount and seeing many bacteria with classic "clue" cells. These cells are vaginal epithelial cells inundated with clusters of bacteria along their surface, giving the cell a granular appearance with obscure cell borders. Such cells are found in about one half of cases. White cells may be present but are generally not seen in large quantities. If they are, other infections, such as chlamydia, should be considered.

An additional test for bacterial vaginosis can be performed by adding a small amount of 10% potassium hydroxide to the secretions of the vaginal speculum and noting a fishy odor. Trichomonas infection may also give this finding.

The specific treatment for this condition is 500 mg metronidazole twice a day for 7 days. Sexual partners should also be treated.

REFERENCES

1. Weir RF: Icthyosis of the tongue and vulva. *New York State Medical Journal* 1875;21:240.
2. Graves WP, Smith GVS: Kraurosis vulvae. *JAMA* 1929;92:1244.
3. Jeffcoate TNA, Woodcock AS: Premalignant conditions of the vulva with particular reference to chronic epithelial dystrophies. *Br Med J* 1961;2127.
4. Friedrich EG Jr: Vulvar dystrophy. *Clin Obstet Gynecol* 1985;28:178.
5. Lynch PJ: Vulvar dystrophies and intraepithelial on neoplasias. *Dermatologic Clinics* 1987;5:789.
6. Harrington CI, Dunsmore IR: An investigation into the incidence of auto-immune disorders in patients with lichen sclerosis and atrophicus. *Br J Dermat* 1981;104:563.
7. Friedrich EG Jr, Kalra PS: Serum levels of sex hormones in vulvar lichen sclerosis and the effect of topical testosterone. *N Engl J Med* 1984;310:488.
8. Jasionowski EA, Jasionowski PA: Further observations on the effect of topical progesterone on vulvar disease. *Am J Obstet Gynecol* 1987;134:565.
9. Chanda JJ: Extra mammary Paget's disease: Prognosis in relationship to internal malignancy. *J Acad Dermatol* 1985;13:1009.
10. Droegemueller W, Herbst AL, Mishell DR, Stenchever MA: *Comprehensive Gynecology*. St. Louis, CV Mosby, 1987.
11. Eschenbach DA: Vaginal infection. *Clin Obstet Gynecol* 1983;26:186.

Chapter **11**

Gynecologic Malignancies in the Elderly

Morton Stenchever, MD

According to the American Cancer Society, of women of all ages who developed cancer in 1989, 28% had breast cancer, 4% ovarian cancer, and 9% uterine cancer (including cervix). Further, cancer deaths occurring in women in 1989 were due to breast cancer in 18%, ovarian cancer in 5%, and uterine cancer in 4%. While cancer was the second most common cause of death overall in the United States, according to census figures in 1985, it was the largest cause of death in women between the ages of 55 and 74 and continued to be the second most common cause of death in women past the age of 75. In the 55 to 74 age group, lung cancer was the most common cause of death followed by cancer of the breast, colon and rectum, ovary, and pancreas. In women past the age of 75, colon and rectal cancer was the most common cause of death, followed by breast, lung, pancreas, and ovary.[1]

While deaths due to cancer of the uterus have dropped in rate from just above 30 per 100,000 female population in 1930 to approximately 7 per 100,000 in 1985, the death rate from ovarian cancer has stayed fairly constant in the 27 to 28 per 100,000 range over the past 55 years. Colon and rectal cancers in women have dropped somewhat from about 22 to 18 per 100,000, but lung cancer has been responsible for a rapidly increasing death rate changing from about 2 per 100,000 in 1930 to above 26 per 100,000 in 1985. Overall there were 106,299 deaths due to cancer reported in women between the ages of 55 and 74 in 1985, and 78,921 deaths due to cancer reported in women past the age of 75.[1] Since cancer is a major cause of disease and mortality in the elderly female, it is important that this population of women be screened annually for cancer and that modern therapy be applied whenever it is diagnosed.

It will be the goal of this chapter to discuss diagnosis, treatment, and prognosis of gynecologic cancers and cancer of the breast as they occur in older women.

Breast Cancer

Breasts are modified sebaceous glands located within the superficial fascia of the anterior chest wall. In the elderly, the largest component of breast tissue is fat, but glandular tissue is present and may vary depending upon whether or not hormone replacement therapy is being used.

Frequency of breast cancer increases with age. While very rare before puberty and uncommon before the age of 40, the incidence increases directly with the woman's age after menopause.[2]

Breast cancer is more common in obese women than in thin women and this may be related to the amount of fat in the diet. It is also more common in women who go through menopause late as compared to women who have had surgical or spontaneous menopause at an earlier age, but also seems to be more common in nulliparous women than women who have had their first child after the age of 35. Positive family history seems to relate directly to the incidence of breast cancer, being highest when there is a family history of first-degree relatives developing the disease prior to menopause, but higher than the general population when first-degree relatives have had the disease. Whereas the risk to a woman in the United States of developing breast cancer is 1 in 17 (6%), it may be as high as 1 in 10 (10%) when one or more of these risk factors are present. Hormone supplementation in the form of birth-control pills premenopausally or estrogen replacement postmenopausally has not been proven to be associated with an increased incidence of breast cancer in the majority of studies performed.[3]

Early detection is the most important measure available for reducing the mortality rate from breast cancer. Breast carcinoma in general is a slow-growing tumor which doubles in volume every 100 days and doubles in diameter every 300 days. Thus, assuming that the breast cancer begins with a single cell it will, on the average, take 6 to 8 years to reach a diameter of 1 cm. In somewhat less than another year, it will be 2 cm in diameter.[4] Women should be trained early in their reproductive lives to perform self breast examinations. Several studies have demonstrated that women can easily find breast masses of 2 cm. In one study by Foster, 424 women performing self breast examinations and 411 who did not were newly diagnosed with breast carcinoma. Women performing monthly self exams detected tumors with an average diameter of 2.1 cm, whereas those performing self examinations less than monthly detected tumors of 2.4 cm in diameter. Tumors discovered in nonexaminers averaged 3.2 cm in size.[5]

Since the earlier the tumor can be discovered the less likely it is to have metastasized and therefore the better the chance of cure, it is obvious that women who do self breast examinations are more likely to survive their cancers than those who do not. Physicians should train patients to do self breast examinations; with practice on models with progressively smaller masses it may be possible to train them to detect even earlier lesions.

The second line of defense in early diagnosis is the annual physical examination. Unfortunately, physicians are probably not much better at detecting breast masses than are patients, and if given only an annual chance to find such a mass will probably detect larger tumors than would be detected by patients themselves.

Mammography is the third technique available and probably the most accurate method for detecting early breast carcinoma (Figure 11.1). It will allow for the discovery of much smaller tumors and therefore those that have less likelihood of having metastasized. For if the tumor is localized to the breast with negative regional nodes, the 5-year survival rate is as high as 85%. However, if axillary nodes are positive for tumor, the survival rate in 5 years is only 53%.[6] Using mammography and annual physical examinations over a 5-year period, the Health Insurance Plan of New York was able to demonstrate a 30% reduction

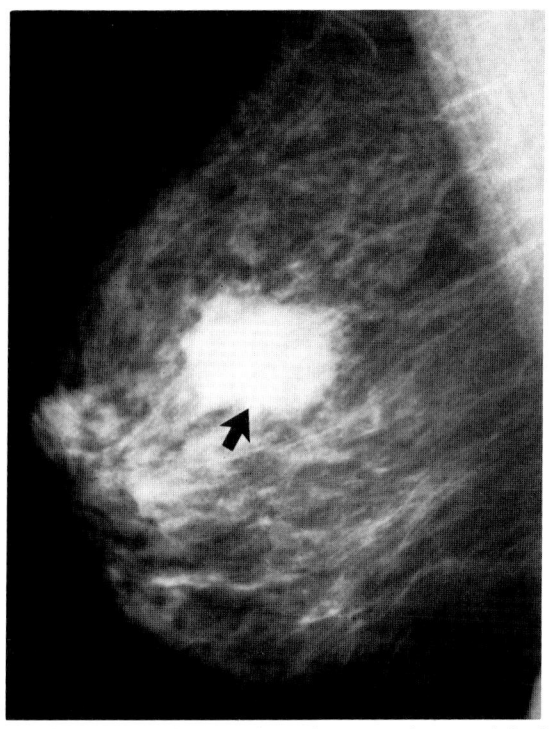

Figure 11.1 Mammography demonstrating a carcinoma of the breast.

in mortality from breast carcinoma compared to control groups.[7] Likewise, in a large Breast Cancer Detection Demonstration Project conducted by the National Institute of Health in the 1970s, 32% of carcinomas discovered were detected by mammography only.[8]

The American Cancer Society guidelines for mammographic screening of asymptomatic women is as follows:

1. Baseline mammogram for all women at age 35 to 40 years.
2. Mammography at 1- to 2-year intervals from 40 to 49 years.
3. Annual mammogram for women 50 years or older.

To date, the use of ultrasound and thermography are still experimental and their place in screening is not established.

Specific diagnosis of breast cancer is made by biopsy. In the case of nonpalpable lesions, x-ray localization of the area to be biopsied is important but, in any case, no therapy should be undertaken until a definitive biopsy is obtained and a diagnosis made. For cystic masses, needle aspiration is appropriate. If the aspiration fluid is clear, it may be discarded, although several breast physicians recommend cytologic evaluation. The chances, however, of discovering malignant cells in clear fluid aspirate is only a fraction of 1%.[9] If the fluid is not clear, it should be sent for cytologic interpretation, but if the cyst recurs rapidly, a biopsy should be considered. When masses are palpated by the patient and physician but not noted on mammography, biopsy should most definitely be performed.

Table 11.1 American Joint Committee on Cancer Staging for Breast Carcinoma*

Primary tumor (T)
- TX   Primary tumor cannot be assessed
- T0   No evidence of primary tumor
- Tis[†]   Carcinoma in situ: Intraductal carcinoma, lobular carcinoma in situ, or Paget's disease of the nipple with no tumor
- T1   Tumor 2 cm or less in greatest dimension
  - T1A   0.5 cm or less in greatest dimension
  - T1B   More than 0.5 cm but not more than 1 cm in greatest dimension
  - T1C   More than 1 cm but not more than 2 cm in greatest dimension
- T2   Tumor more than 2 cm but not more than 5 cm in greatest dimension
- T3   Tumor more than 5 cm in greatest dimension
- T4[‡]   Tumor of any size with direction extension to chest wall or skin
- T4A   Extension to chest wall
- T4B   Edema (including peau d'orange) or ulceration of the skin of the breast or satellite skin nodules confined to the same breast
- T4C   Both (T4A and T4B)
  - Inflammatory carcinoma

Regional lymph nodes (N) (clinical)
- NX   Regional lymph nodes cannot be assessed (eg, previously removed)
- N0   No regional lymph node metastasis
- N1   Metastasis to movable ipsilateral axillary lymph node(s)
- N2   Metastasis to ipsilateral axillary lymph node(s) fixed to one another or to other structures
- N3   Metastasis to ipsilateral internal mammary lymph node(s)

Distant Metastasis (M)
- MX   Presence of distant metastasis cannot be assessed
- M0   No distant metastasis
- M1   Distant metastasis (includes metastasis to ipsilateral supraclavicular lymph node[s])

Stage grouping			
Stage 0	Tis	N0	M0
Stage I	T1	N0	M0
Stage IIA	T0	N1	M0
	T1	N1[§]	M0
	T2	N0	M0
Stage IIB	T2	N1	M0
	T3	N0	M0
Stage IIIA	T0	N2	M0
	T1	N2	M0
	T2	N2	M0
	T3	N1, N2	M0
Stage IIIB	T4	Any N	M0
	Any T	N3	M0
Stage IV	Any T	Any N	M1

* T, primary tumor; N, regional lymph nodes; M, distant metastasis.

[†] Paget's disease associated with a tumor is classified according to the size of the tumor.

[‡] Chest wall includes ribs, intercostal muscles, and serratus anterior muscle but not pectoral muscle.

[§] The prognosis of patients with pN1a is similar to that of patients with pN0.

Pain is not a common finding in early breast cancer, being present in perhaps no more than 10% of women.[10] Induration and dimpling of the skin, ulceration, signs of inflammation, or edema leading to a skin that appears like an orange peel, is generally a late finding or a finding in a rapidly growing inflammatory type of carcinoma, where malignant cells infiltrate the lymphatics producing such findings.

The majority of carcinomas of the breast are adenocarcinomas; in postmenopausal women, they are generally intraductal carcinomas. While they may begin as carcinoma in situ, and indeed stay in this condition for a number of years, they frequently become infiltrating and may be multifocal. Lobular carcinomas of the breast may also occur in postmenopausal women, but the majority are seen in premenopausal women. Overall, lobular carcinoma is responsible for about 10% to 12% of all carcinomas of the breast, as compared to ductal carcinoma being responsible for 80% to 85%.[10]

Paget's disease, which resembles eczema or dermatitis of the nipple, makes up about 1% of breast cancers. It occurs in older women and is the result of infiltrating ductal carcinoma invading the skin.[10]

Decision for treatment of breast cancer depends upon the staging of the cancer, and determination of survivor rates must relate to this. Table 11.1 is a current staging system for breast cancer.

In general, treatment is based upon the histology of the tumor, the presence or absence of positive lymph nodes, and the hormone receptor status of the tumor. Carcinoma of the breast may metastasize both by lymphatic and hematogenous spread, and roughly half of the women diagnosed with carcinoma of the breast eventually die of the disease. Positive nodes are often found without palpable adenopathy, and distant metastases eventually develop in about two thirds of all patients regardless of therapy. Thus, breast cancer is essentially a systemic disease in many women and therapy needs to be designed with this in mind.[11] Surgical removal of the tumor, local irradiation, and chemotherapy are all part of the management for most tumors. Chemotherapy is useful both in women with metastatic disease and those at high risk for this condition. Surgical intervention and irradiation is appropriate to control local tumors. Therapy should also be designed with the quality of the patient's life in mind.

Knowledge of estrogen and progesterone receptors has an important prognostic and therapeutic implication. Approximately 60% of breast cancers that are estrogen-receptor-positive will respond to hormone therapy, such as progesterone and androgen. Indeed, up to 80% response is noted when both estrogen and progesterone receptors are present in the tumor. In the face of negative receptors, less than 10% of tumors will respond.[12]

Multiple drug chemotherapy, using such agents as cyclophosphamide, methotrexate, adriamycin, 5-fluorouracil, and vinblastine, has been tried in a number of individuals with as many as 10% to 20% experiencing a complete remission for about 1.5 years.[13]

Specific recommendations for surgical treatment, irradiation, and chemotherapy are beyond the scope of this book.

Vulvar Cancer

Through the years, carcinoma of the vulva has accounted for between 3% and 5% of all female genital malignancies. However, this condition has been traditionally more common in older women. The majority of tumors are histologically

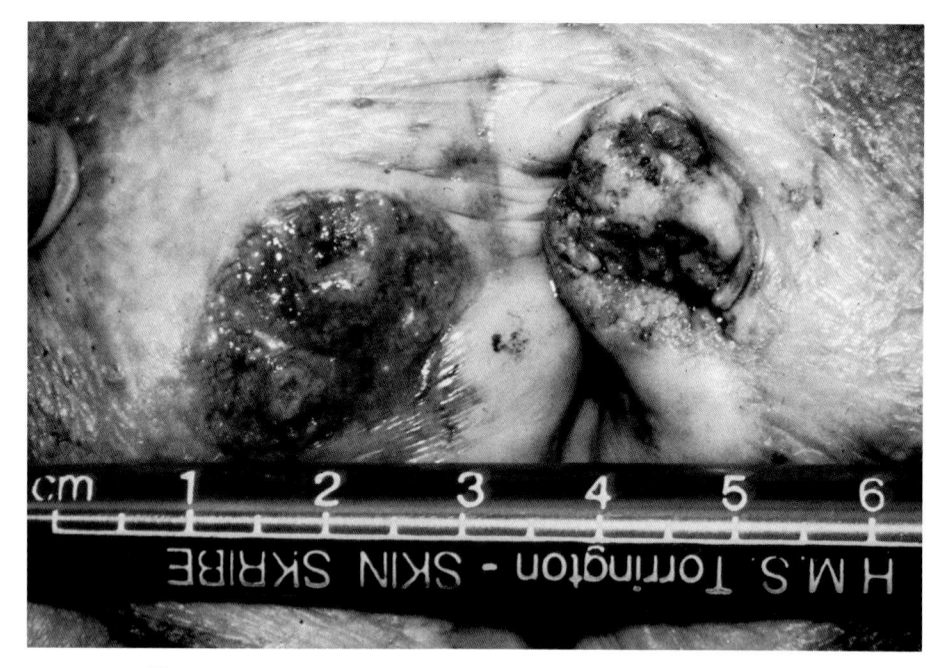

Figure 11.2 Vulva of an elderly woman demonstrating carcinoma.

squamous cell but a small percentage include melanomas, sarcomas, Paget's disease, and adenocarcinomas of the Bartholin gland. The etiology of vulvar carcinoma is unknown. It is seen in every race and has a similar incidence worldwide. In at least 50% of the cases, vulvar itching is the first symptom. Often there is a small painless mass present for a considerable period of time. Occasionally, the lesion resembles a wart. It is likely that some carcinomas of the vulva are first present as carcinoma in situ and many develop from dysplastic skin.[14]

Delays in biopsing the lesions are the responsibility of both the patient and the physician. Since the symptoms are minimal, many patients will ignore the findings until the lesion is quite large or has ulcerated. On the other hand, elderly women consulting physicians for vulvar itching are frequently treated with local medications and not appropriately biopsied for prolonged periods of time. Women who do complain of chronic vulvar itching should be evaluated usually with biopsy (Figure 11.2).

Squamous cell carcinoma of the vulva generally spreads locally to inguinal lymph nodes first, and then to deep pelvic lymph nodes. Distant metastases are unusual. Tumors are staged with respect to the size of the lesion and the presence of palpable lymph nodes. Table 11.2 outlines the method of staging. Multiple authors report positive groin and pelvic nodes in anywhere from 21% to 50% of patients at the time of operation.[15–17]

Diagnosis is made by biopsy. If a lesion is present, a wide excision should be performed. In the case of vulvar pruritus or dystrophy without an obvious lesion, colposcopy may help to outline an area for biopsy (Figure 11.3).

Management is primarily surgical and consists of radical vulvectomy and superficial and deep inguinal lymph node dissection. This is performed in an on-block fashion, and the inguinal nodes are submitted for frozen section. If positive, a pelvic lymphadectomy is performed on the side on which positive

Table 11.2 FIGO Staging (Clinical) of Invasive Cancer of the Vulva

Stage I	T1	N0	M0	All lesions confined to vulva, with maximal diameter of 2 cm or less and no suspicious groin nodes
	T1	N1	M0	
Stage II	T2	N0	M0	All lesions confined to vulva, with diameter greater than 2 cm and no suspicious groin nodes
	T2	N1	M0	
Stage III	T3	N0	M0	Lesions extending beyond vulva but without grossly positive groin nodes
	T3	N1	M0	
	T3	N2	M0	Lesions of any size confined to vulva, with suspicious groin nodes
	T1	M2	M0	
	T2	N2	M0	
Stage IV	T3	N3	M0	Lesions extending beyond vulva, with grossly positive nodes
	T4	N3	M0	
	T4	N0	M0	Lesions involving mucosa of rectum, bladder, or urethra or involving bone
	T4	N1	M0	
	T4	N2	M0	
	T1	N3	M0	
	T2	N3	M0	
	M1a			All cases with distant or palpable deep pelvic metastases
	M1b			

nodes are found. An alternative to deep pelvic node dissection is irradiation of these nodes. In a study by the Gynecologic Oncology Group, a group of patients who were treated with irradiation had a 75% 2-year survival as compared to a matched group who were treated by pelvic node dissection and had a 56% 2-year survival.[18] In general, radical vulvectomy with inguinal and pelvic lym-

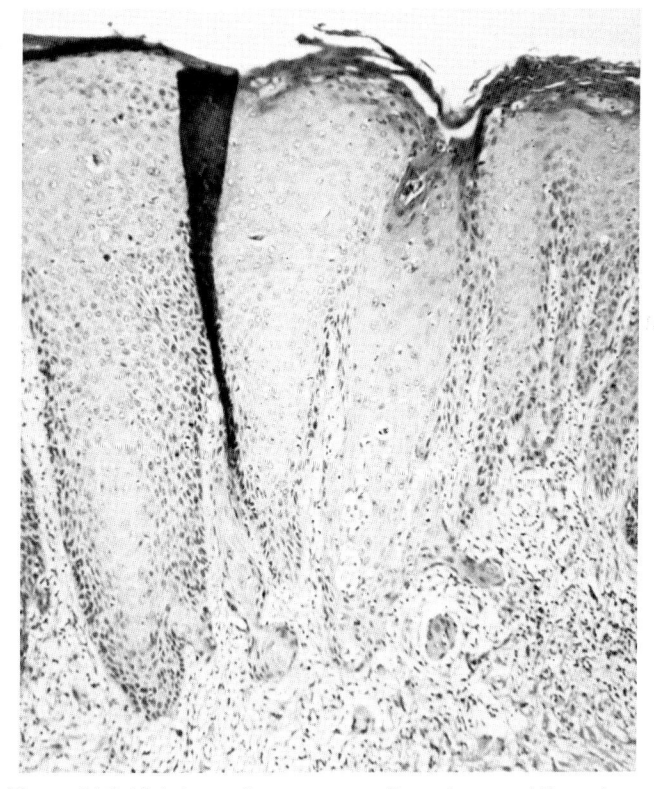

Figure 11.3 Histology of squamous cell carcinoma of the vulva.

phadenectomy as indicated will yield an overall corrected 5-year survival rate in stage I and II disease of approximately 90%.[14] Operative mortality is dependent on the patient's general condition but it is rarely more than 1% or 2%. The procedure can frequently be carried out in very elderly women with satisfactory results. Complications involve wound breakdown, the development of a lymphocyst in the groin, and lymph edema of the leg. Occasionally, women will complain of stress urinary incontinence because of interference with urethral support.

Recurrences generally occur within the first 2 years and are frequently local, although metastatic lesions are known to occur. If the recurrence is local, it may be treated with surgical removal or irradiation. Chemotherapy has not been found to be useful to this point in the treatment of this condition.[14]

Cancer of the Vagina

Cancer of the vagina is a rare gynecologic tumor. It is usually of the squamous cell variety and occurs more commonly in the upper half of the vagina. When it occurs it is usually a disease of older women and often begins as an intraepithelial lesion. As it becomes invasive, it spreads most commonly by local extension. It may be discovered by screening pap smears of the vagina.

Early symptoms of invasive carcinoma of the vagina consist of vaginal bleeding and vaginal discharge. As the tumor increases in size, the lesion may become inflamed and infected, leading to pain or, if situated near the bladder or urethra, may cause urinary symptoms. Since many elderly women are sexually inactive, the lesion may grow to a fairly significant size before it is detected, as the vagina is basically distensible and bleeding and discharge may not occur or be noticed in the sexually inactive woman. Staging of a carcinoma of the vagina is depicted in Table 11.3.

The spread of the carcinoma that is not by direct extension is generally through lymphatics. Carcinomas of the upper vagina will spread through pelvic lymph node distributions similar to carcinoma of the cervix. Carcinomas in the lower portion of the vagina will often spread to the inguinal nodes.

Although the majority of carcinomas of the vagina are of the squamous (epidermoid) type, an occasional adenocarcinoma, sarcoma, or melanoma may be seen.

Therapy for carcinoma of the vagina that is in situ or early invasive may be by wide excision. While radical removal of the vagina and pelvic lymph nodes may be appropriate for later or more advanced lesions, the majority will respond well to irradiation therapy, generally in the form of radium implants, often with supplemental external beam therapy. In the patient who has been treated with

Table 11.3 Staging of Carcinoma of the Vagina

Stage 0	Intraepithelial carcinoma
Stage I	Limited to the vaginal mucosa
Stage II	Involving the subvaginal tissue but not extending on to pelvic sidewalls
Stage III	Extending to the pelvic sidewalls or pubic symphysis
Stage IV	Extending beyond the true pelvis or involving the mucosa of the bladder or rectum

irradiation therapy, recurrence generally occurs locally, and may be managed by exenterative procedures.

The prognosis with therapy in carcinoma of the vagina is related to the stage of the disease. Numerous reports during the last decade note an apparent 5-year cure rate of between 65% and 100% in stage I lesions treated by surgical excision or irradiation. This success rate falls off for stage II lesions to about 50% to 60%, and to about 30% to 35% for stage III lesions. Five-year survival rates with stage IV lesions are close to 0 in just about every study.[19-22]

Cancer of the Cervix

Although cancer of the cervix is a fairly common cancer of the reproductive organs, its peak incidence occurs in women between the ages of 45 and 55. It does occur in older women and, therefore, screening tests for cancer of the cervix should be continued into the advanced age groups. Ninety percent of carcinomas of the cervix are squamous cell type, and about 10% are adenocarcinoma.[23] In most situations, squamous cell carcinoma arises from cells in the transitional zone of the cervix, generally going through a process of dysplasia, carcinoma in situ, and finally invasive carcinoma. The process may take anywhere from months to years. Adenocarcinoma arises from the endocervical gland cells, and may only briefly be present as an in situ tumor.

The typical patient with squamous cell carcinoma of the cervix gives a history of first intercourse during her adolescence, has had multiple partners, and is generally parous often at an early age. There is usually an association epidemiologically with other sexually transmitted diseases, and there may be a biological association with some strains of the human papilloma virus. Squamous cell carcinoma of the cervix is usually not associated with a familial cancer history, and is not an endocrine-sensitive tumor. Adenocarcinoma of the cervix does not seem to follow the same patient profile. It may occur in any age group including the elderly.[23]

The Papanicolaou smear has been an excellent means of screening for dysplasia, as well as in situ carcinoma and invasive lesions. Early in the disease, the patient is usually asymptomatic. As the lesion becomes larger, vaginal spotting and discharge may be noted. Pain is rarely a symptom in early lesions but in more advanced lesions it may be present as the tumor invades more deeply and spreads to the vagina and possibly becomes infected. These tumors spread by local extension and by lymphatic spread. Advanced cases may be associated with obstruction of the ureters or infiltration of nerve roots.[23]

Clinical staging of carcinoma of the cervix is illustrated in Table 11.4.

Diagnosis is established by biopsy, and staging is clinically established before therapy.

Basic treatment for cancer of the cervix is either surgical or irradiation therapy. The choice of which modality depends upon the stage of the tumor, the age of the patient, and her general condition. Basically, advanced stages of carcinoma of the cervix (ie, stage IIB and greater) are best treated by irradiation therapy. Dysplastic lesions and carcinoma in situ may be managed by local destruction with laser or cryo techniques, or by excision using cone biopsy of the cervix. While carcinoma in situ may be treated in the same fashion, a simple hysterectomy either by the vaginal or abdominal route may be appropriate. For

Table 11.4 FIGO Staging and Classification of Cancer of the Cervix

Stage 0	Carcinoma in situ
Stage I	The carcinoma is strictly confined to the cervix (extension to the corpus should be disregarded)
Stage IA	Preclinical carcinomas of the cervix; ie, those diagnosed only by microscopy
Stage IA1	Minimal microscopically evident stromal invasion
Stage IA2	Lesions detected microscopically that can be measured. The upper limit of the measurement should not show a depth of invasion of more than 5 mm taken from the base of the epithelium, either surface or glandular, from which it originates, and a second dimension, the horizontal spread, must not exceed 7 mm. Larger lesions should be staged as IB
Stage IB	Lesions of greater dimensions than Stage IA2 whether seen clinically or not. Preformed space involvement should not alter the staging but should be specifically recorded so as to determine whether it should affect treatment decisions in the future
Stage II	Involvement of the vagina but not the lower third, or infiltration of the parametria but not out to the sidewall
Stage IIA	Involvement of the vagina but no evidence of parametrial involvement
Stage IIB	Infiltration of the parametria but not out to the sidewall
Stage III	Involvement of the lower third of the vagina or extension
Stage IIIA	Involvement of the lower third of the vagina but not out to the pelvic sidewall if the parametria are involved
Stage IIIB	Involvement of one or both parametria out to the sidewall
Stage III (urinary)	Obstruction of one or both ureters on intravenous pyelogram (IVP) without the other criteria for stage-III disease
Stage IV	Entension outside the reproductive tract
Stage IVA	Involvement of the mucosa of the bladder or rectum
Stage IVB	Distant metastasis or disease outside the true pelvis

women with very early stage-I lesions, which have been designated microinvasive lesions, a simple hysterectomy is still acceptable since rarely do these metastasize to lymph nodes. These are generally described as locally invasive tumors of no more than 3 mm depth beneath the basement membrane and without the invasion of vascular spaces.[24]

For frankly invasive stage-I lesions and stage-IIA lesions, a radical hysterectomy with pelvic lymph node dissection or irradiation therapy is appropriate. The decision is generally made on clinical ground and, for most women beyond menopause, the choice is often irradiation therapy. Such therapy generally involves the implantation of radium or cesium sources into the cervical canal and uterus as well as into the upper vaginal fornices in the hopes of delivering a cancerocidal dose of irradiation to the local tumor. Such a dose of irradiation is generally in the neighborhood of 6000 rads, but higher doses are given locally in order to be sure of irradicating the entire tumor. In order to protect the bladder, which can tolerate only between 5000 and 7000 rads, and the rectum, which can tolerate only 5000 rads, the vagina is packed with gauze in order to move the bladder and rectum away from the source of radium. Since the intensity of irradiation from radium or cesium is determined by the inverse square law, the greater the distance the less the irradiation by a matter of the square of the distance between the source and the tissue to be protected. Because of the inverse square law, a significant amount of irradiation to the lateral pelvic lymph nodes is not achieved by radium or cesium sources alone and, therefore, external

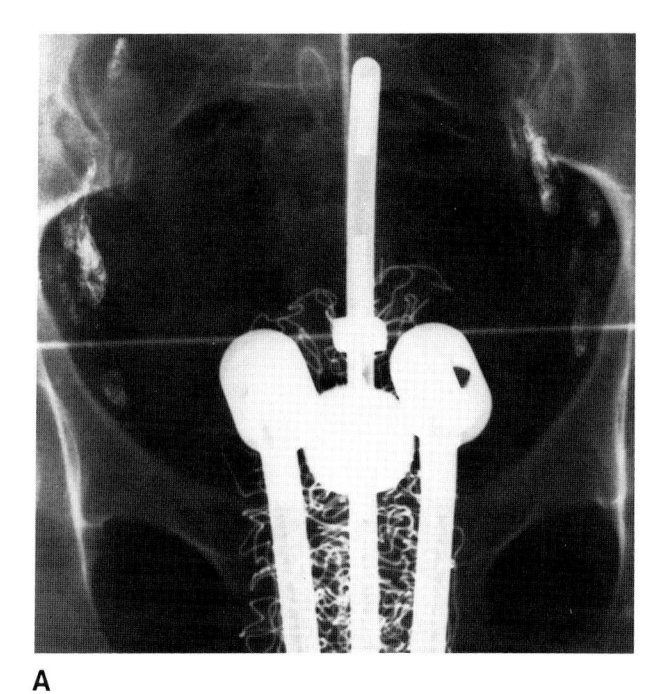

Figure 11.4 X-ray views of the female pelvis, demonstrating the presence of a cesium applicator in the vagina, cervix, and uterus. Dummy sources are present in the applicator so that the isodose measurements can be made. Since the applicator is an after loader, cesium sources are added after localizing films are taken. Barium in the colon and radio-opaque packing material demonstrate the proper positioning of the applicator. (A) Anterior/posterior view; (B) lateral view.

beam irradiation of about 4000 rads is necessary to ensure adequate irradiation of the lateral pelvic lymph nodes. Local irradiation may be given in divided doses, and external beam therapy may be given following local irradiation over a period of time. This allows for recovery of normal tissue while cancer cells are killed.[23] (See Figure 11.4.)

Five-year survival rates for stage-I and stage-IIA cancers are similar between women treated with irradiation or surgery, being between 85% and 90% for stage-I lesions and 75% and 85% for stage-IIA lesions. Five-year survivorship with irradiation therapy in stages IIB, IIIA, IIIB, and IV have been reported in the neighborhood of 65%, 45%, 36%, and 14%, respectively.[24,25]

Complications seen with radical surgery, although relatively rare, include: hemorrhage, infection, lymphedema of the leg, and ureterovaginal fistula. Complications with irradiation therapy include: irradiation damage to the bladder, leading to vesicovaginal fistula, irradiation damage to the rectum, leading to proctitis or rectovaginal fistula; and irradiation damage leading to necrosis of the head of the femur. In addition, sexual dysfunction is a relatively common finding with irradiation therapy.[26]

Overall, the incidence of recurrence or persistence of tumor in all patients with carcinoma of the cervix is about 35%. The majority will recur within the first 2 years after therapy, but some will recur much later. Symptoms and signs of recurrence include weight loss, leg edema, pain in the pelvis or thigh, vaginal discharge and bleeding, obstruction of the ureter, and distant findings, such as lymphadenopathy, cough, hemoptysis, and chest pain. While the tumor generally recurs locally, it can certainly recur at distant sites.[27] Treatment of recurrence may consist of exenterative procedures for locally recurrent tumors, irradiation, and a variety of chemotherapeutic agents, many of which are under protocol for study. Responses have been seen with alkylating agents, such as cyclophosphamide and melphalan; antimetabolites such as 5-fluorouracil and methotrexate; antibiotics such as mitomycin-C, bleomycin, and adriamycin, and cisplatinum.[27]

Carcinoma of the Endometrium

Endometrial carcinoma often arises from areas of hyperplasia of the endometrium, which may exist for varying periods of time before carcinomatous change occurs. Most hyperplasia of the endometrium is a result of either endogenous or exogenous estrogen activity. A mild form of hyperplasia, designated by most pathologists as cystic glandular hyperplasia, is a fairly inactive form commonly seen in postmenopausal women and generally not felt to be a precancerous lesion. A more active form of hyperplasia with proliferation of the endometrial cells is glandular adenomatous hyperplasia. In such situations, although hyperactive, the cells are normal. Adenomatous hyperplasia in which the cells become atypical is felt to be a potential precancerous lesion. Adenocarcinoma of the endometrium is frequently seen in conjunction with areas of atypical adenomatous hyperplasia. In the past, atypical adenomatous hyperplasia had been designated by some as carcinoma in situ. Not all hyperplasia progresses to cancer and some is reversible with progestational agents. Nonetheless, atypical adenomatous hyperplasia is considered a precancerous lesion and should be treated in older women either with hysterectomy or with intensive progestational therapy and close surveillance.[28]

Adenocarcinoma of the endometrium is the most common carcinoma seen in the endometrium, and in the vast majority of cases occurs in postmenopausal women. Unlike cervical cancer, there is no known relationship to coital or reproductive epidemiologic factors, although it is apparently more common in cancer-prone families. Women using unopposed estrogen-replacement therapy or those with estrogen-secreting tumors, such as granulosal cell tumors and thecomas, are at higher risk for developing adenocarcinoma of the endometrium.[29,30] In addition, obese women seem to be at greater risk, probably because of the increased conversion of androgens to estrogens in body fat.[28]

There are no early symptoms or signs of endometrial cancer, and screening tests using the Papanicolaou smear only detect about 50% of adenocarcinomas of the endometrium. Fortunately, however, carcinomas of the endometrium frequently bleed relatively early in their course. Therefore, vaginal bleeding in a perimenopausal or postmenopausal woman must be investigated with endometrial sampling. This may be accomplished either by performing a dilatation and curettage or an endometrial biopsy. Both have about equal likelihood of detecting a cancer. If the endometrial biopsy is performed, a paracervical block is used with sampling of all quadrants of the uterine cavity. It is an office procedure and is less costly than a D&C. When performing an endometrial biopsy, it is also important to perform an endocervical curettage to rule out the possibility of a tumor extending to the cervix.[28] Table 11.5 demonstrates the clinical staging of carcinoma of the endometrium.

The majority of endometrial cancers are stage-I. In a recent report from a combined center study, 75.5% of more than 12,000 patients had stage-I, 13.9% stage-II, 6.2% stage-III, and 3.3% stage-IV.[31] Although the stage of the disease is important in determining appropriate therapy and prognosis, other considerations are equally important. These include: histologic typing and degree of differentiation, size of the uterus, degree of myometrial invasion, the presence of positive peritoneal cytology, and the presence of lymph node and adnexal metastases. Of the histologic types, adenocarcinoma or adenoacanthoma (adenocarcinoma with benign squamous metaplasia within the glands) have the best 5-year survival rates.[28] Other variants, such as papillary carcinoma, adenosquamous carcinoma, and clear cell carcinoma, have a poorer prognosis stage

Table 11.5 FIGO Classification of Endometrial Carcinoma

Stage I	The carcinoma is confined to the corpus
	Stage IA: The length of the uterine cavity is 8 cm or less
	Stage IB: The length of the uterine cavity is more than 8 cm
	Stage I cases should be subgrouped with regard to the histologic type of adenocarcinoma as follows:
	G1: Highly differentiated adenomatous carcinoma
	G2: Differentiated adenomatous carcinoma with partly solid areas
	G3: Predominantly solid or entirely undifferentiated carcinoma
Stage II	The carcinoma involves the corpus and cervix
Stage III	The carcinoma extends outside the corpus but not outside the true pelvis (it may involve the vaginal wall or the parametrium but not the bladder or rectum)
Stage IV	The carcinoma involves the bladder or rectum or extends outside the pelvis

From *Manual for Staging of Cancer 1978,* Chicago, 1978, American Joint Committee for Cancer Staging and End Results Reporting.

for stage. Within the histologic differentiation of adenocarcinoma, three grades are recognized. Grade I is a well-differentiated carcinoma with mostly glandular elements. Grade II is a combination of glandular elements and sheets of malignant cells. Grade III is a poorly differentiated carcinoma consisting of solid sheets of tumor only (Figure 11.5).

All things being equal, myometrial invasion can be a determinant of prognosis. Women who have myometrial invasion in the inner third only do better than those with deeper invasion. Positive peritoneal cytology, lymph node metastases, or metastases to the adnexae decrease the chances of cure as the disease becomes more systemic.[32-34]

The patient with stage-I carcinoma of the endometrium that has a well-differentiated tumor limited to the endometrium or the inner third of the myometrium, and in whom there is negative peritoneal cytology and negative lymph node involvement, has the best chance of having a 5-year survival. In such cases, the 5-year survival is probably in excess of 90%. On the other hand, poorly differentiated tumors, which have invaded more deeply into the myometrium and which may have positive cytology or lymph node findings, will have a much poorer prognosis, perhaps no more than 55% to 60% 5-year survival even in stage-I lesions that are properly treated.[32]

Bokhman has suggested that there are two pathogenic types of endometrial cancer. The first is seen in women with the typical historical features for endometrial cancer (ie, obesity, hyperlipidemia, hyperestrogenism, and other epidemiologic factors—such as a history of anovulatory uterine bleeding, infertility, late onset of menopause, or with ovarian disease which leads to hyperestrogenism). These generally are of the well-differentiated type, and often at the time of discovery have minimal myometrial involvement. The second pathogenic type is seen in women without the epidemiologic features mentioned, is frequently of a poorly differentiated type of tumor, and often at the time of discovery has deep myometrial invasion and may have positive peritoneal cytology and positive lymph nodes. It may be that the former groups relate to hyperestrogenism and the latter group does not.[35] Perhaps supporting this theory is the fact that the majority of women who develop adenocarcinoma in relation to unopposed estrogen therapy fall into the former category.

The histologic grade is important as demonstrated by the fact that the FIGO Study (Pettersson) demonstrated a 79.6% 5-year survivorship in stage I, grade I lesions, as compared to 73.4% for stage I, grade II lesions, and 58.7% for stage I, grade III lesions.[31]

The overall size of the uterus is probably of prognostic importance. Jones demonstrated that women with normal-size uteri had an overall 5-year survivor rate of 84.5% and women with enlarged uteri had an overall survivor rate of 66.6%.[36] From a prognostic standpoint, stage is probably still the most important criteria with overall survivor rates listed in Table 11.6.

A number of studies have shown that the percentage of women with positive pelvic lymph nodes is about 10% in stage-I lesions.[37-39]

Treatment is primarily surgical, with a total abdominal hysterectomy and bilateral salpingo-oophorectomy being performed. Peritoneal cytology and pelvic lymph node sampling is often carried out as part of the procedure. It is appropriate to open the specimen in the operating room to assess size of tumor and the degree of myometrial spread. If the myometrial invasion is deeper than the inner third, it is generally considered appropriate to give irradiation therapy

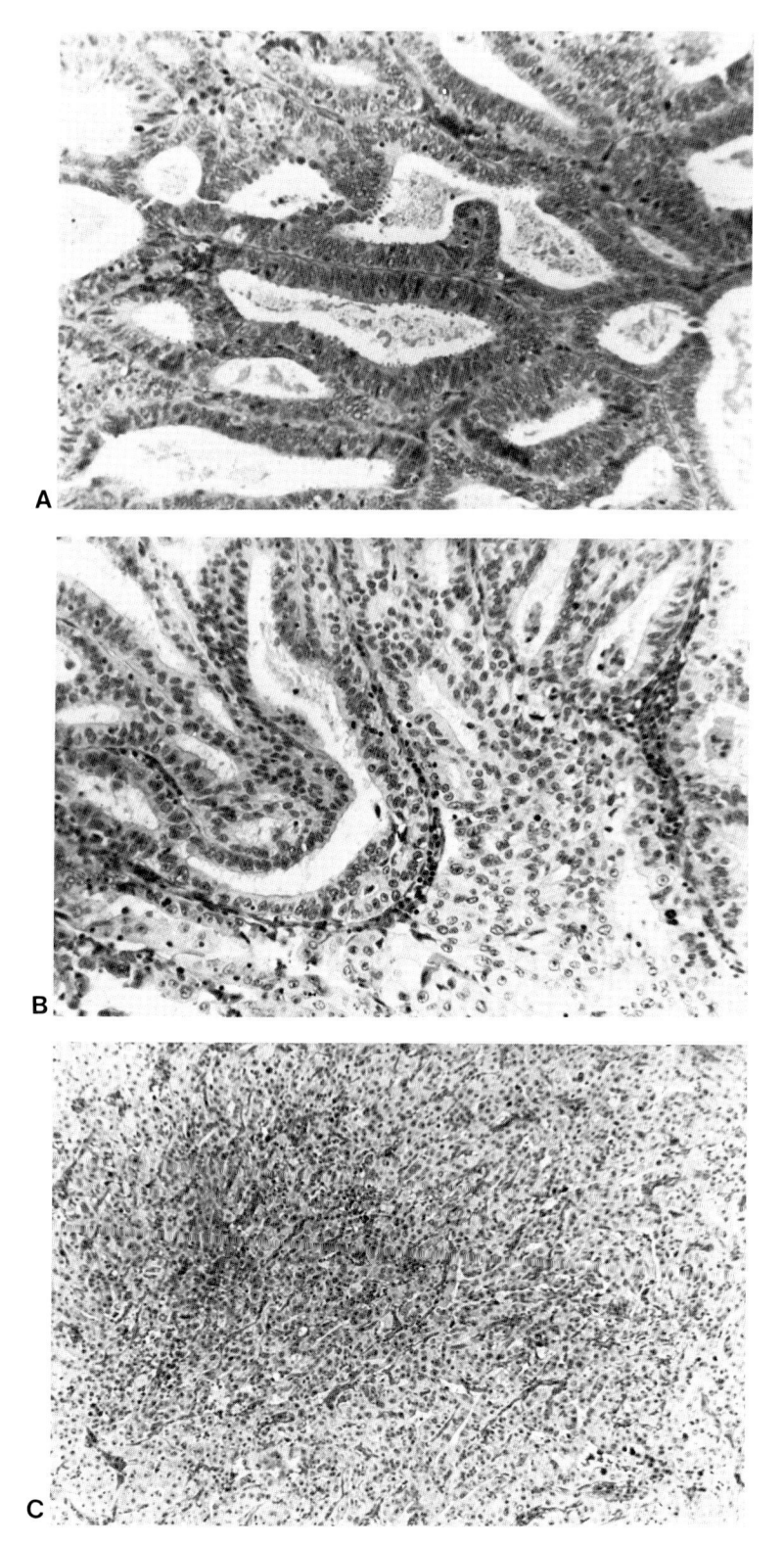

Figure 11.5 (A) Grade-I well-differentiated adenocarcinoma; (B) grade-II intermediate differentiation; (C) grade-III poorly differentiated adenocarcinoma.

Table 11.6 Five-Year Survivor Percentage for Endometrial Cancer by Stage*

Stage I lesions	75.1%
Stage II	51.8%
Stage III	30.0%
Stage IV	10.6%

* See Ref. 31.

to the pelvis. Likewise, most authorities feel that supplemental irradiation therapy is appropriate for individuals with poorly differentiated lesions. In several centers in the world, preoperative irradiation therapy using radium or cesium packing of the uterus is given just prior to hysterectomy. Combined 5-year survivorship using these techniques are similar.[36] For larger uteri or for tumors which are anaplastic, preop irradiation is often given. If the disease is outside the uterus or associated with a recurrence, chemotherapy and progestin therapy may be useful.[40]

It is possible to perform estrogen and progesterone receptor analyses on endometrial cancer. Kauppila et al have demonstrated that patients with cells that contain few estrogen and progesterone receptors had a better response rate to a combined cytoxic therapy, including doxorubicin, cyclophosphamide, 5-fluorouracil, and vincristin.[40] Several authors have demonstrated that if positive receptors are present, progestins offer reasonable response rates.[41-47]

Other less common tumors (such as leiomyosarcoma, mixed mullerian sarcoma, and endometrial stromal sarcoma) can occur in older women but are very rare. Therapy is basically surgical with total abdominal hysterectomy and bilateral salpingo-oophorectomy and node sampling being recommended. Some centers suggest the use of adjunct pelvic irradiation, but the efficacy of this has not been proven. Likewise, chemotherapeutic protocols have been used in these tumors, although their value is also still to be demonstrated.

Carcinoma of the Fallopian Tube

Carcinoma of the fallopian tube is a rare gynecologic malignancy, making up less than 1% of all gynecologic cancers. While it can occur in any age group, it is more commonly seen in the elderly with an average age in the 50s. Few signs and symptoms are noted in early stages of the disease, and discovery is generally by accident at the time of performance of another abdominal procedure. As the tumor grows there may be bleeding. Since most patients are postmenopausal, the usual postmenopausal bleeding evaluation may fail to reveal the tumor. Therefore, in a patient with postmenopausal bleeding in which no diagnosis of endometrial disease is found, and in whom the bleeding persists after endometrial sampling, the diagnosis of carcinoma of the fallopian tube must be considered. At times a fallopian tube will obstruct because of the tumor and fill with fluid. The patient may then experience crampy pain on one side of the lower abdomen accompanied by watery or watery blood-tinged discharge. The combination of pain with a watery vaginal discharge in the presence of carcinoma of the fallopian tube is referred to as hydrops tubae profluens. At times it is possible to identify cancer cells in cervical cytology, and this has been reported as occurring in between 10% and 60% of patients.[48] Often the tumor is diagnosed when the patient is discovered to have an adnexal mass, being part of the differential diagnosis for such a problem, but the specific diagnosis is not usually made until the time of operation. Although ultrasound, CT scan, and MRI offer an opportunity to diagnose an adnexal mass, differentiating these from masses arising from other structures is not always possible.

Although there is no staging protocol for tubal carcinoma, it has been suggested that the staging guidelines used for ovarian carcinoma could be applied, and would be equally useful for management decisions. Therapy is basically surgical, with total abdominal hysterectomy and bilateral salpingo-oophorectomy being the usual therapy. Peritoneal cytology, selective lymph node sampling, inspection of the entire peritoneal cavity and subdiaphragmatic region, and a partial omentectomy comprise the very least therapy that should be offered. For more advanced lesions, debulking procedures, as are performed with ovarian carcinoma, are indicated. If residual disease is left in the pelvis, 5000 rads of whole pelvic irradiation plus cis-platinum-containing chemotherapeutic regimens and progesterone therapy are suggested for 1 year. If no residual disease is noted and the lymph nodes are negative, intraperitoneal P_{32} is a reasonable choice. Where there is residual disease and positive lymph nodes noted, a chemotherapeutic regimen as outlined with a second-look laparotomy in 1 year is suggested.[48]

Prognosis depends upon the extent of the disease and is difficult to determine because few institutions have a very wide experience. Roberts and Lifshitz have demonstrated a 60% 5-year survivorship in patients who had disease limited to the fallopian tubes and/or pelvic structures.[49] Prognostic data are not available when adjunctive therapy is used in advanced lesions.

Cancer of the Ovary

For women ages 55–74, deaths due to cancer of the ovary are the fourth most common cause of cancer deaths in women in the United States. Even in women in the age groups of 75 and over, cancer death due to ovarian cancer ranks fifth. Not all ovarian neoplasms are malignant; in fact, in a series by Bennington et al, benign adnexal tumors outnumbered malignant tumors 2 to 1 in the 55-and-over age group.[50] Likewise, in a small series of 16 patients reported by Hernandez and Miyazawa, of 16 patients with pelvic tumors only 9 (56%) had cancer.[61] Thus, the presence of an adnexal mass in an older woman does not necessarily foretell the diagnosis of malignancy. In the Bennington et al series, the majority of benign tumors were serous cystadenomas, although mucinous cystadenomas and benign cystic teratomas were also seen in the advanced age group. Thecomas and fibromas were also reasonably prevalent, particularly in the 55 to 65 age group. Among the malignant tumors seen in this series, the majority were serous cystadenocarcinomas, mucinous cystadenocarcinomas, and endometriod carcinomas. Granulosal cell carcinoma and metastatic lesions were also seen.[50]

There are no epidemiologic factors supporting the fact that one group of women is more susceptible to ovarian cancer than another, although prolonged use of birth control pills has been found in some studies to be related to a lower incidence of carcinoma of the ovary.[52–53] Since early stages of ovarian tumors are generally silent, such tumors are often found by accident at the time of pelvic examination or when ultrasound examinations are performed for other reasons. Larger tumors are often palpable abdominally, may cause pelvic discomfort or, if torsion occurs, may cause acute pelvic pain. Ascites is often associated with ovarian cancer, and the first presenting symptom may be increased abdominal girth.

When an adnexal mass, be it cystic or solid, is found in a woman past menopause, it must be investigated. In the average postmenopausal woman, the ovary is no more than 2 cm in diameter and retracted quite high toward the pelvis brim. Therefore, any palpable adnexal mass should be investigated as a potential tumor. Both pelvic examination and ultrasound examination (particularly vaginal ultrasound) should be able to differentiate a cystic from a solid lesion. If cystic, it should be determined whether or not the lesions are unilocular or multilocular and whether or not solid components are present. Uniloculated cystic adnexal tumors without appreciable solid components in a postmenopausal woman will often be benign. However, they may be malignant and, therefore, must be investigated. Functioning ovarian tumors (particularly granulosal cell tumors and thecomas) may produce enough estrogen to cause vaginal bleeding due to endometrial hyperplasia. Rare androgen-secreting tumors (such as Sertoli-Leydig and hilus cell tumors) can occur in the older age group and may cause androgenizing symptoms.

The workup of an adnexal mass includes chest x-ray and blood chemistries for distant metastases; barium enema to rule out primary bowel disease or disease which has become metastatic to the pelvis or diverticulitis which may masquerade as a pelvic mass; and intravenous pyelogram to assess the status of the kidneys and the positions of the ureters. In addition, it is helpful to obtain tumor markers, including CA 125, HCG, and α-feto-protein. These may indicate the presence of a malignant tumor and are good prognostic signs to measure the benefits of therapy.

The specific diagnosis of an ovarian lesion is made surgically. In an older woman, a mid-line incision should be made so that adequate evaluation of the pelvis and abdomen can be carried out. Upon entering the abdomen, peritoneal fluid is obtained for cytology. If no fluid is present, peritoneal washings are taken. These should be taken from all four quadrants of the abdominal cavity as well as the pelvis. The lesion is then either removed intact or biopsied, depending upon its characteristics, and sent for frozen section. In the event of a benign cystic or solid adnexal mass, it is usually appropriate to perform a bilateral salpingo-oophorectomy and total abdominal hysterectomy. If the lesion is malignant, it should be staged. Appropriate staging for carcinoma of the ovary is outlined in Table 11.7.

Surgical management of ovarian cancer is as follows: total abdominal hysterectomy; bilateral salpingo-oophorectomy and a debulking procedure which should include a partial omentectomy; a dissection of pelvic and paraortic lymph nodes; multiple sampling of peritoneal surfaces, including subdiaphragmatic surface; inspection of the entire bowel and its mesentery, and inspection of the subdiaphragmatic regions. All attempts should be made to remove as much cancer tissue as possible. The dissection of pelvic and paraortic lymph nodes is important because they may be positive for disease in as many as 10% to 20% of cases in stage-I disease.[54–55]

Adjunct chemotherapy in stage-IA and stage-IB lesions is controversial. Pro-

Table 11.7 Carcinoma of the Ovary: Staging Classification Using the FIGO Nomenclature

Stage I	Growth limited to the ovaries
Stage IA	Growth limited to one ovary; no ascites; no tumor on the external surfaces; capsule intact
Stage IB	Growth limited to both ovaries; no ascites; no tumor on the external surfaces; capsules intact
Stage IC*	Tumor either stage IA or stage IB, but with tumor on the surface of one or both ovaries; or with capsule ruptured; or with ascities present containing malignant cells or with positive peritoneal washings
Stage II	Growth involving one or both ovaries with pelvic extension
Stage IIA	Extension and/or metastases to the uterus and/or tubes
Stage IIB	Extension to other pelvic tissues
Stage IIC*	Tumor either stage IIA or stage IIB, but with tumor on the surface of one or both ovaries; or with capsule(s) ruptured; or with ascities present, containing malignant cells or with positive peritoneal washings
Stage III	Tumor involving one or both ovaries with peritoneal implants outside the pelvis and/or positive retroperitoneal or inguinal nodes; superficial liver metastasis equals stage III; tumor is limited to the true pelvis but with histologically verified malignant extension to small bowel or omentum
Stage IIIA	Tumor grossly limited to the true pelvis with negative nodes but with histologically confirmed microscopic seeding of abdominal peritoneal surfaces
Stage IIIB	Tumor of one or both ovaries; histologically confirmed implants of abdominal peritoneal surfaces, none exceeding 2 cm in diameter; nodes negative
Stage IIIC	Abdominal implants 2 cm in diameter and/or positive retroperitoneal or inguinal nodes
Stage IV	Growth involving one or both ovaries with distant metastasis; if pleural effusion is present, there must be positive cytologic test results to allot a case to stage IV; parenchymal liver metastasis equals stage IV

From *Am J Obstet Gynecol* 1987; 156:263.

* In order to evaluate the impact on prognosis of the different criteria for alloting cases to stage IC or stage IIC, it would be of value to know if rupture of the capsule was (1) spontaneous or (2) caused by the surgeon and if the source of the malignant cells detected was (a) peritoneal washings or (b) ascites.

spective studies by the Gynecologic Oncology Group have not, to date, offered conclusive evidence for any value of such therapy,[56] but some institutions will utilize intraperitoneal installation of radioactive P_{32} or a variety of chemotherapeutic regimens, generally including an alkylating agent such as melphalan or chlorambucil. In such cases, the medication is continued for about 1 year and a second-look procedure carried out. Stage-IIA and stage-IIB disease is handled in different institutions by a variety of regimens, including abdominal or pelvic irradiation with or without systemic chemotherapy. Stage-III disease also varies and may include pelvic and abdominal irradiation and/or chemotherapy. While single-agent therapy using an alkylating agent is the standard in some institutions, most centers now utilize multiple-agent chemotherapy utilizing an alkylating agent and cis-platinum.[56]

For the most part, long-term survival is related to the amount of cytoreduction that can be achieved but, generally, 5-year survival rates for stage-I epithelial ovarian cancer are about 70%. This falls to 25% for stage-II lesions, 12% for stage-III lesions, and 0% for stage-IV lesions.[56] A variety of therapies are available for recurrent disease, including multiple-agent chemotherapy. It is beyond the scope of this text to discuss these, but the role of such regimens in the management of recurrent disease must be taken in the context of time of survival and quality of life.

References

1. Cancer Statistics 1989. *CA* 1989;39:3–20.
2. Seidman H, Mushiski MH: Breast cancer: Incidence, mortality, survival and prognosis, in Feig SA, McLelland R (eds.): *Breast Carcinoma: Current Diagnosis and Treatment.* New York, Masson Publishing, 1983.
3. U.S. Department of Health and Human Services: Long-term oral contraceptive use and the risk of breast cancer. *JAMA* 1983;249:1591.
4. Droegemueller W: Breast diseases, in Droegemueller W, Herbst AL, Mishell DR, Stenchever MA (eds.): *Comprehensive Gynecology.* St. Louis, CV Mosby, 1987, p 339.
5. Foster RS, Constanza MC: Self breast examination practices in breast cancer survivals. *Cancer* 1984;53:999.
6. Droegemueller W: Breast diseases, in Droegemueller W, Herbst AL, Mishell DR, Stenchever MA (eds.): *Comprehensive Gynecology.* St. Louis, CV Mosby, 1987, p 341.
7. Shapiro S, Venet W, Strax T, et al: Selection followup and analyses in the Health Insurance Plan study: A randomized trial of breast cancer screening. *National Cancer Inst Monograph* 1985;67:65–74.
8. Seidman H, Gel VS, Silverberg E, LaVerda N, Lubera J: Survival experience in the breast cancer detection demonstration project. *Cancer* 1987;37:258–290.
9. Vorherr H: Breast aspiration biopsy. *Am J Obstet Gynecol* 1984;148:127.
10. Droegemueller W: Breast diseases, in Droegemueller W, Herbst AL, Mishell DR, Stenchever MA (eds.): *Comprehensive Gynecology.* St. Louis, CV Mosby, 1987, p 348.
11. DiSaia PJ, Creasman WT: *Clinical Gynecologic Oncology*, ed. 3. St. Louis, CV Mosby, 1989, p 485.
12. Sundaram GS, Manimekalai S, Wenk RE, et al: Estrogen and progesterone receptor assays in human breast cancer: A brief review of the relevant terms, methods, and clinical usefulness. *Obstet Gynecol Surv* 1984;39:719.
13. Droegemueller W: Breast diseases, in Droegemueller W, Herbst AL, Mishell DR, Stenchever MA (eds.): *Comprehensive Gynecology.* St. Louis, CV Mosby, 1987, p 353.
14. DiSaia PJ, Creasman WT: Invasive cancer of the vulva, in *Clinical Gynecological Oncology*, ed. 3. St. Louis, CV Mosby, 1989, p 241.
15. Rutledge F, Smith JP, Franklin EK: Carcinoma of the vulva. *Am J Obstet Gynecol* 1970;106:1117.
16. Krupp PJ, Bahm JW: Lymph gland metastases in invasive squamous cell cancer of the vulva. *Am J Obstet Gynecol* 1978;130:943.
17. Simonsen E: Invasive squamous cell carcinoma of the vulva. *Ann Surg Chir Gynaecol* 1984;73:331.
18. Homesley HD, Bundy BN, Sedlis A, Adcock L: A randomized study of radiation therapy versus pelvic node resection for patients with invasive squamous cell carcinoma of the vulva having positive groin nodes (A GOG Study Group). *Obstet Gynecol* 1986;68:733.
19. Nori D, et al: Radiation therapy of primary vaginal carcinoma. *Int J Radiat Oncol Biol Phys* 1983;9:1471.
20. Perez CA, Camel HM: Long-term follow-up in radiation therapy of carcinoma of the vagina. *Cancer* 1982;49:1308.
21. Benedet JL, et al: Primary invasive carcinoma of the vagina. *Obstet Gynecol* 1983;62:750.
22. Gallup DG, et al: Invasive squamous cell carcinoma of the vagina: A 14 year study. *Obstet Gynecol* 1987;69:783.

23. DiSaia PJ, Creasman WT: Invasive cervical cancer, in *Clinical Gynecologic Oncology*, ed. 3. St. Louis, CV Mosby, 1989, p 67.
24. Fletcher GH, Rutledge FN: Extended field technique in the management of cancers of the uterine cervix. *Am J Roentgenol* 1972;114:116.
25. Curry DDW: Operative treatment of carcinoma of the cervix. *J Obstet Gynecol Br Commonwealth* 1971;78:385.
26. Droegemueller W, Herbst AL, Mishell DR, Stenchever MA: *Comprehensive Gynecology*. St. Louis, CV Mosby, 1987, p 767.
27. DiSaia PJ, Creasman WT: *Clinical Gynecologic Oncology*, ed. 3. St. Louis, CV Mosby, 1989, p 67.
28. Droegemueller W, Herbst AL, Mishell DR, Stenchever MA: *Comprehensive Gynecology*. St. Louis, CV Mosby, 1987, p 800.
29. Ingram JM Jr, Novak E: Endometrial carcinoma associated with feminizing ovarian tumors. *Am J Obstet Gynecol* 1951;61:774.
30. Emge LA: Endometrial cancer in feminizing tumors of the ovary. *Obstet Gynecol* 1953;1:511.
31. Pettersson F (ed.): *Annual Report on the Results of Treatment in Gynecological Cancer*, vol 19. Stockholm, FIGO, 1985.
32. Creasman WT, Morrow CP, Bundy L: Surgical pathological spread patterns of endometrial cancer. *Cancer* 1987;60:2035.
33. Creasman WT, Rutledge FN: The prognostic value of peritoneal cytology in gynecologic malignant disease. *Am J Obstet Gynecol* 1971;110:773.
34. Creasman WT, et al: Adenocarcinoma of the endometrium in metastatic lymph node potential: A preliminary report. *Gynecol Oncol* 1976;4:239.
35. Eokhman JV: Two pathogenic types of endometrial carcinoma. *Gynecol Oncol* 1983;15:10.
36. Jones HW: Treatment of adenocarcinoma of the endometrium. *Obstet Gynecol Surv* 1975;30:147.
37. Creasman WT, et al: Adenocarcinoma of the endometrium—Its metastatic lymph node potential: A preliminary report. *Gynecol Oncol* 1976;4:239.
38. Morrow CP, DiSaia PJ, Townsend DE: Current management of endometrial carcinoma. *Obstet Gynecol* 1973;42:399.
39. Boronow RC, et al: Surgical staging of endometrial cancer: Clinical pathological findings of a prospective study. *Obstet Gynecol* 1985;63:825.
40. DiSaia PJ, Creasman WT: *Clinical Gynecologic Oncology*, ed. 3. St. Louis, CV Mosby, 1989, p 161.
41. Ehrlich CE, Young PCM, Cleary RE: Cytoplasmic progesterone and estradiol receptors in normal hyperplastic and carcinomatous endometria: Therapeutic implications. *Am J Obstet Gynecol* 1981;141:539.
42. Benraad TJ, et al: Do estrogen (ER) and progesterone (PR) receptors in metastasizing endometrial cancer predict the response to progestin therapy? *Acta Obstet Gynecol Scand* 1980;59:155.
43. Creasman WT, McCarty KS Sr, McCarty KS Jr: Clinical correlation of estrogen progesterone binding proteins in human endometrial adenocarcinoma. *Obstet Gynecol* 1980;55:363.
44. Martin PM, et al: Estrogen and progesterone receptors in normal and neoplastic endometrium: Correlations between receptors, cytopathologic examination and clinical response under progesterone therapy. *Int J Cancer* 1979;23:321.
45. Kauppila A, et al: Treatment of advanced endometrial adenocarcinoma with combined cytoxin therapy. *Cancer* 1980;46:2162.
46. Pollow K, Manz B, Grill JH: Estrogen progesterone receptors, in Jasonni VM (ed.): *Steroids and Endometrial Cancer*. New York, Raven Press, 1983.
47. Quinn MA, Kouchi M, Fortune V: Endometrial carcinoma steroid receptors in response to medroxyprogesterone acetate. *Gynecol Oncol* 1985;21:314.

48. DiSaia PJ, Creasman WT: *Clinical Gynecologic Oncology*, ed. 3. St. Louis, CV Mosby, 1989, p 450.
49. Roberts JA, Lifshitz S: Primary adenocarcinoma of the fallopian tube. *Gynecol Oncol* 1982;13:301.
50. Bennington JL, Ferguson BR, Haber SL: Incidence and relative frequency of benign and malignant ovarian neoplasms. *Obstet Gynecol* 1968;32:627.
51. Hernandez E, Miyazeawa K: The pelvic mass: Patient's ages and pathologic findings. *J Reprod Med* 1988;33:361.
52. Newhouse ML, et al: Case control study of carcinoma of the ovaries. *Br J Prevent Soc Med* 1977;31:148.
53. Rosenburg L, et al: Epithelial ovarian cancer and combination oral contraceptives. *JAMA* 1982;247:3210.
54. Knapp RC, Friedman EA. Aortic lymph node metastases in early ovarian cancer. *Am J Obstet Gynecol* 1974;119:1013.
55. Piver MS, Barlow JJ, Lele SB: Incidence of subclinical metastases in Stage I and II ovarian carcinoma. *Obstet Gynecol* 1978;52:100.
56. DiSaia PJ, Creasman WT: *Clinical Gynecologic Oncology*, ed. 3. St. Louis, CV Mosby, 1989, p 325.

Chapter **12**

Hormone Replacement

Morton Stenchever, MD

Although the aging process is a continuum throughout life, a major event for women is menopause. Through the centuries this has been noted to occur on an average at about age 50. Some variations have been noted, primarily associated with nutrition, with malnourished women achieving menopause at a somewhat earlier age than well-nourished women. The only specific correlates to earlier menopause seem to relate to living at high altitude and heavy smoking.[1]

Menopause is a physiologic condition that is best described as a failure of the ovarian follicle to develop, mature, and produce estrogen. The actual reason for this is unknown but could be related to changes related to aging in the brain, hypothalamus, and pituitary gland. It does not seem to be influenced by a history of hypothalamic amenorrhea, pregnancy, or suppression of ovulation by such means as birth-control pills. It may be related to the decreasing number of ova that are present in the aging ovary. It has been demonstrated that after the age of 40, as many as 30% to 50% of menstrual cycles are abnormal when basal body temperature records are evaluated. This and the findings of several investigators that fertility declines after age 35 support the fact that ovarian function diminishes over a period of time. Dysfunctional uterine bleeding, therefore, becomes more common as women approach the perimenopausal period. Mean estrogen values become drastically reduced after menopause as do values of androstenedione and testosterone. Estrone levels remain similar to premenopausal levels because of the conversion of androstenedione to estrone by aromatase, an enzyme present in several body tissues, predominantly adipose tissue, muscle, and bone marrow. Although androstenedione production is less in postmenopausal women than it is in premenopausal women, the conversion of this substance to estrone is increased. The adrenal glands contribute about one half of the plasma testosterone and two thirds of the plasma androstenedione in circulation. The conversion is more efficient in women with large amounts of adipose tissue than in thin women. This site of aromatization in adipose tissue has been localized to stroma and vascular cells rather than adipose cells themselves. Conversion is often not affected by sudden weight loss.[2]

Follicular stimulating hormone (FSH) and luteinizing hormone (LH) are elevated after menopause and remain elevated into old age. LH may decrease somewhat with advancing age but the pulsatile release of gonadotropins persists after menopause. Gonadotropin concentrations seem related to nutritional status in aging women, and may be found to be reduced with chronic illness or weight loss.[2]

Effects of Estrogen Withdrawal on the Organ Systems

Figure 12.1 attempts to relate the pathological changes in the various organ systems brought about by estrogen withdrawal over a time frame measured in years. Since estrogen supports a number of organ systems in one way or another, withdrawal leads to symptoms and pathology directly related to the affect of its withdrawal on each of these systems. Table 12.1 summarizes these findings. While estrogen replacement at any time may alleviate or at least modulate many of these symptoms or changes, several may be irreversible. The effects of estrogen withdrawal on bone (osteoporosis) and on the cardiovascular system (arteriosclerotic heart disease) are the most obvious examples of the latter circumstance. Estrogen replacement will have its maximum effect if started shortly after menopause.

Vasomotor Instability

Vasomotor instability is noted with the withdrawal of estrogen at the time of natural menopause or castration and is manifested by peripheral vasodilation and hot flushes. Peripheral vasodilation may be measured by noting augmented digital profusion of fingers and indirectly by measuring peripheral temperature. While peripheral temperature rises in relation to the hot flush, central core temperature, as measured by probes in the esophagus or on the tympanic membrane of the ear, demonstrates no elevation—and indeed a slight decrease in body temperature shortly after the flush begins. Generally, augmented digital perfusion can be measured as occurring about 1.5 minutes before the hot flushes are appreciated and a decrease in core temperature approximately 4 minutes after the flush begins. Some patients complain of chills at that point in time.[3]

Hot flushes are more likely to occur in women immediately after the loss of estrogen than in older women who have been through menopause for a long period of time. Interestingly, they do not occur in women who have had gonadal failure and have not been replaced with estrogen but may occur in women who have been replaced and then have undergone estrogen withdrawal (ie, women with Turner's syndrome). Hot flushes will be a complaint of 50% to 75% of women who undergo physiologic or surgical menopause and 85% will suffer from these problems for more than 1 year, while one fourth to one half will experience the symptoms for more than 5 years. Hot flushes may occur at any time but are more frequent during the night, often awaking the patient. They are often accompanied by palpitation, and heart rate increase of as much as 15% may be noted.[4-9]

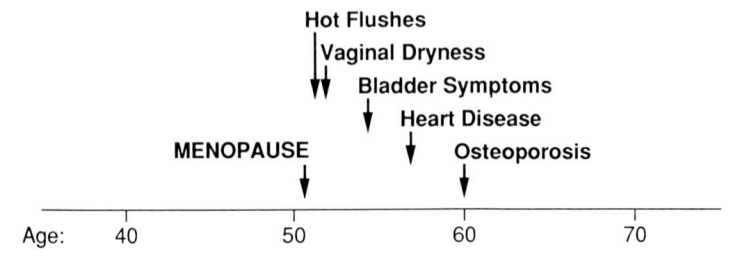

Figure 12.1 Pathologic changes in various organ systems due to estrogen withdrawal measured in years.

Table 12.1 Organs and Organ System Effects of Estrogen Withdrawal

Organ or organ system	Symptoms
Vasomotor	Hot flushes, night sweats, nervousness, headaches, insomnia
Vulva and vagina	Dryness, pruritus, atrophy, dyspareunia
Urinary tract	Frequency, urgency, dribbling, bladder dysfunction, incontinence
Uterus and pelvic supports	Atrophy, prolapse
Breasts	Atrophy, drooping
Cardiovascular	Angina, arteriosclerotic heart disease
Skeleton	Osteoporosis, pain, fracture
Skin and mucus membranes	Pruritus, dryness, loss of subcutaneous tissue, minor hirsutism, voice changes, dry mouth

Measurable physiologic changes involving temperature and vasodilation can be seen in all menopausal women, although not all experience hot flushes. The specific reason for this is unknown but may be influenced in part by secretions from the adrenal gland, specifically epinephrine, and thus may be related to the degree of patient sensitivity to psychic and emotional stimuli. Significant increases in plasma epinephrine and decreases in norepinephrine were described as accompanying hot flushes by Casper et al in carefully timed studies.[10]

Whatever the etiology, relief can often be obtained with very small doses of estrogen replacement. Clonidine in minimal doses of 0.1 to 0.2 mg per day has also been noted to reduce hot flush occurrence in as much as 46% over placebo.[11]

Vaginal Changes

The vaginal epithelium and indeed the vascular supply to it are sensitive to estrogen. Withdrawal will lead to a thinning of vaginal epithelium, decrease in blood supply with subsequent decrease in normal secretions of the vagina, and loss of vaginal rugae. In addition, the upper third of the vagina will retract and shorten, leading to a shorter vagina overall. Vaginal pH increases allowing for change in vaginal flora and senile vaginitis may occur. The patient often complains of dryness of the vagina and dyspareunia. As time goes on the supports of the uterus, vagina, bladder, and rectum become weakened because of the lack of estrogen, elasticity of tissues is diminished, and a relaxation of these organs can take place leading to cystocele, rectocele, or uterine and vaginal prolapse. These changes occur relatively rapidly after the cessation of menses. Vaginal pH change and thinning of the epithelium is quite rapid. Further symptomatology may be noted in the first few months after menses cease but may require up to 5 years to become a clinical problem. These changes can be reversed by estrogen therapy but not by other means.[12]

Urologic Changes

As with the vagina, the epithelium of the urethra, the tone of the urethral sphincter, and the vascular supply of the urethra and bladder are sensitive to estrogen. With estrogen withdrawal, urethral epithelium thins, vascular supply decreases, and α receptors in the urethral musculature decrease. These changes lead to decrease in urethral closing pressure and eventually may contribute to incontinence. At the very least, postmenopausal women often complain of difficulty in completely emptying the bladder and dribbling. This may be made worse by the development of a cystocele as bladder and vaginal supports relax. If the bladderneck loses its firm attachment to the pubic symphysis, stress incontinence may occur. Symptoms related to menopausal changes occurring in the urinary tract may occur at any time after cessation of menses but frequently occur within the first 5 years. The severity may increase as time goes on. Estrogen-replacement therapy will increase the number of α receptors, improve the epithelium of the urethra, improve the blood supply to the urethra and bladder, and help the supports of the bladder and the bladderneck.[13]

Cardiovascular Disease

Cardiovascular disease is one of the major causes of death in the United States. Premenopausal women seem to be at much less of a risk than men of comparable ages when death rates from coronary artery disease are compared by decade. This protection disappears rapidly, and by age 65 the two sexes are at about equal risk. For instance, in 1979 the death rate due to coronary artery disease and stroke for men between the ages of 45 and 49 was 160.6 per 100,000 as compared to 34.8 per 100,000 for women. At age 55 through 59, the rate was 468.1 for men to 131.9 for women. By age 65 they were about equal.[14] Most of the data points to the fact that menopause, whether natural or surgically induced, in some way has an effect on increasing the risk of coronary artery disease in women. Increased risk may be related partly to biochemical changes, particularly those related to serum lipids; however, most authorities do not feel that this reason explains the magnitude of the change seen.[15] It is logical to ask whether or not estrogen replacement allows for a degree of protection from coronary artery disease in women. Data from the Framingham study indicate that at menopause there is an elevation in high-density lipoprotein, low-density lipoprotein, and very-low-density lipoprotein (HDL, LDL, and VLDL). Studies in women who had undergone menopause because of oophorectomy demonstrated an elevation in serum cholesterol and phospholipids, primarily involving LDL but not HDL.[16] Not all studies have demonstrated these specific findings.[17] With estrogen therapy LDL is reduced and HDL seems to be increased.

Although a number of case-control studies have been carried out, which seem to show that estrogen replacement reduces the risk of cardiovascular disease in users, confounding factors such as hypertension, diabetes, and smoking have made it difficult to clearly compute potential benefits. In a recent study by Henderson et al,[18] evaluating users and nonusers of estrogen in a retirement community of predominately middle-class white women, there was a reported reduction in all cause mortality rates and in mortality rates for acute myocardial infarction among estrogen-replacement users when compared to never-users. These authors corrected for previous myocardial infarction, previous hypertension, and smoking, and in each instance showed an improvement. On the other hand, evidence from the Framingham study seems to demonstrate a more than 50% elevation of risk of cardiovascular morbidity and a twofold risk for cerebral vascular disease in users over nonusers. However, when correcting for smoking, the increased rates of myocardial infarction reached statistical significance only for smokers, whereas nonsmokers reached a statistically significant difference for stroke in estrogen-users as compared to nonestrogen-users. In most studies smoking was a confounding issue that, when corrected for, removed all or most of the risk implied.[19]

Osteoporosis

The aging process with respect to the skeletal system begins in the fourth and fifth decades in women and continues throughout life. At the time of menopause, however, there is a rapid acceleration and by age 60 as many as 50% of women will have reached a decrease in bone mass that makes fracture, at least theoretically, possible. If there are questions about whether or not estrogen-replacement therapy decreases the risk of coronary artery disease, there is little doubt that it significantly modulates the development of osteoporosis.

While 85% of all hip fractures occur in women and the incidence rises from 9 per 100,000 person years for women between the ages of 35 and 44 to 3317 per 100,000 person years for women ages 85 and over, there is good evidence that this increase can be greatly modulated if not removed with estrogen-replacement therapy.[20–22] Figure 12.2 reveals the difference in bone density be-

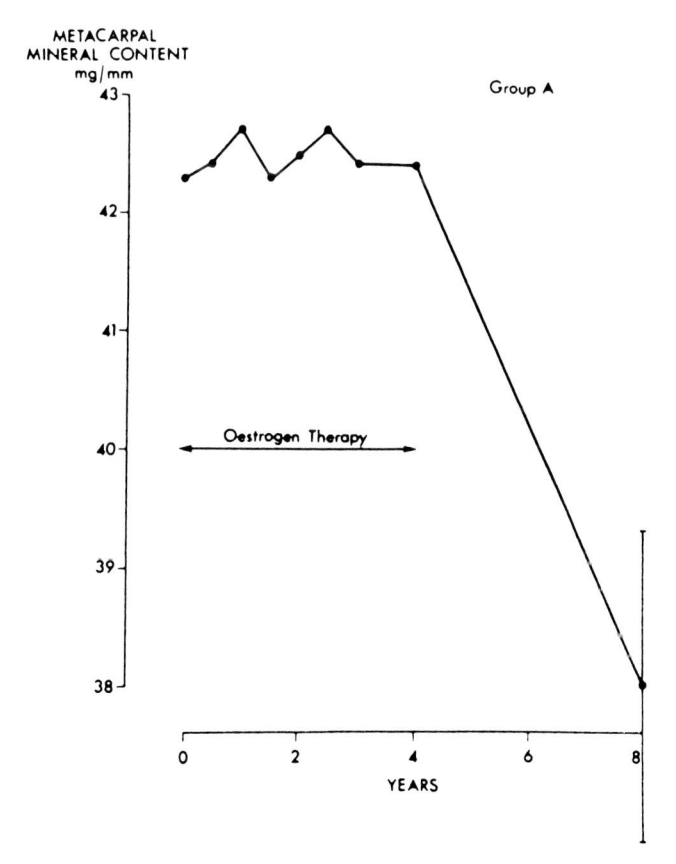

Figure 12.2 Bone loss after removal of estrogen treatment. Patients had been treated with 25 μg mestranol daily for 4 years. Therapy was discontinued after bone loss ensued at a rate equivalent to that observed in the immediate postmenopausal or postoophorectomy period. (From Mishell DR Jr: *Menopause: Physiology and Pharmacology*. Chicago, Year Book Medical Publishers, 1987, p 83.)

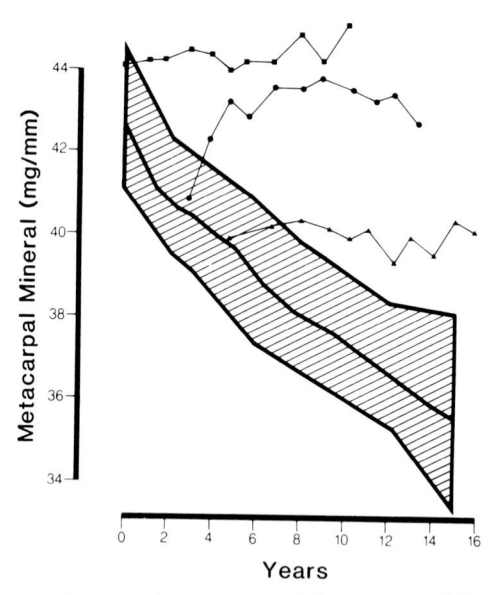

Figure 12.3 Metacarpal content in women receiving mestranol (24µg/day) or placebo. (From Mishell DR Jr: *Menopause: Physiology and Pharmacology*. Chicago, Year Book Medical Publishers, 1987, p 171.)

tween two groups of patients treated with estrogen replacement and placebo, respectively, after bilateral oophorectomy. Figure 12.3 indicates the decrease in metacarpal mineral content in a group of patients first treated for 4 years in whom treatment was then discontinued. A number of other studies have been performed, which demonstrate bone mineral loss accelerates with menopause or with bilateral oophorectomy and is halted and even reversed with estrogen therapy.

A recent study from Great Britain, which followed bone density using dual-photon absorptiometry in 284 healthy female volunteers between the ages of 21 and 68, demonstrated the peak adult bone density was obtained shortly after the end of linear skeletal growth. From then on there was a decline in density of proximal femur over time, but with a major fall in all bone density after menopause. Generalized risk factors in this study were low body weight, alcohol and cigarette consumption, nulliparity, lack of previous use of oral contraceptives, and lack of regular exercise. None of these factors could satisfactorily predict which women were at risk for osteoporosis.[23] Other risk factors for developing osteoporosis relate to: Caucasian and Asian race; positive family history; slight build; lifelong low-calcium intake; high protein, caffeine, sodium, and phosphate intake history; and low vitamin D intake history.

Although the exact action of estrogen on the skeletal system is unknown, it does seem to be involved with the control of calcium metabolism via the parathyroid hormone, calcitonin, and the vitamin D system. A popular theory until recently was that estrogen increased plasma calcitonin, thereby inhibiting osteoclast activity and reducing the amount of bone resorption occurring. Recent work by Hurley et al could demonstrate no stimulatory effect on calcitonin secretion by estrogen, suggesting that the beneficial actions of estrogen on preventing bone reabsorption were not mediated, at least directly, through the calcitonin pathway.[24]

Even though the specific effects of estrogen in preventing osteoporosis are still not clear, there is little question that estrogen replacement slows the process of osteoporosis in women who are postmenopausal. Also, in women in whom estrogen replacement had not been given until the process of demineralization was under way, this process could be reversed at least in part.

Problems Related to Estrogen-Replacement Therapy

Cancer

Women and their physicians alike fear that there may be a relationship between the development of cancers of the breast or female reproductive tract and the use of replacement estrogen. To date, there is no epidemiologic data to support a relationship between estrogen use and cancer of the vulva, vagina, cervix, ovary, or fallopian tube.

The question of whether or not the risk of breast cancer is increased in users of replacement estrogen has not yet been clearly answered. The majority of studies do not demonstrate an increase in relative risk for such women. However, in a few studies, long-term use seems to have been associated with increased relative risk of between 1.3 and 2.[25-29] Several authors have suggested that there may be subgroups of women who are more susceptible to the carcinogenic effects of estrogen, if such be the case, than others. However, epidemiological literature in this respect is confusing and contradictory. Several models have been constructed using epidemiologic data which imply that the risk of breast cancer may be increased in a direct relationship to dose of estrogen used and duration of use. Henderson et al point out that when these models are used, long-term users of estrogen may increase their risk of cancer over a period of ages 50 to 80 years by as much as 7% to 9.5% but quickly point out that these risks must be balanced against the benefits of estrogen replacement on other organ systems.[30]

Adenocarcinoma of the endometrium is an entirely different problem. While rates for endometrial cancer in the United States remained unchanged between 1930 and 1970,[31] shortly thereafter a number of studies demonstrated a sharp increase in incidence. One such study by Weiss et al[32] from Washington State paralleled this increase with the use of exogenous estrogen-replacement therapy with an increased relative risk for long-time users of 8.2. Several other studies performed between the mid-1970s and the mid-1980s reported similar findings.[33-35] It has since been shown that these risks can be reduced to close to 1 by adding progesterone to the replacement regimen.[36] For the most part, the endometrial cancer that was produced secondary to estrogen replacement was a well-differentiated adenocarcinoma of low grade (grade 1), which was generally discovered in an early stage (stage 1) and easily treatable. Minimum effects were noted on mortality rates secondary to the disease. While Gambrell demonstrated that the incidence of endometrial cancer in women using estrogen alone was 359 per 100,000 women years compared with 248 per 100,000 in women not receiving estrogen,[37] Nachtigall showed no increased risk in 84 matched pairs of women in New York City in whom the controls used no hormones and the study subjects used both estrogen and progesterone therapy in a cyclic manner.[38] Likewise, 72 women treated by Hammond with estrogen and progesterone were found to develop no endometrial cancer.[39]

Carbohydrate Metabolism

Although carbohydrate metabolism has been known to be altered somewhat, in some studies, by estrogen and progesterone, a perspective study by Nachtigall et al in both normal and diabetic menopausal women, who were treated with estrogen and progesterone replacement, could demonstrate no adverse effects on carbohydrate metabolism.[38]

Cholecystitis and Cholelithiasis

It has been suggested that the use of birth-control pills and replacement estrogen increases the incidence of gallstones and cholecystitis. Since estrogen replacement affects hepatic lipid metabolism, and because small increases in bile saturation of cholesterol which may occur with estrogen replacement may lead to an increase in gallstones, the risk is certainly there. Nachtingall et al, in their prospective study over 10 years, discovered a higher, although statistically non-significant, incidence of cholelithiasis in the estrogen-treated group when compared to the controls. Four of the 84 women in the patient group and two in the control group actually had cholelithiasis. Although there may be an increased risk, the risk is probably a small one.[38]

Thromboembolic Disease

Estrogen exerts several effects on the clotting mechanism, both because of its effect on hepatic function and by a direct effect on the clotting factors. A number of clotting factors are increased with estrogen administration, including VII, IX, X, and X complex. While some more potent estrogens will reduce antithrombin III, usual estrogen-replacement doses do not have such an effect. Thus, whereas oral contraceptives are related epidemiologically to an increased risk of thromboembolic disease, this has not been noted with the usual doses of estrogen used in estrogen-replacement therapy.[40,41]

Treatment Philosophy

Estrogen Therapy

There is little doubt that the most effective pharmacologic agent for treating the symptoms and problems of menopause is estrogen. Estrogen can be administered using a number of different compounds, both synthetic and naturally occurring, and by a variety of routes of administration, including oral, sublingual, nasal, vaginal, transdermal, subcutaneous, and intramuscular. Table 12.2 lists the commonly used estrogens, both naturally occurring and synthetic. Basically, synthetic estrogens (including ethinyl estradiol, its C-3 methylated derivative mestranol, its cyclophenyl ether quinestrol, and its stilbene derivative diethylstilbestrol) are examples of such substances. In general, the synthetic estro-

Table 12.2 Commonly Used Estrogen Compounds*

Natural and equine estrogens
   Estrones
      Conjugated equine estrogens
      Piperazine estrone sulfate
   Estradiols
      Micronized estradiol
      Estradiol valerate
Synthetic estrogens
   17α-ethinyl estrogens
   17α-ethinyl estradiol
   17α-ethinyl estradiol-3-methyl ether (mestranol)
   Stilbene derivatives
      Diethylstilbestrol

* See Ref. 42.

gens are more potent than the naturally occurring estrogens in such areas as increasing the production of hepatic globulins, sex hormone binding globulins, and substrait corticosteroid binding globulin and thyroid binding globulin. They are also far more potent in reducing FSH levels, since their effect is many-fold higher than that of the natural occurring estrogens, and lowering the dose or changing the route of administration does not seem to alter these factors.

Naturally occurring estrogens are most often administered orally, although there are vaginal, subdermal, and transdermal preparations available and in common use. Perhaps the most commonly used naturally occurring estrogens are the conjugated equine estrogens. After ingestion of a typical 0.625 mg dose of conjugated equine estrogen, serum levels of estradiol will be about 30 to 40 pg/mL and of estrone 150 to 250 pg/mL in approximately 4 to 6 hours. Significant levels will remain present for 24 hours and will not fall off until 48 hours. Similarly, vaginal application of 1.25 mg of conjugated estrogen will yield peak serum levels of 25 pg/mL estradiol and 120 pg/mL estrone. Transdermal estradiol given in a 50 μg patch will yield serum levels of estradiol of 60 pg/mL and 50 pg/mL of estrone. One favorable aspect of the effect oral conjugated estrogen on hepatic globulins is the fact that it stimulates an increase in high-density lipoprotein cholesterol (HDL) which is not a constant finding in the transdermal delivery system.[42]

Of importance is the fact that naturally occurring estrogens in the appropriate pharmacological doses, such as described here for conjugated estrogen and transdermal estradiol, are effective in reducing postmenopausal symptoms; and, since they produce estrogen levels similar to that of the early follicular phase, they are responsible for normalizing the calcium–creatinine ratio to premenopausal levels.[42]

The cyclic or continuous use of estrogen by itself to treat postmenopausal symptoms will increase the occurrence of hyperplasia of the endometrium to 3.7 per 100 women months for continuous therapy and 4.5 per 100 women months with cyclic therapy. This was noted when the dose of conjugated estrogen was 0.625 mg daily.[43] That progesterone modulates this hyperplastic effect was seen in a prospective study which histologically sampled the endometria of women treated with unopposed estrogen for 2 years. In this series, the incidence of endometrial hyperplasia was 18% to 32%, with up to one third of the hyperplasias being atypical. When progesterone was added for 7 days each cycle, the incidence dropped to 3% to 4%.[44,45] Studd et al demonstrated that continuing progesterone administration for 10 days decreased the incidence to 2%, and with progesterone therapy of 12 to 13 days, reduced the incidence of hyperplasia to 0. In addition, Gambrell has shown that not only is the endometrial carcinoma risk lower in women using estrogen and progesterone versus women using estrogen alone to combat postmenopausal symptoms, but also that the rate of endometrial cancer occurrence is actually lower than it is in the general population of women not on combined therapy.[46]

Although a number of progestins are available for use in counteracting the hyperplastic effects of estrogen on the endometrium, Whitehead et al have recently suggested that norethindrone (1 mg/day for 12 days/cycle) or medroxyprogesterone acetate (10 mg/day for 12 days) appear to cause minimal lipid disturbance and do not oppose the beneficial effects of estrogen in preventing osteoporosis.[47] Alternately, 300 mg/day of oral progesterone has also been seen to be effective.

Progestogens

Progestogens have been shown to relieve both vasomotor symptoms and to correct urinary calcium–creatinine ratios. Therefore, some authors believe that progesterone-alone therapy can be used to successfully treat menopausal symptoms and prevent osteoporosis. Lobo et al have demonstrated this to be the case using depo-medroxyprogesterone acetate in a dose of 150 mg every 3 months. From their experiences, this was as effective as the use of conjugated equine estrogen in a dose of 0.625 mg/day.[48,49] Symptomatic relief has been noted with other progestins in varying dosage schedules, making this means of therapy appropriate for women with contraindications to estrogen therapy.

Cyclic Versus Continuous Estrogen and Progesterone Therapy

A number of regimens for delivering estrogen and progesterone in postmenopausal women have been suggested (Figure 12.4). Most of those in common use are effective in preventing menopausal symptoms and reducing the risk of osteoporosis and other complicating features of menopause. Two common protocols in use today are: conjugated equine estrogen 0.625 mg for 25 days with medroxyprogesterone acetate 10 mg per day during the last 10 to 14 days and transdermal estriol 0.050 µg applied in patch form every 3 days with 10 mg medroxyprogesterone acetate given for 10 to 14 days each month. Other regimens using different estrogens and progesterones work equally as well. Recently, continuous estrogen and progesterone therapy has been tried in order to overcome withdrawal bleeding found to be distasteful by many patients, especially the more elderly ones. These regimens, for the most part, yield an atrophic type of endometrium and, therefore, breakthrough bleeding is a rare phenomenon. An example of such a regimen would be conjugated equine estrogen 0.625 mg plus 2.5 or 5 mg of medroxyprogesterone acetate daily. Alternatively, this may be given on weekdays only. Trials of conjugated equine estrogen using doses of norethindrone 0.35 to 2.1 mg daily have also been found to be effective.

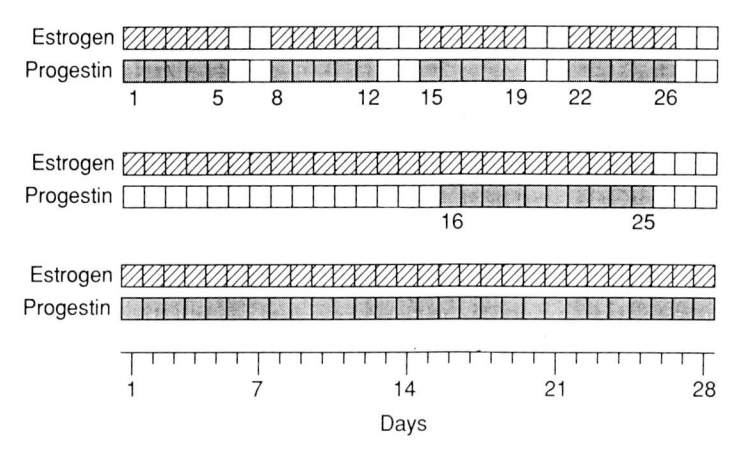

Figure 12.4 A number of different estrogen and progesterone regimens in use for the treatment of postmenopausal women.

Other Therapies

In patients who cannot be given or cannot tolerate estrogen and/or progesterone, there are a few other therapies which may be tried. One of these is clonidine, a centrally acting α-adrenergic agonist/antagonist. There is some evidence that in doses of 0.1 to 0.2 mg bid that some relief of hot flushes can be obtained. However, its effectiveness is not as much as that seen with estrogen and progesterone, and patients who were normotensive often complained of dizziness due to lowering of blood pressure.

A second alternative medication is bellergal. This drug is a combination of ergotamine tartrate, belladonna, and phenobarbital. Most patients will report some relief on this compound, and when compared to a placebo it seemed to be more effective. Symptoms of nervousness, palpitations, nausea, insomnia, dizziness, and irritability were often relieved. The physician must consider whether or not the patient should be exposed to ergotrate, belladonna, and phenobarbital for a prolonged period of time. The drug is contraindicated because of the presence of ergotrate in such conditions as coronary artery disease and hypertension, and because of belladonna in glaucoma.

Contraindications to Estrogen Therapy

There are a number of contraindications to estrogen therapy, and these relate to the specific effect of estrogen on various disease states. (Table 12.3 lists these.)

With the advent of low-dose estrogen-replacement therapy, some of the contraindications may be waived at the discretion of the physician. One such example might be seen in an individual with carcinoma of the breast who was found to have negative lymph nodes, and who is now many years posttherapy without evidence of disease. Another would be a patient with a history of traumatic thrombophlebitis not related to hormonal change (ie, pregnancy, use of birth-control pills, etc.). In such situations, the physician will need to decide

Table 12.3 Contraindications to Estrogen Therapy

Absolute contraindications
    Previous or suspected carcinoma of the breast
    Previous or suspected carcinoma of the endometrium
    Acute liver disease
    Acute thrombophlebitis or thromboembolic disorder
Relative contraindication
    Other types of liver disease
    Large leiomyoma
    Endometriosis
    History of estrogen-related thromboembolism or thrombophlebitis

whether or not the benefits that the patient may derive from the use of hormone replacement outweight the small potential risk of using these agents.

References

1. Weg RB: Demography, in Mishell DR (ed.): *Menopause: Physiology and Pharmacology.* Chicago, Yearbook Medical Publishers, 1987, pp 23–40.
2. Sherman BM: Endocrinologic and menstrual alterations, in Mishell DR (ed.): *Menopause: Physiology and Pharmacology.* Chicago, Yearbook Medical Publishers, 1987, pp 41–51.
3. Mashchak CA, Kletzky OA, Artal R, et al: The relations of physiologic change to subjective symptoms in postmenopausal women with and without hot flushes. *Maturitas* 1985;6:301–308.
4. Neucarten DL, Kriner RG: Menopausal symptoms in women of various ages. *Psychosom Med* 1965;27:26–27.
5. Bar W: Problems related to postmenopausal women. *S Afr Med J* 1975;498:437–439.
6. Thompson B, Heart SA, Durno D: Menopausal age and symptomatology in general practice. *J Biol Sci* 1973;5:71–82.
7. Jaszmann L, VanLith ND, Zaat WCA: The perimenopausal symptoms. *Med Gynecol Soc* 1969;4:268–276.
8. Molnar GW: Body temperature during menopausal hot flushes. *J Appl Physiol* 1975;38:499–503.
9. Sturdee DW, Wilson KA, Pipili E, et al: Physiological aspects of menopausal hot flushes. *Br Med J* 1978;2:79–80.
10. Kasper RF, Yen SSC, Wilkes MM: Menopausal flushes: A neuroendocrine link with pulsatile LH secretions. *Science* 1979;205:823–825.
11. Laufer LR, Erlik Y, Meldrum DR, Judd HL: Effective clonidine on hot flushes in postmenopausal women. *Obstet Gynecol* 1982;60:583.
12. Bergman A, Brenner PF: Alterations in urogenital system, in Mishell DR (ed.): *Menopause: Physiology and Pharmacology.* Chicago, Yearbook Medical Publishers, 1987, pp 67–75.
13. Stenchever MA: Gynecologic urology, in Droegemueller W, Herbst AL, Mishell DR, Stenchever MA (eds.): *Comprehensive Gynecology.* St. Louis, CV Mosby, 1987, pp 538–566.
14. Johansson S, Vedin A, Wilhelmsson C: Myocardial infarction in women. *Epidemiol Rev* 1983;5:67–95.
15. Kannel WB, Gordon T: Cardiovascular effects of the menopause, in Mishell DR (ed.): *Menopause: Physiology and Pharmacology.* Chicago: Yearbook Medical Publishers, 1987, pp 91–102.

16. Kannel WB, Hjortland MC, McNamara PM, et al: Menopause and risk of cardiovascular disease: The Framingham study. *Ann Intern Med* 1976;85:447–452.
17. Robinson RW, Higano N, Cohen WD: Increased incidence of coronary heart disease in women castrated prior to menopause. *Arch Intern Med* 1959;104:908–913.
18. Henderson BE, Ross RK, Paganini-Hill A, Mack TM: Estrogen use and cardiovascular disease. *Am J Obstet Gynecol* 1986;154:1181–1186.
19. Wilson PWF, Garrison RJ, Castelli WP: Postmenopausal estrogen use, cigarette smoking, and cardiovascular morbidity in women over 50: The Framingham study. *N Engl J Med* 1985;313:1038–1043.
20. Melton LJ III, Riggs BL: Epidemiology of age related fractures, in Avioli LV (ed.): *The Osteoporotic Syndrome*. New York, Grune & Stratton, 1983, p 54.
21. Gotfredsen A, Riis BJ, Christiansen C: The total and local bone mineral during estrogen treatment: A placebo controlled trial. *Bone Mineral* 1986;1:167–173.
22. Lindsay R, Tohme JF: Alterations in skeletal homeostatis with age and menopause, in Mishell DR (ed.): *Menopause: Physiology and Pharmacology*. Chicago, Yearbook Medical Publishers, 1987, pp 77–90.
23. Stevenson JC, Lees B, Davenport M, et al: Determinance of bone density in normal women: Risk factors for future osteoporosis. *Br Med J* 1989;298:924–928.
24. Hurley DL, Tiegs RD, Barta J, et al: Effects of oral contraceptives in estrogen and menstruation on calcium, calcitonin in pre- and postmenopausal women. *J Bone Miner Res* 1989;4:89–95.
25. Hoover R, Gray L, Cole P, et al: Menopausal estrogens and breast cancer. *N Engl J Med* 1976;295:401.
26. Ross RK, Paganini-Hill A, Gerkins VR, et al: A case controlled study of menopausal estrogen therapy and breast cancer. *JAMA* 1980;243:1635.
27. Briton LA, Hoover RN, Szklow M, et al: Menopausal estrogen use and risk of breast cancer. *Cancer* 1981;47:2517.
28. Hoover R, Glass A, Finkel WD, et al: Conjugated estrogens and breast cancer risk. *J Natl Cancer Inst* 1981;67:812.
29. Hiatt RA, Bawol R, Friedman GD, et al: Exogenous estrogens in breast cancer after oophorectomy. *Cancer* 1984;54:139.
30. Henderson BE, Ross RK, Pike MC: Breast neoplasia, in Mishell DR (ed.): *Menopause: Physiology and Pharmacology*. Chicago, Yearbook Medical Publishers, 1987, pp 261–274.
31. Cramer DW, Cutler SJ, Christine B: Trends in the incidence of endometrial cancer in the United States. *Gynecol Oncol* 1974;2:130.
32. Weiss NS, Szekely DR, English DR, Schweid Al: Endometrial cancer in relation to patterns in menopausal estrogen use. *JAMA* 1979;242:261–264.
33. Horwitz RI, Feinstein AR, Horwitz SM, et al: Necropsy diagnosis of endometrial cancer in detection bias in case control studies. *Lancet* 1981;2:66.
34. Gray LA Jr, Christopherson WM, Hoover R: Estrogens in endometrial cancer. *Obstet Gynecol* 1977;49:385.
35. Antunes CMF, Stolley PD, Rosenshein MB, et al: Endometrial cancer and estrogen use: Report of a large case control study. *N Engl J Med* 1979;300:9.
36. Gambrell RD Jr, Bagnell CA, Greenblatt RB: The role of estrogen and progesterone in the etiology and prevention of endometrial cancer: Review. *Am J Obstet Gynecol* 983;146:696–707.
37. Gambrell RD Jr, Massey FW, Castaneda TA, et al: Use of progestin challenge test to reduce the risk of endometrial cancer. *Obstet Gynecol* 1980;55:732.
38. Nachtigall LE, Nachtigall RH, Nachtigall RD, Beckman EM: Estrogen replacement therapy: II. Prospective study in the relationship of carcinoma and cardiovascular and metabolic problems. *Obstet Gynecol* 1979;54:74–79.
39. Hammond CB, Jelovsek FR, Lee KL, et al: Effective long-term estrogen replacement therapy: II. Neoplasia. *Am J Obstet Gynecol* 1979;133:537.

40. VonKaulla E, Droegemueller W, VonKaulla KN: Conjugated oestrogens and hypercoagulability. *Am J Obstet Gynecol* 1975;122:688.
41. Bonnar J, Haddon M, Hunter DH, et al: Coagulation system changes in postmenopausal women receiving oestrogen preparations. *Postgrad Med J* 1976;52(Supp 6):30.
42. Barnes RB, Lobo RA: Pharmacology of estrogens, in Mishell DR (ed.): *Menopause: Physiology and Pharmacology*. Chicago, Yearbook Medical Publishers, 1987, pp 301–315.
43. Schiff I, Sela K, Kramer D, et al: Endometrial hyperplasia in women on cyclic and continuous estrogen regimen. *Fertil Steril* 1982;37:79–85.
44. Whitehead MI, King RJB, McQueen J, et al: Endometrial histology and biochemistry in climateric women during oestrogen and oestrogen/progesterone therapy. *J R Soc Med* 1979;72:322–327.
45. Studd JWW, Thom MH, Patterson MEL, et al: The prevention and treatment of endometrial pathology in postmenopausal women receiving exogenous estrogen, in Paoletti R, Ambrus JL (eds.): *Menopause and Postmenopause*. Lancaster, England, MTP Press, 1980, pp 127–139.
46. Gambrell RD: Clinical use of progestins in the menopausal patient. *J Reprod Med* 1982;27:531–538.
47. Whitehead MI, Siddle N, Blaine G, et al: The pharmacology of progestins, in Mishell DR (ed.): *Menopause: Physiology and Pharmacology*. Chicago, Yearbook Medical Publishers, 1987, pp 317–334.
48. Lobo RA, McCormick W, Singer F, et al: Depo-medroxyprogesterone for the treatment of postmenopausal women. *Obstet Gynecol* 1984;63:1.
49. Lobo RA, Roy S, Shoupe D: Estrogen and progesterone effects on urinary calcium calitrophic hormones in surgically induced postmenopausal women. *Horm Metab Res* 1985;17:370.

Index

A

Abscess, liver, 48, 49t
Abuse, screening for, by gynecologist, 4
Acceptance stage of death and dying, 6
Acetaminophen, side-effects, 98
Acetylcholine, 139
Achlorhydria, 58
Acknowledgement phase of grief reaction to organ loss, 5
Actinic keratosis, 78
Acyclovir, for herpes zoster, 50
Adenocanthoma, endometrial, 195
Adenocarcinoma
  breast, 187
  cervical, 191
  endometrial, 194, 195
    estrogen replacement therapy related, 211–212
Adenomatous hyperplasia, endometrial, 195
Adenomatous polyp, 75
Adnexal mass, 199, 200
  diagnosis of, 200
Adrenal glands, 205
Adrenergic inhibiting drugs, *See also* specific drug
  for hypertension, 130, 131t, 132–134
Adverse drug reactions (ADR), 61–62
Age, salience of, 16–17
Age composition, of population, 1, 2t
"Aged hearing," *See* Presbycusis
"Ageism," self-directed, 10
Ageist attitudes, 10–11
  related to autonomy and beneficence, 11, 12, 13
  related to quality of life, 14–16
  self-directed, 10
    related to decision to forgo care, 12–13
Aging
  biological definitions of, 21–22
  biology of, *See* Biology of aging
  pharmacodynamics of, 59–60
  pharmacokinetic effects of, 58–59
  subjective experience of, 17
Alcoholic dementia, 90
Aldosterone antagonists, 130
Alkaline drugs, dissolution rate of, 58

Alpha-receptor stimulating drugs, for stress incontinence, 152
Alzheimer's disease, dementia of, 30, 89
Amantidine, for influenza, 80
  for prophylaxis, 50
Aminoglycoside, 46, 49
Ampicillin, 147
Ampicillin-sulbactam (Unisyn), 46
Androstenedione
  plasma levels, 205
  production of, 205
Anemia
  pernicious, 90
  symptoms of, 103
Anger stage of death and dying, 5
Angiotensin-converting enzyme inhibitors (ACEI), *See also* specific agent
  adverse effects, 136
  for hypertension, 132t, 135–136
Antagonistic pleiotropy, 22
Antibiotics, *See also* specific agent for lower urinary tract infection, 147
Antibody response, 40
Anticholinergic drugs
  adverse effects of, 61
  for detrusor dyssinergia, 153
Antigen, 40
Antigen-DR complex, 40
Antigenic drift, 80
Antihistamines, side-effects, 97
Antihypertensive medications, 68–69, 129–130
  adrenergic-inhibiting drugs, 130, 131t, 132–134
  angiotensin-converting enzyme inhibitors, 132t, 135–136
  calcium channel blockers, 132t, 135
  diuretics, 130
  efficacy of, 124
  lower urinary tract effects, 142t
  myocardial infarction risk from, 124–125
  side-effects, 68
  vasodilators, 132t, 134–135
Antiinflammatory drugs, nonsteroidal (NSAID), 97–98
  adverse response to, 61
  for osteoarthritis, 82
  side-effects, 98

219

Atherosclerosis, infection and, 45
Atypia, in vulvar dystrophy, 174
Audiogram, 86
Autoantibodies, incidence of, age-related changes in, 44
Autonomic nervous system, feedback loops, related to voiding, 140, 142t, 142
Autonomy
  beneficence and, 8
  defined, 7
  ethics and, 11–14
Aztreonam, 46

B

B-cells, 40
  age-related changes in, 43–44
Bacteremia
  incidence of, 38
  pneumococcal, 80–81
Bacteriuria, 146
  asymptomatic, 38, 103
  catheter-associated, 47
  incidence of, 45, 47
  treatment of, 47
Bargaining stage of death and dying, 5–6
Bartholin glands, 171
Basal cell cancer, 78
Behavioral methods, for hypertension treatment, 128–129
Bellergal, 215
Beneficence
  assigning priority to, 8
  autonomy and, 8
  ethics and, 11–14
  principle of, 7
Best interest, promotion of, 7
Beta-adrenergic agents
  for detrusor dyssinergia, 153
  lower urinary tract effects, 142t
Beta-adrenergic blockers, *See also* specific agent
  cardioselective, 132
  for hypertension, 131t, 132–134
  side-effects, 132–133
Beta receptors, pharmacodynamics and, 59–60
"Big bang" reproduction, 22
Biliary tract infection, 49t
Biofeedback, 128
Biology of aging, 21
  clonal senescence, 27–28
  definitions, 21–22
  evolutionary, 22–23
  glycation of proteins and DNA, 27
  longevity differential between males and females, 32
  molecular and cell, 14–17
  organ system changes during aging, 29–31
  protein synthesis error catastrophe theory, 27
  quantity of genes involved in, 23–24
Biopsy, for breast cancer, 185
Birth control pills, 212
Bladder, 141
  age-related changes in, 31
  diverticula, 161
  drainage of, postoperative, 162–163
  dyssynergia, 145
  emptying, inadequate, 144
  innovation of, 140f
  tumors, 161
Bladder retraining and drills, 153
Bladderneck, 149
  plication of, for stress incontinence, 150, 151
Blood pressure, 67
  diastolic, 121, 122, 123
  evaluation of, 67, 121
  increase in, *See* Hypertension
  inheritance of, 71
  labile, 67
  lowered, 122
  systolic, 121, 123
  variations in, 67, 121
Blood pressure cuff, 67
Bone
  density
    decrease in, 83
    estrogen replacement therapy effects, 209–210
    maximum, 82
  mass, premenopausal, 85
  mineral loss, 101
Bonney test, 145
Bowel function, 96
Brain, structural abnormalities, dementia from, 90
Breast
  cancer, 73, 185–186
    diagnosis of, 184–185
    estrogen replacement therapy related, 211
    incidence of, 184
    risk factors for, 73–74
    screening techniques, 74, *See also* Mammography
    staging for, 186t
    symptoms of, 187
    treatment of, 187
  disease, screening for, 3–4
  self examination, 3, 74, 184
Bulbocavernosus muscle, 158
BUN, 102
Butoconazole (Femstat), 180

C

Calcitonin, 210
Calcium
  absorption, 83–84
  content of foods, 93, 94t
  deficiency, 93
  intake of, 84
    recommended, 93
  metabolism, 210
  screening of, in hyperparathyroidism, 101
  supplementation of, 94
    for osteoporosis, 84
Calcium channel blockers, *See also* specific agent
  adverse effects, 135
  for hypertension, 132t, 135
Cancer, *See also* specific body area, specific type of cancer

INDEX   221

estrogen replacement therapy related, 211–212
gynecologic, *See* Gynecologic malignancies
incidence of, in American women, 72t, 72
preventive health care for
  for breast cancer, 73–75
  for colorectal cancer, 75–77
  family cancer syndrome, 77
  for lung cancer, 72–73
  for skin cancer, 77–78
Candida, 87
  vaginitis (moniliasis), 180
Captopril, for hypertension, 132t, 136
Carbohydrate, metabolism of, estrogen replacement therapy effects on, 212
Cardinal ligaments, pelvic, 158
Cardiovascular disease, *See also* specific disease
  estrogen withdrawal and, 208–210
  from hypertension, 122
  preventive health care for
    for coronary artery disease, 66, 66t
    diabetes and, 71
    for hypercholesterolemia, 69–70
    for hypertension, 67–69
    life style and, 71
    obesity and, 71, 72
    positive family history and, 71
    smoking cessation, 69
    for stroke, 66
Cardiovascular system, age related changes in, 30–31
Cartilage, irregularities of, 82
Catalase, 24
Cataract, 85–86
  congenital, 85
  formation of, 85
  risk factors, 86
  senile, 85
Catheter
  Foley, 163
  lower urinary tract infection from, 147
Cavernous plexus, submucosal, 143
Cell biology of aging, 24–27
Cellulitis, 47–48
  etiologtic organisms and empiric treatment, 47t
Central nervous system, feedback loops, related to voiding, 139–140, 142t
Cephalosporin, 46, 147
Cerebral infarction, dementia from, 89, 90
Cerebrovascular disease, *See also* Stroke
  infection of, 45
Cervix, cancer of, 191
  diagnosis of, 191
  prognosis of, 195
  recurrence or persistence of, 195
  staging of, 191, 192t
  treatment for, 191, 192–195
Cesium implantation, for cervical cancer, 192
Chemoattractants, 40
Chemoprophylaxis, against infection, 51
Chemotherapy
  for breast cancer, 187
  for ovarian cancer, 200, 201
  patient's decision for, 14

Chest x-ray, 104
  for lung cancer, 73
Cholecystitis, 48
  estrogen replacement therapy related, 212
Cholelithiasis, *See* Gallstones
Cholesterol, 93, 208, *See also* Hypercholesterolemia
  levels
    inheritance of, 71
    screening for, 70
Cholinergic agents, lower urinary tract effects, 142t
Chromosomes, mutations, 26
Chronic disease, 8
Chronic obstructive pulmonary disease, 31
Cimetidine
  adverse effects of, 61
  interaction with other drugs, 62
Clitoris, anatomy of, 171
Clonal senescence
  aging and, 27–28
  defined, 27
Clonidine, 215
  adverse effects of, 133
  for hypertension, 133
Clotrimazole (Lotrimin, Mycelex), 180
Clotting factors, estrogen administration effects on, 212
Coccygeus muscle, 157, 158f
Cognitive impairment, drug-induced, 61
Collagen, aging effects on, 44
Colles' fracture, 83
Colon, infection of, 49
Colonoscopy, for colorectal cancer, 75, 76
Colorectal cancer, 183
  risk factors for, 75, 75t
  screening for, 75, 76
Colpocleisis, for uterine prolapse, 168–169
Colporrhaphy, 161, 162
  for rectocele, 164
  for stress incontinence, 150, 151
Colposcopy, 188
Competence, *See also* Incompetence
  assessment of, 12
Complement
  activation of, 40
  aging and, 42
  components of, 40
Complete blood count (CBC), 102–103
Compliance
  differences in, 57
  noncompliance, 16
Conceptions of elderly, negative, 9–11
Congestive heart failure, infection and, 45
Constipation, 96
Constraints, internal, absence of, 7
Coronary artery disease
  death rate from, 208
  diabetes and, 71
  hypercholesterolemia and, 69–70
  hypertension and, 67–68
  life-style and, 71
  preventive health care for, 66
  risk factors for, 66, 66t
Corticosteroids, for vulvar dystrophy, 174–175
Cost factors, related to treatment decisions, 12

Counseling
  diet, 95–96
  for smoking cessation, 92
Creatinine, 102
  clearance values, 102
Cystadenoma, ovarian, 199
Cystic masses, breast, 185
Cystocele, 160, 208
  diagnosis of, 160–161
  incontinence and, 149, 150
  symptoms of, 160
  therapy for, 161–163
Cystometry, 146
  office, 145
Cystoscopy, 146
Cystourethrocele, incontinence and, 149
Cystourethrogram
  in stress incontinence, 149
  for urethral diverticulum, 148
Cystourethroscopy for urethral diverticulum, 148

D
Death
  impending, management of, 5–6
  physician's fear of, 11
  premature, early menopause and, 29, 30
  sudden, 66
"Death hormones," 29
Decongestants, side-effects, 97
Decubitus ulcers, 47, 48
Degenerative joint disease, *See* Osteoarthritis
Dementia, 89
  alcoholic, 90
  of Alzheimer's disease, 30, 89
  causes of, 89, 90
  testing for, 90
Denial process, in grief reaction to organ loss, 5
Denial stage of death and dying, 5
Dentures, ill fitting, 87
Depomedroxyprogesterone acetate, 214
Depression, 89
  cognitive deficits in, 90
  diagnosis, criteria for, 89, 89t
  related to autonomous choices, 13–14
Depression stage of death and dying, 6
Detrusor dyssinergia, 152–153
Diabetes, diabetes mellitus
  cardiovascular disease and, 71
  in elderly, symptoms, 99
  infection and, 45
  noninsulin-dependent (type II), 99
  screening tests for, 99–100
Diagnosis, in elderly, 16
Diazepam, interaction with other drugs, 62
Dienestrol, 179
Diet, *See also* Nutrition
  changes, for hypertension, 68
  counseling for, 95–96
  cholesterol lowering, 70
Diethylstilbestrol, 212
Diphenhydramine, 97
Dipstick, 103
Diptheria, immunization against, 78–79, 79t

Disease
  aging as, 11, 14
  prevention of, *See* Preventive health care
Distigmine bromide, for stress incontinence, 150
Ditropan, *See* Oxybutynin chloride
Diuretics, *See also* specific agent
  for hypertension, 130, 131t
  loop, 130, 131t
  potassium-sparing, 130, 131t
Diverticula
  bladder, 161
  urethral, 147–148
Diverticulitis, 49t
Diverticulosis, 48
DNA, 25
  damage to, 26
  glycation of, 27
  synthesis, interruption of, 26
Do Not Resuscitate (DNR) orders, 9
Dopaminergic agents, lower urinary tract effects, 142t
Drugs, 57, *See also* specific agent
  absorption of, 58
  adverse effects of, 60–62
  affecting lower urinary tract, 142t
  compliance, differences in, 57
  distribution of, 58–59
  -drug interaction, 62
  excretion of, renal, 59
  free, 58
  metabolism of, 59
  optimal therapy, in older women, 62–63
  over-the-counter, use of, 97–98
  sensitivity to, increased, 59–60
Dyspareunia, 3

E
EKG, 104
Elastic tissue, aging effects on, 44
Elderly
  negative conceptions of, 9–11
  population of, 1, 2t, 21
Emotions, blood pressure effects, 128
Empathy, 14
Endocarditis, 49
  incidence of, 38
Endometrium
  carcinoma of, 84, 194–198
    classification of, 195–196, 197f
    diagnosis of, 194–198
    estrogen replacement therapy related, 211–212
    pathogenic types, 196
    prognosis of, 196
    treatment of, 196, 198
  hyperplasia of, 194
    estrogen therapy related, 213–214
Endopelvic fascia, 158, 159
Endoscopy, for colorectal cancer screening, 75, 76–77
Enterocele, 165
  symptoms of, 165
  treatment of, 165–166
Entropy, 21

Environment, changes in, infection and, 45–46
Ephedrine sulfate, 153
Equine estrogen, 213
  conjugated, 214
Erythroplakia, 87
Esophagus, age-related changes in, infection and, 44
Estradiol, transdermal, 213
Estrogen, 141
  action on skeletal system, 210, 211
  feedback role of, 30
  urethral closure effects, 143
  vaginal effects, 179
  withdrawal
    effects on organ systems, 206–211
    pelvic support structures effects, 160
  tumors secreting, 195
Estrogen receptors
  breast cancer and, 187
  endometrial cancer and, 198
Estrogen replacement therapy (ERT), 3
  for atrophic vaginitis, 179–180
  cardiovascular benefits of, 84
  cardiovascular disease risks and, 208
  contraindications to, 84–85, 215–216
  cyclic versus continuous, 214, 215f
  for detrusor dyssynergia, 153
  natural estrogens, 213t, 213
  for osteoporosis, 84
  problems related to, 211–212
  for stress incontinence, 150
  synthetic estrogens, 212, 213t, 213
  treatment philosophy, 212–214
  for urethrocele and cystocele, 161
Ethanol, 90
Ethical issues in the care of older women, 7
  cases illustrative of, 7–9
  interpreting and utilizing ethical principles, 11–14
  negative conceptions of the elderly, 9–11
  quality of life and, 14–16
  salience of age, 16–17
Ethinyl estradiol, 212
Evolutionary biology, aging and, 22–23
Exercise
  bone mass and, 85
  for hypertension, 68, 128–129
  preventive health care by, 92–93

F
Fallopian tube, carcinoma of, 198–199
Family cancer syndrome, 77
Family history
  breast cancer and, 75, 184
  cardiovascular disease and, 71
Fat, dietary, 93
Femstat, See Butoconazole
Fertility, 205
Fever
  absence of, 39
  without known underlying disease, outcome of, 39t, 39
Fiber, dietary, 93, 96
Finger-rub test, 87

Fistula
  incontinence and, 153
  ureterovaginal, 153
  urethrovaginal, 148, 153
  vesicovaginal, 153
Flavoxate (Uripas), 153
Flu, See Influenza
Fluid intake, recommended, 96
Fluoride supplementation, osteoporosis prevention by, 85
Fluorinated compounds, for vulvar dystrophy, 174–175
Foley catheter, 163
Fourchette, posterior, 171
Fracture
  Colles', 83
  hip, 209
Free drug, 58
Free radical theory of aging, 24–27
FSH, 205
Future, planning for, 104–106

G
Gallstones, 48
  estrogen replacement therapy related, 212
Gastric fluid, pH of, 58
Gastrocolic reflex, 96
Gastrointestinal system, age-related changes in
  drug absorption and, 58
  infection and, 44–45
Gender differences, in longevity, 32
Genes
  dosage, alterations in, 25
  life span and, 22–23
    quantity involved in, 23–24
Genetic loci, alleles at, 22
Genitourinary tract, See also Urinary tract
  changes in, 31, 139, 208, See also Incontinence
    anatomy and physiology of micturition, 139–144
    diagnostic tests and procedures, 144–148
    infection and, 45
    urethral diverticulum, 147–148
  infection, 47t, 47, 103, See also Bacteriuria
    incidence of, 38
Gentigel, See Gentigen violet jelly
Gentigen violet jelly (Gentigel), 180
Germ line, mutations in, 26
Glaucoma, 85
Glomerular filtration rate (GFR), 102
Glucose
  excretion of, 99
  -mediated glycation of proteins, 27
Glucose tolerance test (GTT), 99–100
Glutathione peroxidase, 24
Glycemia, test for, 99
Glycosylated hemoglobin level (HbA1C), 100
Glycosylation reactions, nonenzymatic, 27
Gonadotropin, 205
Grief, management of, 4–5
Growth potential, deficiencies of, 28
Guanabenz, 134
Guanethidine
  for hypertension, 134
  side-effects, 134

Guanfacine, 134
Gynecologic malignancies, 183
  breast cancer, 183–187
  cervical cancer, 191–194
  endometrial carcinoma, 194–198
  fallopian tube carcinoma, 198–199
  ovarian cancer, 199–202
  vaginal cancer, 190–191
  vulvar cancer, 187–190
Gynecologist, *See also* Physician
  role in care for older women, 1, 2
    primary care goals, 3–6

H

"Hayflick limit," 28
Health history
  annual up-dating of, form for, 106f
  initial, form for, 105f
Hearing
  loss, 86, 87
  testing of, 86–87, 88f
Hematocrit, 103
Hematuria, 103
Hemoglobins
  glycation of, 27
  glycosylated, level of, 100
  measurement of, 103
Herpes zoster, 49–50
Hip, fracture, 209
History, *See also* Family history; Health history
  drug, 62
Home care, 15
Hormone replacement, 3, 205
  estrogen, *See* Estrogen replacement therapy
  philosophy, 212–215
Host-defense mechanisms
  changes in, 51–52
  normal, infection and, 39–40
Hot flushes, 3, 206
Husband, *See* Spouse
Hydralazine
  for hypertension, 132t, 134
  side-effects, 132t, 134–135
Hydrocortisone, for vulvar dystrophy, 174
Hydrops tubae profluens, 198
Hypercholesterolemia, cardiovascular disease and, 69–70
Hyperparathyroidism
  diagnosis of, 101
  screening for, 101–102
Hypertension, 121–122, 136
  diastolic, 67
  drug treatment of, *See* Antihypertensive medications
  hygienic method of treatment, 68, 125
    body weight reduction, 125–126
    dietary salt restriction, 68, 126–127
    exercise, 68, 127–128
    psychological and behavioral methods, 128–129
  prevalence of, 122
  preventive health care for, 67–69
  pseudohypertension, 121–122
  risks to health of, 122–124
  systolic, 67

withdrawal, 133
Hyperthyroidism
  apathetic, 100
  screening for, 100–101
Hypotension, postural, 134
Hypothalamus, age related changes in, 30
Hypothyroidism
  complications of, 100
  screening for, 100
  symptoms of, 100
Hypoxanthine guanine phosphoribosyltransferase (HPRT), 26
Hysterectomy
  for cervical cancer, 192
  for endometrial cancer, 196
  for stress incontinence, 150
  for uterine prolapse, 168

I

IgG, 40
IgM, 40
Iliococcygeus muscle, 157
Imidazoles, 180
Imipramine (Tofranil), 153
  for stress incontinence, 150
Immune response, to viruses, 80
Immune system, defects, with aging, 40–44
Immunization, immunoprophylaxis, against infectious disease, 50–51, 78–81
Immunosenescence, 37
Impact phase of grief reaction to organ loss, 5
Incompetence, judgment of, 12
Incontinence, urinary, 31
  detrusor dyssynergia in, 152–153
  diagnostic tests and procedures for, 144–148
  evaluation and treatment of, by gynecologist, 4
  lower urinary tract infection and, 146
  motor urge, 152
  overflow, 144, 154
  stress, *See* Stress incontinence
  sensory urge, 152
  true, 153–154
Individual, value of, old age and, 10
Infection, infectious diseases, 46, 51–52, *See also* specific type of infection; specific organ system
  age-related changes in organ structure and function, 44–45
  endocarditis, infective, 49
  environmental changes and, 45–46
  epidemiology, age-related, 37–39
  etiologic organisms and empiric treatment, 47t
  herpes zoster, 49–50
  immune defects with aging, 40–44
  increased incidence of underlying disease, 45
  intraabdominal, 48, 49t
  neutrophilic response to, 41, 42
  normal host-defense mechanisms and, 39–40
  pneumonia, 46–47
  prevention and treatment
    chemoprophylaxis, 51
    immunoprophylaxis, 50–51, 78–81

skin and soft-tissue, 47–48
tuberculosis, 48
urinary tract, 47
    lower urinary tract, 146–147
of vagina and vulva, 172
Influenza
A, 80
bacterial pneumonia from, 80
immunoprophylaxis for, 50, 79t, 80
Information, disclosing of
autonomy and, 14
effects of, 8
INH, 48
Integument, See Skin
Interleukin-1 (IL-1), 40
    production of, 42
Interleukin-2, 40
Intraabdominal infections, 38, 48
    etiologic agents and treatment, 49t
Intraabdominal pressure, increase in
    incontinence and, 144
    urethral closure pressure and, 148
Irradiation therapy
    for cervical cancer, 191, 192–194
    for endometrial cancer, 196, 198
    for vulvar cancer, 22

J
Joint, osteoarthritis, 81–82

K
Kegal exercise, 161
Kegel exercises, 150
Kelly procedure, 150
Keratosis, actinic, 78
Kidney
    age related changes in, 31
        drug excretion and, 59
    disease, screening for, 102
Kraurosis, 172

L
Labetolol (Normodyne)
    adverse effects of, 133
    for hypertension, 131t, 133
Labia
    majora, 171
    minora, 171
Lactic acid, 179
Lavator ani muscle, 157, 158f
Lefort operation, for uterine prolapse, 168
Legitimation, 14
Leukoplakia, 87
    vulvar, 171, 172
Levator muscle, vaginal, 139
LH, 205
Lichen sclerosis, vulvar, 173t, 173, 175–177
Life
    prolongation of, 8
    quality of, See Quality of life
    subjective satisfaction with, 15
    value of, old age, and, 10
Life expectancy, 1, 2t, 21
    for women, 7

Life-extending care, elderly patient's claim to, 12–13
Life-span
    genes and, 22–23
        quantity involved in, 23–24
    maximum, 23
    mean, 23
Life-style
    changes, preventive health care by, 90–93
    coronary artery disease and, 71
Ligaments, pelvic, 158, 159
Lipofuscin pigments, 24–25
Lipoprotein
    high-density (HDL), 70, 84, 208
    low-density (LDL), 69, 70, 208
    very low-density (VLDL), 208
Liver
    abscess, 48, 49t
    age-related changes in, drug metabolism and, 59
Longevity
    differential between males and females, 32
    trends in, 1, 2t
Loss, management of, 4–5
Lotrimin, See Clotrimazole
Lung cancer
    incidence of, in women, 72–73
    screening for, 72–73
Lymphadenectomy, pelvic, 189, 190
Lymphocyte count, age-related changes in, 43
Lymphokines, 40
    biologic effects of, 42t

M
Mackenrot's ligaments, 158
Macrophages, age-related changes in, 42
Mammography, 3, 74, 184–185
    age and, 74–75
    guidelines for, 185
Manchester procedure, 168
Marshall-Krantz suprapubic urethrovesicle suspension operation, for stress incontinence, 151–152
Measles (rubeola), immunization against, 79, 79t, 80
Medical problems, general, gynecologist's screening for, 4
Medical resources, distribution of, 10
Meditation, 128
Medroxyprogesterone, 214
Melanoma, 77
    risk factors, 77–78
Menopause, 205
    early, premature death and, 29, 30
Menses, cessation of, 29, See also Menopause
Mestranol, 212
Metacarpal mineral content, estrogen withdrawal and, 209–210
Methyldopa, for hypertension, 133–134
Metoclopramide, adverse effects of, 61
Metronidazole, 181
Miconazole (Monistat), 180
Micturition, 154
    anatomy and physiology of, 139–144
Midodrine, for stress incontinence, 150

Mini Mental State Exam (MMSE), 90
Minipress, *See* Prazosin
Minoxidil, for hypertension, 132t, 135
Molecular biology of aging, 24–27
Molecular disorder, degree of, 21
Mon pubis, 171
Moniliasis, 180
Monistat, *See* Miconazole
Monoclonal proteinemias, 44
Monocytes, age-related changes in, 42
Mouth, preventive health care for, 87, 89
Musculoskeletal disease, preventive health care for
   for osteoarthritis, 81–82
   for osteoporosis, 82–85
Mutations, 25–27
Mycelex, *See* Clotrimazole
Myocardial infarction, 66
   risk of, from antihypertensive medications, 124–125
Myometrial invasion, by endometrial carcinoma, 196

N

Nafcillin, 49
Narcotics, for osteoarthritis, 82
Natriuretics, 130
Natural killer (NK) cells, 40
   function, age-related changes in, 44
NegGram, 147
Neuroendocrine system
   age-related changes in, 30
   mechanisms of aging, 28–29
Neuroleptics, lower urinary tract effects, 142t
Neutrophils, 40
   age-related changes in, 41, 42
   function of, 40–41
Nevi
   acquired, 78
   congenital, 77–78
   dysplastic, 78
Night sweats, 3
NK cells, *See* Natural killer cells
Nocturia, 152
Noncompliance, 16
Norepinephrine, 139
   age related changes in, 30
Norethidrone, 214
Normodyne, *See* Labetolol
Nose drops, 97
Nosocomial infections, incidence of, 38
Nutrition, 46, *See also* Diet
   preventive health care and, 93–94

O

Obesity, 94–95
   breast cancer and, 73, 74
   cardiovascular disease and, 71, 72
   hypertension and, 68
Opsonins, 40
Oral contraceptives, 212
Organ, *See also* specific organ
   loss of, grief reaction from, 5
   structure and function, age-related changes in, 44–45
Organ system, *See also* specific system
   changes during aging, 29–31
   effect of estrogen withdrawal on, 206–211
Oropharyngeal bacteria, aspiration of, 46
Osteoarthritis, 81–82
   symptoms of, 82
   treatment of, 82
Osteoclast activity, 210
Osteopenia, screening for, 83
Osteophyte, growth, 82
Osteoporosis, 82
   causes, 93
   following estrogen withdrawal, 209–211
   hyperparathyroidism and, 101
   risk factors, 82–83
   screening for, 83
   treatment of, 83–85
Ovarian aging, 29, 29f
Ovarian follicle, primary, depletion of, 29, 29f
Ovary, cancer of, 199–200
   diagnosis, 199–200
   epidemiologic factors, 199
   prognosis of, 201–202
   staging classification, 200, 201t
   surgical management of, 200, 201
Oxybutynin chloride (Ditropan), 153
Oxygen-free radicals, 26

P

Paget's disease
   of breast, 187
   vulvar, 177–179
Pain, in osteoarthritis, 82
Papanicolaou smear, 191, 195
Papillary necrosis, 103
Parkinsonism, drug-induced, 61
Partnership, 14
Paternalism, concept of, 7–8
Pelvic diaphragm, anatomy of, 157, 158f
Pelvic node, dissection, 189
Pelvic support, loss of, 148, 149, 157
   anatomic considerations
      pelvic diaphragm, 157, 158f
      supporting ligaments, 158–160
      urogenital diaphragm, 157, 158, 159f
   changes with estrogen withdrawal, 160
   conditions occurring in
      enterocele, 165–166
      rectocele, 163–165
      ureterocele and cystocele, 160–163
      uterine prolapse (descensus, procidentia), 166–167
Penicillin G, 49
Pereya procedure, 162
Perineorrhaphy, for rectocele, 164–165
Perineum, schematic view of, 159f
Periodontal disease, 87
Peripheral vascular disease, infection and, 45
Pernicious anemia, 90
Pessary, for uterine prolapse, 167
pH
   of gastric fluid, 58
   vaginal, 179

INDEX 227

Phagocytosis, 40
Pharmacodynamics of aging, 59–60
Pharmacokinetic effects of aging, 58–59
Pharmacotherapeutics, See Drugs
Phospholipids, 208
Physician, See also Gynecologist
  decision to treat, 11
  fear of death, 11
  responsibilities in care for elderly, 16
Physiologic functions, declining, 10
Pigments, lipofuscin, 24–25
Plasma
  drugs in, 58
  glucose levels, 100
Plasma proteins
  drugs bound to, 58
  exudation of, 40
Pleiotropy, antagonistic, 22
Pneumococcus, vaccination against, 51, 80–81
Pneumonia, 45, 46–47
  bacterial, 80
  in elderly, incidence of, 37–38
  etiologic organisms in, 46, 46t
  postinfluenza, immunoprophylaxis for, 50
  treatment of, 46, 47t
Pneumovax, 51t
Point mutations, 26
Polio, immunization against, 79, 79t
Polyp
  adenomatous, 75
  hyperplastic, 76
Population, age composition of, 1, 2t
Potassium, 94
Pouch of Douglas, obliteration of, 169–170
Prazosin (Minipress)
  for hypertension, 134
  side-effects, 134
Prednisone, for herpes zoster, 50
Premarin, 179
Presbycusis ("aged hearing"), 86
Presbyopia, 86
Pressure sores, See Decubitus ulcers
Preventive health care, 65–66
  for bowel functions, 96
  for cancer, 72–78, See also Cancer
  for cardiovascular disease, 66–73, See also Cardiovascular disease
  for depression and dementia, 89–90
  diet counseling, 95–96
  EKG and chest x-ray, 104
  goals of, 65
  for infectious diseases, 78–81, See also Infectious disease
  life style changes for, 90–93
  medication use, 97–98
  for mouth, 87, 89
  for musculoskeletal disease, 81–85, See also Musculoskeletal disease
  nutrition for, 93–94
  obesity and weight loss, 94–95
  planning for the future, 104–106
  screening techniques, 66, 98–104, See also Screening tests
  summary of recommendations, 107t–108
  for vision and hearing, 85–87
Pro-Banthine, See Propantheline

Procidentia, See Uterus, prolapse
Progeria of the adult, See Werner syndrome
Progeroid syndrome, 26
Progesterone, 141
  therapy
    cyclic versus continuous, 214, 215f
    endometrial hyperplasia effects, 213–214
    for lichen sclerosis, 177
Progesterone receptors
  breast cancer and, 187
  endometrial cancer and, 198
Progestogens, replacement, 214
Propantheline (Pro-Banthine), 153
Protein
  glycation of, 27
  synthesis, error in, 27
Protein calorie malnutrition, 46
Proteinemias, monoclonal, 44
Proteinuria, 104
Pruritis, vulvar, 188
Pseudoephedrine, 97
Pseudohypertension, 121–122
Psychiatric symptoms, drug-induced, 61
Psychological methods, for hypertension treatment, 128–129
Psychoses, drug-induced, 61
Pubococcygeal muscles, 157
  contraction of, 150
Puborectalis muscle, 157
Pudendal artery, 171
Pudendal vein, 171
Pulmonary system, age-related changes in, infection and, 31, 44
Pyuria, 103, 146
  sterile, 103–104

Q
Q-tip test, 149
Quality of life
  conceptions of, 8–9
  ethics and, 8, 9, 14–16
  evaluation of, 15
Quinestrol, 212

R
Radium implantation, 190
  for cervical cancer, 192
Recessive mutations, in aging, 26–27
Reconstruction phase of grief reaction to organ loss, 5
Rectal cancer, 183
Rectocele
  diagnosis of, 163, 164f
  symptoms of, 163
  treatment of, 163, 164–165
Relaxation, 128
  for hypertension, 68
Reproduction
  iteroparous types of, 22
  semelparous types of ("big bang" reproduction), 22
Reproductive system, age changes in, 29–30
Resources, medical, 10
Respect, 14

Respiratory system, *See* Pulmonary system
Rete pegs, 174
Retreat phase of grief reaction to organ loss, 5
Retroperitoneal fascia, 158
Rifampin, 48
Rimantidine, 80
Rubeola, *See* Measles

S
Salt, *See* Sodium
Screening tests, 98–99, *See also* under specific heading; specific test
    biochemical, multi-item, 98
    for breast disease, 3–4
    complete blood count, 102–103
    for diabetes mellitus, 99–100
    for hyperparathyroidism, 101–102
    for renal disease, 102
    for thyroid disease, 100–102
    urinalysis, 103–104
Sedatives, 97
Senescence, 21, 22
    clonal, 27–28
Senses, age related changes in, 30
Serotonin, age related changes in, 30
Sexual dysfunction, drug-induced, 61
Sexual standard, related to aging, 11, 14, 15
Sigmoidoscopy, for colorectal cancer, 75, 76–77
Skene's glands, 171
    inflamed, 161
Skin
    aging effects on, infection and, 44
    cancer, 78
        melanoma, 77–78
    infections, 47–48
Smoking
    abstention from, benefits of, 91, 92
    disease risks from, 69, 91, 91t
Sodium
    concentrating and conserving abilities, 102
    content of foods, 127t
    intake, 93
        restriction of, 68, 126–127
Soft-tissue infections, 47t, 47–48
Somatic cells, diploid, 28
Somatic mutational theories of aging, 25–27
Somatic nervous system, feedback loops, related to voiding, 140, 142t
Somatic symptoms, in depression, 89
Speech discrimination test, 87
Spironolactone, 130
Spouse, cognitive function in, 90
Sputum tests
    in pneumonia, 46
    in tuberculosis, 48
Squamous cell cancer, 78
    cervical, 191
    of vulva, 188, 189f
Staphylococcal endocarditis, 49
Staphylococcus aureus, 46

Starling mechanism, 31
Stereotyping, of elderly, negative, self-directed, 10
Stomach, age-related changes in, infection and, 44–45
Stool, testing of, for occult blood, 75, 76
Streptococcal endocarditis, 49
Stress, hypertension and, 128
Stress incontinence, 152, 162
    causes of, 148–149
    defined, 148
    genuine, 148–152
    tests for, 145
    therapy for, 150–152
Stroke
    death rate from, 208
    preventive health care for, 66
Subjective experience of aging, 17
Sudden death, 66
Sulfonamide, adverse effects of, 61
Sun, exposure to, melanoma and, 77, 78
Superoxide dismutase, 24
Support, 14
Suprachiasmatic nucleus, age related changes in, 30
Surgery, *See also* specific procedure
    for endometrial cancer, 196
    for ovarian cancer, 200, 201
    for rectocele, 163, 164
    for stress incontinence, 150
    for urethrocele and cystocele, 161, 162–163
    for uterine prolapse, 167–170
Suspensory sling operation, for stress incontinence, 150
Swimming, 128
Sympathetic receptors, 141
Syphilis, 90

T
T4, *See* Thyroxine
T-cells, 40, 42–43
    function of, 40
        age-related changes in, 43
    helper, 40, 43
    somatic mutation and, 26
T-suppressor cells, 40, 43
Temperature (body), estrogen withdrawal and, 206, 207
Terazol, *See* Terconazole
Terconazole (Terazol), 180
Terminal care, discussion of, 104
Testosterone
    for lichen sclerosis, 177
    plasma levels, 205
Tetanus, immunoprophylaxis, 51, 78–79
Tetracycline, 147
Thermography, 185
Thromboembolic disease, estrogen replacement therapy related, 212
Thrush, 87

Thymus gland, age-related changes in, 43
Thyroid gland, disease, screening for, 100–101
Thyroid stimulating hormone (TSH), 100, 101
Thyroxine (T4), 100, 101
Tofranil, See Imipramine
Travel immunizations, 81
Treatment, See also specific treatment
    foregoing of, ageist assumptions and, 12–13
  inadequate, 10
  life extending, 12–13
  physician's decision for, 11
  prolongation of, 8
  withdrawal of, 9
Trichomonas vaginitis, 180–181
Trigonitis, 103
Triiodotyronine resine uptake (T3RU), 101
Triodurin, for stress incontinence, 150
Tuberculosis, 48
  incidence of, 38
  treatment of, 48
Turner's syndrome, 206

U

Ultrasound, 185
Unisyn, See Ampicillin-sulbactam
Ureter, 158
Urethra, 141
  closure, factors affecting, 139
  closure pressure, 139–140, 141, 143, 148
    decrease in, 151, 208
    maximum, 141, 142, 143–144
    in stress incontinence, 148
  diverticulum, 147–148
  innovation of, 140f
  shortening of, 148–149
  vesicle angle, stress incontinence and, 149
Urethrocele, 160
  diagnosis of, 160–161
  symptoms of, 160
  therapy for, 161–163
Urethropexy, for stress incontinence, 151–152
Urethroscopy, 145–146
Urethrovaginal fistula, 148, 153
Urethrovesicle suspension operations, for stress incontinence, 150
Urinalysis
  abnormalities found on, 103–104
  for urinary tract symptoms and incontinence, 144
Urinary bladder, See Bladder
Urinary tract, See also Genitourinary system
  lower
    drugs affecting, 142t
    infections of, 146–157
Urine
  residual
    accumulation of, 45
    test for, 144
  voiding of, See Micturition
Uripas, See Flavoxate
Urogenital diaphragm, anatomy of, 157, 158, 159f

Urologic changes, from estrogen withdrawal, 207t, 207–208
Uterine bleeding, dysfunctional, 205
Uterine descensus, See Uterus, prolapse
Uterosacral ligaments, 158
Uterus
  cancer of, death rate from, 183
  prolapse, (descensus, procidentia), 161, 165f, 166–167
    grading of, 166–167
    treatment of, 167–170

V

Vaccine-associated polio, 79
Vagina
  cancer of, 190–191
  changes in
    age-related, 179
    from estrogen withdrawal, 207t, 207
  infectious diseases of, 172
  levator muscle, 139
  prolapse of, repair of, 169–170
Vaginal wall, sacrospinous ligament fixation of, 170
Vaginitis
  atrophic (senile), 45, 179–180
  candida (moniliasis), 180
  nonspecific, 181
  trichomonas, 181
Vaginosis, bacterial, 181
Vancomycin, 49
Varicella-zoster virus, reactivation of, 49–50
Vasodilation, 207
  peripheral, 206
Vasodilators, See also specific agent for hypertension, 132t, 134–135
Vasomotor instability, from estrogen withdrawal, 206, 207t, 207
Vasomotor symptoms, 3
  progestogens for, 214
VDRL test, 90
Vertebral fracture, 83
Vesicovaginal fistula, 153
Vision, impairment of, 85–86
Vitamins, 94
  D, levels, calcium absorption and, 83–84
Vulva
  anatomy of, 171, 172f
  cancer of, 187–188
    diagnosis of, 188
    management of, 188, 189, 190
    staging of, 188, 189t
  dystrophy, 171, 172–175, 188
    hyperplastic, 173, 173t, 174–175
    lichen sclerosis, 173t, 173, 175–177
    mixed, 177
  infectious diseases of, 172
  nerve supply to, 171
  Paget's disease of, 177–179
  pruritis, 188
Vulvectomy, for vulvar cancer, 188, 189, 190

W

Walking, 128
Warfarin, increased sensitivity to, 60
Weight (body)
  gain, acceptable, 94
  loss, 94–95
    diet counseling for, 95–96
    for hypertension, 125–126
Werner syndrome, 26, 28
Whispered voice test, 87

X

X chromosome, 32
X-rays, chest, 73, 104
Xanthines, lower urinary tract effects, 142t

Y

Youth, loss of, 15

Z

Ziel-Nielsen staining, 48

RG 103 .C27 1991

Caring for the older woman